Eating Expectantly

Eating Expectantly

A Practical and Tasty Guide to Prenatal Nutrition

Bridget Swinney, M.S., R.D.

with

Tracey Anderson, R.N., B.S., F.A.C.C.E.

Vermilion
LONDON

1 3 5 7 9 10 8 6 4 2

First published in the USA by Meadowbrook Press
www.meadowbrookpress.com

This UK edition first published in 2002 by Vermilion, an imprint of Ebury Press
Random House, 20 Vauxhall Bridge Road, London SW1V 2SA

Random House Australia (Pty) Limited
20 Alfred Street, Milsons Point, Sydney,
New South Wales 2061, Australia

Random House New Zealand Limited
18 Poland Road, Glenfield,
Auckland 10, New Zealand

Random House South Africa (Pty) Limited
Endulini, 5A Jubilee Road,
Parktown 2193, South Africa

The Random House Group Limited Reg. No. 954009

www.randomhouse.co.uk

A CIP catalogue for this book is available from the British Library

ISBN: 0 09 188293 1

Papers used by Vermilion are natural, recyclable products made from wood grown in sustainable forests.

Printed and bound by Scotprint, Haddington

Dedication

This book is dedicated to the memory of two people:
my mother, Marjorie Morgan Swinney,
and my friend and mentor, Robert Chambers.
It is also dedicated to the three special men
in my life: Frank, Nicolas, and Robert.

Acknowledgements

Thanks to my family for sticking by me through yet another revision: to Robert and Nicolas for late-night hugs and help around the house and to my personal MIS consultant (and husband), Frank, for helping me through major techno-problems and for being Mr. Mom when I was doing 'book stuff'. Thanks to colleagues Cathy Fagen, M.S., R.D., at the California Diabetes and Pregnancy Program; Dr. Barbara Luke at the University of Michigan Multiples Clinic; and Sandy Eardley for their assistance and kind words. Thanks to my writer friends who are always willing to lend an ear or give advice: Connie Evers, Amy Tracy, and Brenda Ponichtera. Thanks to my friends who offered meals, helped with the kids, and provided encouragement: Alicia and John Barrera, Leo and Wanda Melendez, Debbie and Bert Navar, and Beatrice and Jose Leyba. Thanks to my dad and my sisters Judy and Colleen for their continued support.

Thank you to all the past readers of *Eating Expectantly* for making a third edition possible.

Thanks to Bruce Lansky for *still* believing in this book as much as I do.

Special kudos to one awesome editor, Christine Zuchora-Walske, whose skillful editing of this edition was outstanding. (And I'm not just saying that because she extended my deadlines!)

Thanks to Danielle White for the easy-to-read typesetting and to Jone Hallmark for another beautiful cover.

Thanks to Steve Linders and Phil Theibert from the Meadowbrook PR department for their enthusiastic promotion of *Eating Expectantly*. And thanks to all the other folks at Meadowbrook Press for helping this book to be.

Contents

Foreword xii
Introduction: *Why You Need This Book* xiii

Section I

Nutrition Needs, Challenges, and Eating Tips

Chapter One: Contemplating Pregnancy **3**
- Why Pre-pregnancy Planning Is Best 3
- Who Should Have Genetic Counselling? 4
- The Importance of Good Nutrition before and during Pregnancy 4
- A Few Words about Infertility 8
- Planning a Healthy Pregnancy 11
- Focus on Folic Acid 13

Chapter Two: The Knowledgeable Pregnancy **17**
- Ten Steps to a Healthy Diet 18
- Everything You Ever Wante\w about Weight Gain during Pregnancy 20
- All about Fat 25
- Changing Your Mindset for Pregnancy 28
- The Essential Guide to Vitamins and Minerals 28
- Vitamin Supplements: You May Need Them 36
- Keeping Your Baby's Environment Safe 39
- Travelling during Pregnancy 44
- The Positives of Pregnancy 46

Chapter Three: The First Trimester **47**
- How Baby Is Growing 47
- Weight Gain and Energy Needs 48
- Protein Needs 48
- Other Nutrient Needs 50
- Focus on Fibre 51
- The Eating Expectantly Eating Plan 53
- Morning Sickness 54
- Other First-Trimester Challenges 56
- Food Planning for the First Trimester 59

Chapter Four: The Second Trimester **61**

• How Baby Is Growing 61
• Weight Gain and Energy Needs 62
• How's Your Diet? 62
• Protein Needs 64
• Other Nutrient Needs 64
• The Power of Soya 66
• Focus on Calcium 66
• Focus on Iron 69
• 'Thrive on Five' 71
• Smart Snacking 73
• Second-Trimester Challenges 75
• Food Planning for the Second Trimester 77

Chapter Five: The Third Trimester **79**

• How Baby Is Growing 79
• Weight Gain and Energy Needs 80
• Other Nutrient Needs 81
• Focus on Vitamin B_6 and Zinc 82
• What about Sugar? 83
• Tips for Keeping Up Your Energy 84
• Third-Trimester Challenges 85
• Food Planning for the Third Trimester 87

Chapter Six: Vegetarian Eating **89**

• Vegetarians: The Healthy Minority 90
• The Pregnant Vegetarian 90
• Nutrients of Special Concern 91
• The Eating Expectantly Vegetarian Eating Plan 94
• Vegetarian Shopping List 96
• Vegetarian Food Planning 98
• Eating Out Vegetarian-Style 98
• Vegetarian Convenience-Food Choices 100
• Eating after Delivery 100

Chapter Seven: Special Care for High-Risk Pregnancies **103**
- Expect the Unexpected 103
- Dealing with Your Emotions 103
- Pre-existing Diabetes 104
- Gestational Diabetes 110
- The Diabetic Eating and Exercise Plan 114
- High Blood Pressure 123
- Multiple Births 128
- Coping with Bed Rest 135
- Older Mothers 139
- Teen Pregnancy 140

Chapter Eight: Considering Breastfeeding **145**
- My Experiences with Breastfeeding 145
- The Feeding Decision: It's Up to You 146
- Why You Should Consider Breastfeeding 147
- Possible Obstacles 148
- A Note to Dad 151
- Preparing for Breastfeeding 152
- Nutrition during Breastfeeding 154
- Nutrients of Special Concern 158
- Drugs and Breastfeeding 159
- Breastfeeding for Special Groups 159
- Tips for Formula Feeding 167
- About Bonding 167

Chapter Nine: The First Weeks with Baby **169**
- What to Expect after Delivery 169
- Menus for the First Week with Baby 170
- Going Back to Work 171
- Your Body Is Changing 172
- Losing that Baby Fat Sensibly 173
- Weight-Loss Plans 175
- Preparing for Your Next Pregnancy 180

Chapter Ten: Fitting Fitness In **181**
- Benefits of Exercise 181
- What Every Pregnant Woman Should Know about Exercise 182
- Fitting Fitness into Your Busy Lifestyle 185
- Exercise after Pregnancy 186
- Tips for Getting with the Programme after Your Baby Is Born 187

Section II

Shopping, Cooking, and Eating Out

Chapter Eleven: Stocking the Pregnant Kitchen **193**

- Check Out Your Kitchen 193
- A Peek in My Kitchen 194
- Reading Food Labels 195
- Eating on a Budget 199
- Stocking the Kitchen Toolbox 201
- Keeping the Vitamins in Your Vegetables 203
- The Essential Guide to Food Safety 204
- How to Lower Your Risk 208
- Food Safety Reports: Who to Believe? 222
- Food Safety in a Nutshell 223

Chapter Twelve: Fast Foods: Eating In and Eating Out **227**

- Tips for Choosing Convenience Foods 227
- Complete, Convenient Meals for One 228
- Convenience Foods for the Whole Family 230
- Healthy Convenience-Food Menus 230
- Last-Minute Meals from the Cupboard 233
- Fifty Quick-and-Easy Meals or Snacks 234
- Choosing Wisely at Restaurants 237
- Choosing Nutritious Fast Foods 239

Chapter Thirteen: Menus and Recipes for the First Trimester **241**

- About the Eating Expectantly Menus 241
- About the Eating Expectantly Recipes 242
- First-Trimester Menus 243
  - Don't Feel Like Eating Menus 243
  - Don't Feel Like Cooking Menus 243
  - Don't Feel Like Cooking or Eating Menu 244
  - Feel Like Staying in Bed but Can't Menu 244
  - Feel Great Menu 245
  - Blender Breakfasts (or Snacks to Go) 245
  - Snack Ideas 245
  - High-Energy Snack Ideas 247
- First-Trimester Recipes 249

Chapter Fourteen: Menus and Recipes for the Second Trimester **275**

   • Second-Trimester Menus 275

     A Month of Breakfast Ideas 275

     Menus for a Hungry Appetite 276

     I Could Cook All Day Menus 277

     Company's Coming! Menus 277

   • Second-Trimester Recipes 279

Chapter Fifteen: Menus and Recipes for The Third Trimester **307**

   • Third-Trimester Menus 307

     Using Leftovers with Flair 307

     Meals in Minutes 309

     Feel Full Menus 310

     Best Bite Snacks 311

     Vegetarian Budget Menus 311

   • The Bean Routine 316

   • Third-Trimester Recipes 317

References **355**

Recommended Resources **367**

Index **371**

Recipe Index **380**

Foreword

Eating Expectantly effectively informs expectant parents of the value (for both mother and baby) of optimal maternal nutrition during pregnancy. The 1990 report of the US Food and Nutrition Board of the National Academy of Sciences entitled 'Nutrition during Pregnancy' played a special role in focusing our attention on nutrition during pregnancy and provided a thorough review of the major issues.

This report came exactly twenty years after the US Food and Nutrition Board's 1970 report on 'Maternal Nutrition and the Course of Pregnancy'. The convening of an expert committee, including leaders in the field of nutrition and obstetrics, to write this report reflects the substantial advances in our knowledge during the intervening years and the need to apply recent findings to prenatal care.

Of the many conclusions reached by this expert committee, two are especially noteworthy. The first is the recommendation for greater maternal weight gain than previously recommended. This recognizes the association between maternal weight gain during the second and third trimesters and the growth of the baby prior to birth. The committee recommends a minimum weight gain of eleven and a half kilograms (twenty-five pounds), unless the mother is overweight prior to pregnancy. For mothers who are underweight prior to pregnancy, even greater weight gain is recommended.

The second recommendation of particular note is that routine micronutrient supplements be limited to a daily iron supplement of 30 milligrams. While other specific micronutrient supplements are advised in a number of special circumstances, a routine prenatal vitamin/mineral supplement is not recommended. Rather, the emphasis is on an optimal diet as the source of micronutrients.

The reasons for emphasizing the foods we eat reach far beyond the simple fact that we don't need to take supplements if we consume an adequate, nutritionally well-balanced diet. One important reason is the very real risk that we will consciously or subconsciously pay less attention to an optimal diet if we take our daily multivitamin/mineral pill. Shortcomings of the latter approach include the risk of nutrient/nutrient interactions and imbalances, an area about which we continue to learn more. 'New' micronutrients that are important for human health continue to be discovered. Not surprisingly, regular consumption of fruits and vegetables results in health benefits far greater than those obtained by vitamin supplements.

One of the most important reasons for selecting an optimal diet rather than a substitute pill is the fact that prenatal vitamins are not prescribed in all countries. We now know, for example, that an adequate intake of folic acid, one of the B vitamins, in the preconceptional period will greatly reduce the risk of spina bifida and other neural tube defects. To be protective, however, adequate folic acid must be taken prior to conception and in those first few weeks of pregnancy. The bottom-line message is that the emphasis on an optimal diet being important to all women of childbearing age at all times—not only during pregnancy—has been confirmed.

I commend Bridget Swinney for this timely and informative guide. You should get your copy now and not wait until you are pregnant.

Michael Hambidge, M.D., Sc.D., Professor of Pediatrics, Director of the Center for Human Nutrition, University of Colorado Health Sciences Center.

Introduction
Why You Need This Book

When a woman became pregnant years ago, she didn't change her lifestyle very much. The baby's health was thought to depend mostly on chance, and the placenta was thought to protect the foetus from all dangerous substances. Things are different today. We have an abundance of knowledge about pregnancy and nutrition, and the amount of research on the subject grows daily. Now we know that the placenta only acts as a screen, and many toxic substances can still get through to the baby. We've learned that mothers are the true gate-keepers.

You will probably find pregnancy more high-tech than it was as recently as ten years ago. But even with all the diagnostic tests and fancy equipment now available, good nutrition is still the most important factor in giving your baby a healthy start in life.

Eating Expectantly puts nutrition and health during pregnancy into perspective. It gives you answers to questions you may want to ask but are not quite sure whom to ask. This book is based on a realistic and practical approach to eating, instead of one that relies on theoretical advice that doesn't work in the real world.

Eating Expectantly not only gives you guidance on what to eat, it provides over 100 delicious recipes developed specifically for each stage of pregnancy. In addition, it has over 300 menus to meet different needs; you'll find Don't Feel Like Cooking Menus, Meals in Minutes, I Could Cook All Day Menus, Healthy Fast-Food Menus, Company's Coming! Menus, and much more.

If you are vegetarian or trying to eat meatless meals more often, you'll find the vegetarian chapter helpful. If you experience one of the unexpected challenges of pregnancy, such as gestational diabetes, high blood pressure, or bedrest, *Eating Expectantly* will explain the facts and provide tips for eating and food preparation.

If you're not pregnant yet, you will benefit even more from this book. You'll know what your eating habits should be and you'll know what to expect during pregnancy. I suggest that you read the entire book, skipping the chapter on high-risk pregnancies (unless you already have a chronic disease such as diabetes). Then, start using the menus and recipes now! This will get you used to eating right, and healthy eating will be easy to keep up when you're pregnant. Just keep in mind that you won't need to increase your calories until you are pregnant.

Eating Expectantly answers the following questions and more:

- What can I do before I get pregnant to help ensure a healthy baby?
- Will pesticides and preservatives in foods affect my baby?
- What if I can't drink milk? Do I really need a lot of calcium?
- I'm vegetarian. How can I meet my nutrient needs?
- Help! I have just been diagnosed with gestational diabetes. What do I do?
- Should I take a vitamin supplement?
- How much weight should I gain?
- How effective is my current eating plan?
- Do I need to reduce salt intake if I start to have high blood pressure?
- How can I eat right when I'm on bedrest?
- I don't feel like cooking. Help!
- What are the best fast-food and restaurant choices for me while I'm pregnant?
- Should I exercise?

This book uses knowledge and experience gathered from hundreds of pregnant women and mothers, including myself. I've also collected answers from scientific experts: those who do nutrition research and who work with pregnant and breast-feeding women daily.

If you have any questions or concerns about what to eat, how much to eat, or how to practise good nutrition—before, during, and after your pregnancy—this book is a must! I hope you enjoy reading it as much as I enjoyed writing it. More importantly, I hope that by reading and following the advice in *Eating Expectantly,* you will give your baby and yourself the gift of good nutrition and good health!

Bridget Swinney

Section I

Nutrition Needs, Challenges, and Eating Tips

CHAPTER ONE

Contemplating Pregnancy

What you will find in this chapter:

- *Why Prepregnancy Planning Is Best*
- *Who Should Have Genetic Counselling?*
- *The Importance of Good Nutrition before and during Pregnancy*
- *A Few Words about Infertility*
- *Planning a Healthy Pregnancy*
- *Focus on Folic acid*

This chapter answers such questions as:

- *How can I cut down on caffeine?*
- *How will I know if I'm healthy enough to have a baby?*
- *How can I stop eating junk food?*

Why Pre-pregnancy Planning Is Best

Thinking about having a baby? If you're thinking about starting a family or having another child and are seeking information about pregnancy, you're making a smart move. In addition to reading about pregnancy on your own, you may also want to visit with your doctor or health visitor when you decide you're ready to become pregnant. Pre-pregnancy counselling is recommended for several reasons:

1. It provides the information you need to change lifestyle habits that may affect your pregnancy, especially smoking, drinking, caffeine intake, and eating habits.

2. It gives you time to start eating a well-balanced diet, build up nutrient stores, start exercising regularly, and lose or gain weight, if needed.

3. It can teach you about foetal development and help you understand the importance of changing your habits before the first weeks of pregnancy. Much critical development takes place during the first weeks after conception, and this is when poor diet or lifestyle habits can damage the foetus the most. Most of a foetus's brain cell division, for example, occurs before most women know they're pregnant.

4. If you have a chronic medical condition, such as high blood pressure, diabetes, or kidney disease, pre-pregnancy counselling can help you get it under control before you become pregnant. This is vital to having the healthiest baby possible!

3

5. If you have had a miscarriage or have delivered a baby with birth defects, pre-pregnancy counselling can teach you how to improve your chances of having a healthier baby next time.

6. If this is your first pregnancy and you have a history of genetic defects in your family, or if you have a genetic condition that you could pass on to your children, pre-pregnancy counselling will give you time to seek genetic counselling.

▼

Who Should Have Genetic Counselling?

According to the March of Dimes of the US, anyone who has unanswered questions about diseases in the family or who is concerned about being at increased risk for having a child with a birth defect or inherited disorder should consider genetic counselling. It is also suitable for:

Couples who . . .

- already have a child with mental retardation, an inherited disorder, or a birth defect.
- have or are concerned that they might have an inherited disorder or birth defect.
- have an infant who has a genetic disease diagnosed by routine newborn screening.
- are concerned that their jobs, lifestyles, or medical histories may pose a risk to pregnancy because of exposure to radiation, medications, chemicals, infections, or drugs.

- would like testing or more information about genetic defects that occur frequently in their ethnic group (such as Tay-Sachs disease, thalassemia, and sickle cell anaemia).
- are first cousins or other close blood relatives.

Women who . . .

- will be thirty-four years old or older at the time of pregnancy.
- have had two or more miscarriages or babies who died in infancy.
- based on tests such as ultrasound or alpha-foetoprotein, have been told that they may be at increased risk for pregnancy complications or birth defects.

For more information on genetic counselling and other helpful information about pregnancy, you can contact the March of Dimes Birth Defects Foundation at www.modimes.org.

▼

The Importance of Good Nutrition before and during Pregnancy

The following examples illustrate the importance of good nutrition and early prenatal care for a healthy pregnancy:

- Folic acid is critical before and during the first trimester of pregnancy for the prevention of neural tube defects (defects of the formation of the spinal column) such as spina bifida. Up to 70 per cent of neural tube defects could be prevented by consuming adequate folic acid before and during the first trimester. The US Institute of Medicine recommends that all women of childbearing potential consume 400 micrograms of folic acid daily from fortified foods or a supplement in addition to the folic acid found in a healthy diet. (An intake of 600 micrograms is recommended during pregnancy.) However, only 7 per cent of women are aware of this recommendation.[1] To reduce your risk for birth defects, you should consider taking a multivitamin containing folic acid.[2] Women who have had a child with a neural tube defect are much more likely to have another child with the same problem; these women should talk to their doctors or health visitors about a larger supplement of folic acid. (See page 28 to learn more about the key nutrients for pregnancy.)

- According to certain studies, your child's health as an adult could be affected by your eating habits during pregnancy. Recent research shows that babies who are born small for their gestational age and who are small during their first year are at higher risk later in life for insulin resistance (which could lead to diabetes), elevated triglycerides, lower HDL cholesterol levels, and heart disease.[3]
- Another study showed that women's lower weight gain between fifteen and thirty-five weeks gestation was related to higher blood pressure when their children were ten to twelve years old. It was also found that the thinner a mother's triceps skinfold (a measure of nutritional status), the greater the chance of her child having higher blood pressure.[4]
- Women with pre-existing diabetes are several times more likely to have a baby with birth defects than non-diabetic women. This fact may be related to glucose control before conception and in the very early weeks of pregnancy.[5] However, this increased risk can be reduced significantly with good control of blood sugars and early prenatal counselling.
- Research shows that iron and folic acid intake are related to increased infant body weight and length – another reason to make sure your diet includes adequate iron and folic acid in pregnancy.[6]
- Anyone who is unknowingly pregnant might drink alcohol or take medication that could harm the foetus. Excessive alcohol intake can cause birth defects and long-lasting problems such as mental and physical retardation, hyperactivity, and smaller birth weight. Because researchers aren't sure what small amounts of alcohol could do to a foetus, the safest strategy is to avoid alcohol during pre-pregnancy and pregnancy.
- According to researcher Michael Crawford of the Institute of Brain Chemistry and Human Nutrition in London, 'The individual responsibility for the development of the brain rests with the mother. Some 70 per cent of the total number of brain cells to last an individual's lifetime have divided before birth.' Crawford also proposes that

The Pre-pregnancy Quiz

The following quiz will help you and your partner determine whether your diet and lifestyle are ready for pregnancy. Circle 'Yes' or 'No' after each statement; then follow the scoring directions on the next page.

1. I eat at least three servings of fruit and three servings of vegetables on most days.   Yes   No

2. I eat a vitamin-C-rich food daily. (Examples include citrus fruit or juice, berries, papaya, mango, pineapple, melon, broccoli, cauliflower, tomato, and vegetable juice.)   Yes   No

3. I eat a wide variety of foods, including many types of protein foods.   Yes   No

4. I do some form of aerobic exercise at least twice each week.   Yes   No

5. I don't smoke and I avoid secondhand smoke.   Yes   No

6. I consume one or fewer caffeinated beverages a day.   Yes   No

7. I avoid taking drugs of any kind: prescription drugs, over-the-counter drugs, herbal preparations, or 'street drugs'.   Yes   No

8. I am at or close to my desirable body weight.   Yes   No

9. I avoid exposure to radiation, pesticides, herbicides, solvents, PCBs, and other chemicals.   Yes   No

10. I limit my consumption of shark, swordfish, or lake whitefish to once a month or less.   Yes   No

11. I usually eat three balanced meals a day and watch my saturated fat intake.   Yes   No

12. I eat three servings of calcium-rich foods daily. (Examples include milk, yogurt, cheese, high-calcium vegetables, tofu made with calcium, and juice fortified with calcium.)   Yes   No

13. I take a multivitamin/mineral supplement containing 400 micrograms of folic acid daily.   Yes   No

14. I avoid taking any single vitamin supplements (such as vitamin A) without my doctor's approval.   Yes   No

15. I avoid drinking alcohol.   Yes   No

16. I avoid eating unpasteurized milk, eggs, shellfish, or foods that are made with these. (Examples include caesar salad dressing, mousse with uncooked egg, and sushi.)   Yes   No

17. I eat three servings of wholegrain breads, cereals, or other wholegrain products on most days.   Yes   No

The Pre-pregnancy Quiz

18. I live a moderately paced lifestyle, get eight hours of sleep most nights, and feel generally happy. **Yes** **No**

19. I have not followed any severe diets or had an eating disorder in the last three months. **Yes** **No**

20. I am a vegetarian who eats no animal products, though I do take vitamin B_{12} and calcium supplements if recommended by my doctor. **Yes** **No**

21. I have visited my doctor and discussed a future pregnancy. **Yes** **No**

How Did You Do?

Count your 'Yes' answers and see how you scored below.

17-21: Congratulations! Your body is ready for pregnancy!

13-16: You're doing pretty well; you have just a few things to work on for the healthiest pregnancy possible.

9-12: Start working; you may need a few months to make the changes necessary to have the healthiest pregnancy possible.

9 or fewer: Oops! Your lifestyle may need an overhaul! Talk to your doctor or health visitor before beginning a pregnancy.

developmental disorders common to low-birth-weight infants (such as mental retardation, cerebral palsy, and blindness) are the result of poor maternal nutrition before and during the first trimester.[7]

• Children of women who have had gestational diabetes are at greater risk for obesity and impaired glucose tolerance. However, by starting pregnancy close to ideal body weight and exercising regularly, a woman can prevent gestational diabetes.[8]

• Evidence shows that smoking during pregnancy is not only related to lower birth weight, but may also affect neurological development and behaviour.[9] Also, smoking by either parent during pregnancy is related to a higher risk of childhood cancer.[10]

• According to a recent US government survey, women's diets need some work. In 1994, only 55 per cent of women ate fruit or drank juice daily. Soft drink consumption for women has surpassed milk consumption. Women are not meeting the Dietary Reference Intakes (DRI) for iron, zinc, calcium, magnesium, and vitamin E. Average fibre intake is 10 grams short of the recommendation, and 44 per cent of women report consuming 15 teaspoons of sugar daily.[11] One out of four adults skips breakfast – a significant source of nutrients, especially folic acid.[12] Based on this information, it could be concluded that many women start their pregnancies a bit malnourished.

- An overweight woman is more likely to lose her foetus late in pregnancy than a woman of normal weight.[13] Also, two studies have recently shown that obese women are two to four times more likely to have a baby with a neural tube defect than women who are not significantly overweight.[14] The solution? If you are overweight, and especially if you are 20 per cent or more over your ideal weight, lose weight before you conceive. (See Recommended Resources for weight-control resources on page 370.)

A few words of advice: Make sure that you don't become pregnant while you are on a weight-loss diet; your intake of certain vitamins may not be enough for the important stages of early foetal development. Taking a vitamin/mineral supplement during the weight-loss period is advisable. (See page 36.)

Eating at least the number of servings of each food listed in the Before-Baby Eating Plan will help you become a healthy future mother. As soon as you find out you're pregnant, you can switch over to the Eating Expectantly Eating Plan on page 53. The two diets are not very different, so your transition will be easy. (If you're wondering how to begin eating a healthy diet, see Chapter Eleven: Stocking the Pregnant Kitchen.)

▼

A Few Words about Infertility

Infertility, defined as not conceiving after one year of unprotected intercourse, affects about one in ten people of reproductive age. Some of these numbers may be a result of delaying pregnancy. Generally, the older we are, the longer we take to conceive. Seeking assistance for infertility can be an emotionally charged venture, to say the least.

Nutrition can and does play a role in fertility. If you are seeking help for infertility, please make sure you are not underweight. If you are underweight when you become pregnant, your chances of having a low-birth-weight infant are much higher. Some fertility treatments greatly increase your chances for having twins or more, and this further increases your chances for having low-birth-weight infants.

Here is an overview of some of the effects body weight, smoking, nutrition, and activity level have on fertility.

The Before-Baby Eating Plan	
Food	**Daily Servings**
Grains/starches	6 or more
Fruits	3 or more
Vegetables Be sure to include at least 1 vitamin-C- and 1 vitamin-A-rich fruit or vegetable daily.	3 or more
Protein or equivalent	100–175 g (4–6 oz)
Dairy or calcium-rich foods	3 or more

Body Weight

The female body appears to be very protective of an unborn baby. Conceiving is more difficult if you are underweight or overweight. Body fat seems to be the synchronizing factor (or the conductor, if you will) for the harmonious hormonal symphony that must take place for pregnancy to occur and be carried to term. Being close to your ideal body weight before you become pregnant can help you conceive and can reduce your risk of complications and of having a low-birth-weight or premature baby.

Overweight

Having too much body fat can affect fertility because part of the body's estrogen is made in the fat of the breasts and abdomen. Excess body fat can affect the amount and types of circulating hormones that influence fertility. Obesity is also related to polycystic ovarian disease, a cause of infertility. Studies show that overweight women have great success in conceiving once they have gotten closer to their ideal body weight.[15]

Underweight

Regular function of ovulation and menstrual cycles requires a minimum weight for height. In fact, body weight changes of just 10 to 15 per cent can disrupt menstrual cycles. A maternal body weight closer to ideal weight is best for conceiving and for carrying a healthy baby to term. It may also help the health of future generations: Women born with low birth weights are more likely to have poor pregnancy outcomes than women with higher birth weights.[16]

Smoking

Smoking is related to decreased sperm quality and infertility in men as well as oxidative damage to sperm, which could be responsible for birth defects and other diseases.[17] Smoking can also deplete antioxidants (especially vitamins C and E), which can result in DNA damage to sperm.[18] It appears that women who smoke also have a higher risk of infertility and other problems associated with pregnancy.[19]

Nutrition

Caffeine

In a large multicountry study, it was found that women who consumed over 500 milligrams of caffeine (the equivalant of about 4 cups of coffee) took 11 per cent longer to become pregnant. The effect was even stronger in women who also smoked.[20]

Vegetarian Diet

A meatless eating plan can be very healthy. (See Chapter Six for more information.) However, one study showed that a low-calorie vegetarian weight-loss diet caused seven out of nine women in the study to stop ovulating. The same study related an abrupt switch to a vegetarian diet to lack of ovulation.[21] If you are vegetarian and are having trouble conceiving, take a very close look at your diet to make sure you are not lacking any nutrients. Compare your diet to the recommended diet in Chapter Six. You may also want to take a multivitamin supplement.

Eating Disorders

Amenorrhoea (lack of menstrual periods) and oligomenorrhoea (infrequent periods) often occur in women with anorexia nervosa and are also seen in about 50 per cent of women with bulimia. Reproductive hormones are also reduced in women who maintain a lower-than-normal body weight.[22] An increase in body weight and a balanced food intake will help restore normal reproductive functions.

If you have an eating disorder, you should try to resolve the underlying causes of the disorder for a permanent recovery. The eating habits and health problems associated with some eating disorders can put your baby at risk for birth defects, low birth weight, or prematurity. So, it is best to normalize your eating habits and make sure you are not below your ideal body weight prior to pregnancy.[23] Comprehensive programmes that involve a psychologist, doctor, and dietitian can be most helpful.

Depleted Iron Stores

Women whose depleted iron stores were supplemented with iron and vitamin C had increased chances of conception.[24] So, make sure your diet includes ample iron from food or a supplement.

Alcohol

For couples trying to conceive, both men and women should avoid alcohol. Even moderate alcohol intake by women (less than five drinks per week) can affect fertility.[25] It has been suggested that alcohol intake by men can affect fertility as well as pregnancy outcome.[26]

Vitamin C

Two different studies demonstrated that vitamin C supplements of 200 milligrams improved fertility in men, in both heavy smokers as well as in non-smokers.[27] Vitamin C may also protect against DNA damage to sperm – all the more reason to make sure both partners follow the Before-Baby Eating Plan. Men may especially want to increase intake of vitamin C foods or take a supplement.

Zinc

Zinc is important in the male and female reproductive systems. A zinc deficiency in men is related to decreased sperm count, decreased sperm motility, and decreased serum testosterone (a sex hormone) levels.[28] All of these factors could have a large impact on fertility. (See page 33 for food sources of zinc.)

Selenium

Inadequate and excess selenium are both related to male fertility. To make sure both partners' intake of selenium is adequate, eat plenty of seafood and whole grains.

Too Many Carrots

Women who ate no red meat and who supplemented their diet of mostly vegetables and salads with up to half a kilogram (a pound) of carrots a day had stopped ovulating. After reducing carrot intake, most women's menstrual function improved, which points to the conclusion that their infertility problem could be completely diet related.[29] Although this conclusion is speculative, it does draw attention to the important concept of moderation.

Activity Level

Women involved in competitive sports sometimes reduce their body fat so much that they stop menstruating. Strenuous exercise and decreased body weight and body fat are related to reproductive problems, including infertility. Regular exercise is important for good health. However, if you take exercise to the extreme and are having trouble conceiving, you may need to slow down.

▼

Planning a Healthy Pregnancy

Several months before you become pregnant, both you and your partner should follow the advice below. Men are often left out of pregnancy planning – but they must also take good care of themselves, since sperm is affected by diet and the environment.

▶ **Don't drink alcohol or take drugs.**

That includes aspirin! If you take a prescription medication, ask your doctor if it is safe to take during pregnancy. If your medicine is not safe, your doctor may substitute one that is. Find out from the doctor or your health visitor which over-the-counter medications are safe during pregnancy, especially during the first trimester.

▶ **Make a pre-pregnancy visit to your doctor or health visitor.**

During this visit you can discuss your current health as well as your immunity to diseases such as chickenpox and rubella. These diseases are fairly harmless most of the time, but if you contract them during pregnancy, they could cause serious problems to the foetus. You may want to get immunized.

▶ **Both you and your partner should follow the Before-Baby Eating Plan.**

Since one cycle of sperm production takes ten weeks, you should both follow the Before-Baby Plan for three months prior to pregnancy.[30] When couples discuss pregnancy, they often ignore the father's diet. However, research shows that the father's diet *can* affect his sperm and, ultimately, the foetus. A joint project at the University of California-Berkeley and the U.S. Department of Agriculture (USDA) Western Human Nutrition Research Center has linked low dietary intakes of vitamin C to increased genetic damage in sperm, which presumably translates into a higher risk for birth defects and genetic disease.[31] (See page 33 for good food sources of vitamin C.)

Study leader Dr. Bruce Ames says, 'All we know now is that if your dietary intake of vitamin C gets below a certain level – about 60 milligrams per day, which is the Recommended Daily Allowance – you get into trouble. This strongly indicates that vitamin C protects against DNA damage.'

▶ **Keep your environment safe.**

For both partners, this means avoiding exposure to pesticides, herbicides, radiation (X-rays), and fumes from paint, extermination chemicals, and glue. Avoid exposure to lead, which can cause premature birth, brain damage, learning disabilities, and kidney and liver damage. More than forty million people in the US have too much lead in their drinking water.[32] (See page 40 for the important details.)

If you smoke, try to quit or reduce your smoking. Avoid or limit exposure to second-hand smoke.

▶ Avoid or limit caffeine.

The pendulum seems to swing back and forth on caffeine and its effects on fertility and other reproductive issues. Low birth weight and birth defects don't seem to be related to caffeine consumption. On the other hand, caffeine intake may be linked to infertility and miscarriage. Common sense says to avoid caffeine or limit your intake to one serving per day.

▶ Take a multivitamin supplement containing 400 micrograms of folic acid and no more than 100 per cent of the RDA of other nutrients...

The main reason is to prevent neural tube defects such as spina bifida. Some evidence shows that vitamin supplementation may also prevent other birth defects, such as heart and limb defects and oral cleft problems. On the other hand, avoid taking supplements of individual vitamins, especially vitamin A; as mentioned earlier, extreme doses of certain vitamins may produce unwanted results.

▶ Reduce stress or learn how to cope with it effectively.

Extreme stress is thought to affect fertility. However, stress is hard to measure because people perceive it differently. Exercise is a good stress reliever.

▶ Avoid exposure to high temperatures.

Sperm production is reduced in men who weld inside storage tanks, who drive a truck and literally sit on a hot seat for hours, and who regularly sit in a hot tub. Tight briefs or pants can also reduce sperm production. However, most experts believe that to have a real effect on fertility, a man's exposure to high temperatures would have to be continuous over a long period of time.[33]

Also, a woman who takes long hot baths or sits in a hot tub or sauna can actually damage her embryo's nervous system during the first thirty days after conception.

▶ Analyze your workplace for reproductive hazards.

Many occupations use chemicals or energy that is dangerous to unborn children. Much controversy surrounded a lawsuit that addressed removing women from jobs involving exposure to lead because of the reproductive hazard. However, your baby or your ability to become pregnant could be affected by what you and your partner are exposed to at work (and in other places, too). One study showed that the wives of men exposed to ethylene oxide, rubber chemicals, solvents used in refineries, and solvents used in the manufacturing of rubber products had increased risk of miscarriage.[34] Other known hazards include exposure to radiation, lead, solvents, paints, anesthetic gases, glues, copper, arsenic, cadmium, solder fumes, polyvinyl chloride, aerosol sprays, and dyes.[35]

The Health and Safety at Work Act 1974 requires an employer to ensure, so far as it is reasonably practicable, the health and safety of employees and others who may be affected by the working activities.

Companies employing five or more people, must prepare a Safety Policy Statement covering all aspects of safety at work, and in which it must show the steps taken to control any work involving harmful substances such as lead and asbestos.

▶ **Be safe at the plate.**

Food safety is essential for the health of the unborn foetus. For example, a food-borne illness caused by the organism *Listeria monocytogenes* can cause miscarriage or stillbirth. Listeriosis has been associated with eating soft white cheeses, prepared meats, hot dogs, and unpasteurized milk. Toxoplasmosis is a parasitic infection that can cause mental retardation and blindness. It has been found in uncooked and undercooked meat, unwashed fruits and vegetables, and cat faeces.[36] For more information on food safety, see page 204.

▼

Focus on Folic Acid

Folic acid, also called folacin, is a B vitamin that is very important during pregnancy; it plays a critical role in making new cells and in making haemoglobin in red blood cells. Folic acid is water-soluble and can be destroyed by cooking, so when you cook vegetables, cook in as little water as possible for as short a time as possible.

People who may need more folic acid in their diet are those who have been on such medications as anticonvulsants and some birth control pills. The U.S. Public Health Service now recommends that all women of childbearing age who are capable of becoming pregnant should consume 400 micrograms of folic acid per day.[37] If you have had a child with a neural tube defect, you will need to take a much higher dose – check with your doctor of health visitor.

? Questions You May Have

Q: I drink about 4 cups of coffee every day. Any advice on cutting down?

A: Caffeine is a stimulant, and as most people know, it is habit-forming. In addition, caffeine is a diuretic: It causes your body to lose fluid, and during pregnancy your need for fluid increases. Substances found in coffee and tea also interfere with the absorption of iron. All of the above are good reasons for reducing coffee, caffeinated soda, and tea intake. Cut down gradually to avoid such side-effects as headaches. You may want to substitute low-caffeine drinks such as decaffeinated tea or coffee, or hot cocoa.

Q: Help! I'm a junk-food junkie! I eat fast food every day and actually crave it. How can I improve my diet?

A: Fast food can fit into a balanced diet if done right. However, if you eat fast food often (and you're not making healthy choices), you are likely to have decreased

Best Sources of Folic Acid

The DRI* for folic acid is 400 micrograms during pregnancy; 500 micrograms for breastfeeding.

Food	Serving sizes	Folic acid (micrograms[†])
Lentils	90 g (3½ oz)	358
Sunflower seeds	175 g (6 oz)	317
Pinto beans	90 g (3½ oz)	294
Asparagus	150 g (5 oz)	262
Haricot beans	90 g (3½ oz)	255
Spinach, frozen, drained	190 g (6½ oz)	204
Sunflower seeds, roasted	75 g (3 oz)	201
Soybean nuts, roasted	90 g (3½ oz)	181
Turnip greens, fresh	150 g (5 oz)	171
Black beans, canned	225 g (8 oz)	158
Artichoke	1	153
Hummus	90 g (3½ oz)	146
Split peas	90 g (3½ oz)	127
Black-eyed peas, canned	225 g (8 oz)	123
Pistachios or peanuts, dry roasted	75 g (3 oz)	123
Baked beans, homemade	225 g (8 oz)	122
Papaya	1 medium	116
Avocado	1 medium	113
Orange juice, from concentrate	250 ml (8 fl oz)	109
Broccoli, frozen	250 g (8 oz)	104
Peas, frozen	190 g (6½ oz)	94
Boysenberries, frozen	190 g (6½ oz)	84
Romaine lettuce, shredded	65 g (2½ oz)	76
Creamed corn	65 g (2½ oz)	74
Beets, canned	250 g (8 oz)	73
Ham and cheese sandwich	1	71
Trail mix	75 g (3 oz)	60
Wakame (seaweed), raw	25 g (1 oz)	55
Kombu (seaweed), raw	25 g (1 oz)	51
Vegetable juice	250 ml (8 fl oz)	51
Blackberries, frozen	190 g (6½ oz)	49

*Formerly known as RDA

†Numbers are rounded to nearest whole number; numbers are for cooked foods, as applicable.

Sources: Pennington, J. *Bowes and Church's Food Values of Portions Commonly Used*, 17th edition. Philadelphia: Lippincott Williams and Wilkins, 1998.

U.S. Department of Agriculture. USDA Nutrient Database for Standard Reference, Release 13, 1999.

intakes of vitamin A, vitamin B₆, vitamin C, and calcium, which are all important nutrients during pregnancy.[38] The other problem is that most restaurant meals are higher in fat and calories than those eaten at home.

Try switching to healthier choices, such as bean burritos, grilled chicken sandwiches, or salads with low-fat meats. Add a salad bar or side salad with lots of fruits and vegetables, drink semi-skimmed or skimmed milk with your meal, and bring along a fruit for dessert. Be sure to eat more fruits, vegetables, and whole grains at other meals to reach your totals. (See page 239 for more information regarding fast-food restaurants.)

Q: I've been taking birth control pills for five years. Is there anything special I should do before I become pregnant?

A: Doctors usually recommend that you have at least two periods off the pill to make sure your hormone levels are back to normal. However, the American College of Obstetricians and Gynecologists no longer has a recommendation regarding this. They state, 'Using birth control pills before you become pregnant does not cause birth defects, no matter how close to conception you stop using them.'[39] However, your periods may be irregular at first, which makes it difficult to determine your fertile times or to calculate your due date when you become pregnant. If you had painful or heavy periods before you started taking the pill, you may experience those types of menstrual cycles again.

Nutritionally, you should make sure your diet is better than average, since any medication taken over a long period of time can affect your nutritional status. Oral contraceptives can increase your need for B vitamins, including folic acid, so be sure to take a multivitamin/mineral supplement containing folic acid.

Q: I am diabetic and always thought trying to have a baby would be dangerous, but I hear things are different now.

A: You're right! The important thing is for your diabetes to be under control before you get pregnant, because high blood sugar could cause birth defects in the first few weeks of pregnancy. Also, during pregnancy your insulin needs will change often, and you will need close monitoring. Visit your doctor and talk about your plan. Your doctor might refer you to an obstetrician who specializes in taking care of diabetic mothers. You may also want to see an eye doctor. (See page 104 for more advice for diabetic mothers-to-be.)

Q: I'm thirty-eight, and my biological clock just went off. Anything I can do before pregnancy to ensure the health of my baby?

A: Visit your doctor to get a checkup and a clean bill of health. Older women who are in good health and who receive early and regular prenatal care can have perfectly healthy babies. Preparing for your pregnancy and establishing good lifestyle habits can start your baby out right. However, older mothers do face increased risks during pregnancy. This is mostly because as women get older, conditions such as diabetes and high blood pressure are more common. (See page 139 for more information.)

Q: Before I realized I was pregnant, I drank too much at a party. What should I do?

A: Your situation is not uncommon; many pregnancies are a surprise. The best thing to do is stay calm. Start following all the advice above and don't think about what you've done in the past. Discuss your concerns with your doctor or midwife, who will help you put them in perspective.

The Knowledgeable Pregnancy

What Every Woman Needs to Know

What you will find in this chapter:

- *Ten Steps to a Healthy Diet*
- *Everything You Ever Wanted to Know about Weight Gain during Pregnancy*
- *All about Fat*
- *Changing Your Mindset for Pregnancy*
- *The Essential Guide to Vitamins and Minerals*
- *Vitamin Supplements: You May Need Them*
- *Keeping Your Baby's Environment Safe*
- *Travelling during Pregnancy*
- *The Positives of Pregnancy*

This chapter answers such questions as:

- *Should I take a vitamin supplement?*
- *What if I'm not gaining enough weight?*
- *How often should I weigh?*
- *How much caffeine is okay during pregnancy?*
- *How can I reduce my exposure to lead?*
- *Should I take individual vitamin supplements?*
- *How much caffeine is in hot chocolate?*

So you're pregnant – or planning to be. Congratulations! You are about to begin the most exhilarating, exhausting, challenging, and special time of your life. No doubt you will find yourself daydreaming in the months to come: 'What will my baby look like? How will I be as a first-time (or second- or third-time) mother? What will my baby grow up to do – discover the cure for cancer or become Prime Minister?' And your thoughts will inevitably drift back to one important question: 'Will my baby be healthy?'

Fortunately, the answer to that question depends mostly on you. Although genetics and pure chance can affect your baby's health, taking good care of yourself gives your baby the best possible odds of being born healthy.

If you are just considering pregnancy, you are one step ahead of the game and have time to get your body and personal habits into great shape. (See Chapter One: Contemplating Pregnancy.) Pre-pregnancy counselling is a popular buzzword among hopeful mothers-to-be, and with good reason. Pre-pregnancy counselling allows your doctor or health visitor to give you important advice on eating, exercise, alcohol, and so on. If you are diabetic or have another medical condition, counselling is an especially good idea.

As a pregnant or soon-to-be-pregnant woman, you have a unique opportunity to make your health the best it can be. The good habits you start now can be with you and your family for life! In fact, exciting research shows that your diet and nutritional status before and during pregnancy and your baby's birth weight can have an effect on your baby's risk of chronic diseases like diabetes, high blood pressure, and cardiovascular disease. Apparently, a poor diet before and during pregnancy leads to lower birth weight and so 'programmes' your baby to have health problems as an adult. (See Chapter One for more specifics.)

Good nutrition is not something you should only worry about during pregnancy. I've seen many a fifty-year-old who needed to change his or her eating habits to lose weight, reduce blood sugar, or lower cholesterol. But it's tough to teach an old dog new tricks. If your children learn good eating habits from the start, they will never have to worry about changing them!

▼

Ten Steps to a Healthy Diet

Because so much conflicting advice is available on nutrition today, I've put together ten easy eating tips to follow, now and after your pregnancy.

1. *Variety provides good balance.* We all know people who eat a tuna sandwich and an apple for lunch day in and day out. What's missing is variety. Variety not only is the spice of life, it also helps provide the right balance of nutrients, vitamins, and minerals you need. Not that a tuna sandwich is a bad lunch. But just think of all the other foods and nutrients you'd miss if you ate one for lunch every day! Variety and balance are especially important during pregnancy to

ensure that you don't get too much of certain vitamins or additives and that you get the right mix of vitamins and minerals for your baby's growth and development.

2. *Moderation is the key* to an enjoyable life, and it's also the key to good health. In a survey of secondary school students, 85 per cent of the students said that you should avoid all high-fat foods, and 77 per cent thought that you should never eat foods that have a lot of sugar.[1] Wrong! There is no food that you should *never* eat, unless you are a diabetic who must strictly control your blood sugar. (The occasional sweet is probably okay, but you should discuss this with your doctor first.) For most people, high-fat and high-sugar foods are harmless in small amounts.

3. *Follow the Food Guide Pyramid.* This is a wonderful visual representation of how our diet should be built. Below is a food pyramid designed especially for pregnancy. Start with a base of whole grains and cereals and add

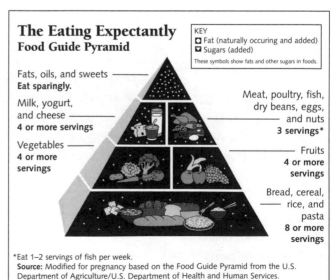

The Eating Expectantly Food Guide Pyramid

KEY
☐ Fat (naturally occuring and added)
☑ Sugars (added)
These symbols show fats and other sugars in foods.

Fats, oils, and sweets — **Eat sparingly.**

Milk, yogurt, and cheese — **4 or more servings**

Vegetables — **4 or more servings**

Meat, poultry, fish, dry beans, eggs, and nuts **3 servings***

Fruits **4 or more servings**

Bread, cereal, rice, and pasta **8 or more servings**

*Eat 1–2 servings of fish per week.
Source: Modified for pregnancy based on the Food Guide Pyramid from the U.S. Department of Agriculture/U.S. Department of Health and Human Services.

fruits, vegetables, protein, milk, and tiny amounts of sugar and fat. If your shopping trolley doesn't reflect the food pyramid, you should reconsider your shopping list.

4. *Bone up on calcium.* Calcium has never been more important in the diet. In fact, a US National Institutes of Health panel recommended calcium intakes above the Dietary Reference Intakes (DRI) for all age and sex groups. During pregnancy, supplemental calcium has been shown to lower blood pressure and reduce the risk of pre-eclampsia (a form of hypertension occurring in pregnancy).[2] But even after pregnancy, you should try to have two or three servings of calcium-rich food every day (more if you're breastfeeding). Research on calcium is promising – higher calcium intake is linked to lower blood pressure and is also related to a lower risk of colon cancer.[3]

Of course, calcium is well known for building bones to their maximum strength and keeping them that way, thus helping to prevent osteoporosis. You start losing bone mass in your thirties, so be sure to consume adequate calcium either in your diet or in supplements throughout your lifetime.

5. *Don't skimp on iron.* Getting enough iron in your diet may be a real challenge: Women need more iron than men, yet we generally eat many fewer calories. Factor in nutritionally unbalanced diets and too many meals eaten on the run, and the result is often iron-deficiency anaemia. One study showed that anaemia during early pregnancy results in a three-times-higher risk of delivering a low-birth-weight baby and a double risk of hav-

ing a premature infant.[4] (See page 33 to learn more about the importance of iron.)

6. *Go for whole grains.* Women often shy away from foods like bread, pasta, and corn, which are seen as fattening. But, because of their nutritional punch, such foods should be the foundation of every meal. They provide energy, fibre, vitamins, and minerals. Recent research links eating more fibre from whole grains with reduced risk of fatal colon cancer, breast cancer, and endometrial cancer. Examples of whole grains are wholegrain (such as wholemeal) breads and cereals, brown rice, and wholemeal pastas.[5]

Whole grains also contain trace minerals that are important for chronic disease prevention, but are in short supply in the Western diet. Some of these minerals are chromium, selenium, zinc, copper, manganese, and magnesium.

7. *Don't forget the exercise.* We've become a nation of couch potatoes, and as the saying goes: Couch potatoes have tater tots! This is changing as people realize the many benefits of exercise: stress reduction, improved endurance, lowered resting heart rate, blood pressure control, cardiovascular efficiency, improved self-esteem and body image, better sleep habits, and lowered risk of heart attack, stroke, diabetes, and even some types of cancer. During pregnancy, staying supple can ease aches and pains, help reduce fatigue, and get you ready for the 'mother's marathon' – labour and delivery. However, you should take care to exercise appropriately during pregnancy. (See Chapter Ten: Fitting Fitness In.)

8. *Get your fill of fluids.* The human body is composed of about 60 per cent water, so drinking plenty of water is common sense. Thirst is the first sign of dehydration, but it lags behind actual need. By the time you feel thirsty, you are already behind in your fluid intake. Eight to ten glasses per day are recommended during pregnancy. With your increased blood supply, amniotic fluid, and extra tissue to support, the more fluids you have, the better. You can drink fluid in the form of juice and decaffeinated tea and soda, but try to drink most of it as clear, clean water.

9. *Focus on fibre.* The US National Cancer Institute recommends consuming 20 to 35 grams of fibre per day,[6] but most of us don't get enough. During pregnancy, you'll find yourself trying to eat more high-fibre foods to combat constipation. Adequate fibre in the diet may reduce risk of colon cancer and breast cancer, and during pregnancy fibre can prevent constipation and haemorrhoids. (See page 51 for more fibre facts.)

10. *Take it easy on the extras.* As mentioned before, no food should be totally off-limits. However, you can easily go overboard with fat, sugar, and even artificial sweeteners if you let your taste buds rule. You should eat extras like candy, junk food, and ice cream as treats only after you have eaten all the 'must' foods. With all the extra nutrients you need during pregnancy, you can't afford to eat many empty-calorie foods.

Everything You Ever Wanted to Know about Weight Gain during Pregnancy

Putting on weight may be a woman's nightmare, but during pregnancy the amount of weight you gain and how you gain it may make the difference between a healthy, full-term baby and one that is born small and premature.

A review of thirteen studies shows that inadequate weight gain and a low rate of weight gain in the latter part of pregnancy are both associated with pre-term delivery.[7] Happily watching yourself gain weight may be tough, but try to get used to it.

Suggested Weight Gain	
Pre-pregnancy Weight	**Suggested Weight Gain**
Underweight (10% below ideal weight)	12.5–18 kg (28–40 pounds)
Normal weight (Average weight for height)	11.5–16 kg (25–35 pounds)
Overweight (20% or more over ideal weight)	6.75–11 kg (15–25 pounds)

Teens and women of African origin should strive for gains at the upper end of the range. Women under 1.6m (5'3") should gain an amount of weight at the lower end of the range.

Source: *Nutrition during Pregnancy: Part I, Weight Gain; Part II, Nutrient Supplements*, Subcommittee on Nutritional Status and Weight Gain during Pregnancy, National Academy of Sciences.

Where the Weight Goes	
Tissue	**Weight**
Breast	450–900 g (1–2 lb)
Placenta	675 g (1½ lb)
Enlarged uterus	900 g (2 lb)
Increased blood and fluids	4 kg (8½ lb)
Baby	3.5 kg (7½ lb)
Fat stores	1.8–6.4 kg (4–14 lb)
Total gained	**11–16 kg (25–35 lb)**

Where the Weight Goes

You have probably seen a life-size picture of a foetus no bigger than a spoon that weighs less than 25 g or an ounce. So why have you gained 2.25 kg/5 pounds? Since the average birth weight is about 3 kilograms/7 pounds and the average weight gain is 13.5 kilograms/30 pounds, pregnancy weight gain is obviously more than just baby. During pregnancy your blood supply increases, your breasts and uterus enlarge, you acquire miscellaneous extra fluids, and – you guessed it – you put on FAT! The fat provides additional calories for breastfeeding. During pregnancy, your body also builds additional muscle to carry the extra weight. The chart above shows where your weight goes.

Weight gain recommendations have changed dramatically over the years. Once, pregnant women were told to gain as little weight as possible and were sometimes reprimanded for gaining weight! Now we know that good nutrition and a specific pattern of weight gain are the keys to having healthier babies.

According to University of California-Berkeley nutritional epidemiologist Barbara Abrams, co-author of a large study that looked at weight gain in pregnant women, 'Our study shows that maternal weight gain is an important factor in pregnancy outcome, especially the baby's birth weight. Since low birth weight is the major cause of infant mortality and mental and physical disability, it can be dangerous to restrict a pregnant woman's weight gains.'[8]

The recommended weight gain for the average woman is 11–16 kilograms/25 to 35 pounds, but many don't fit the average mould. The amount of weight you should gain depends on your weight before you

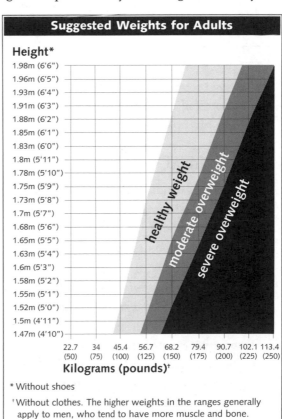

Suggested Weights for Adults

Height*

1.98m (6'6")
1.96m (6'5")
1.93m (6'4")
1.91m (6'3")
1.88m (6'2")
1.85m (6'1")
1.83m (6'0")
1.8m (5'11")
1.78m (5'10")
1.75m (5'9")
1.73m (5'8")
1.7m (5'7")
1.68m (5'6")
1.65m (5'5")
1.63m (5'4")
1.6m (5'3")
1.58m (5'2")
1.55m (5'1")
1.52m (5'0")
1.5m (4'11")
1.47m (4'10")

healthy weight *moderate overweight* *severe overweight*

22.7 (50) 34 (75) 45.4 (100) 56.7 (125) 68.2 (150) 79.4 (175) 90.7 (200) 102.1 (225) 113.4 (250)

Kilograms (pounds)†

* Without shoes

† Without clothes. The higher weights in the ranges generally apply to men, who tend to have more muscle and bone.

Note: This chart refers to *prepregnancy* weights.

Source: *Report of the Dietary Guidelines Advisory Committee on the Dietary Guidelines for Americans*, 1995, pages 23–24.

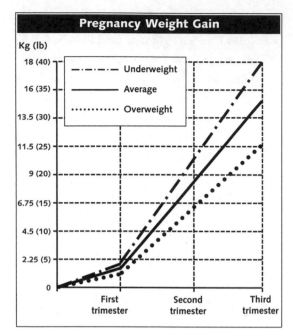

Pregnancy Weight Gain

Kg (lb)

- · – · · – · Underweight
- ——— Average
- · · · · · · Overweight

were pregnant and on whether you are having twins or more. (See page 128 for information on multiple births.) Refer to the chart above to see how much you should gain.

What's 'Ideal Weight'?

Ideal weight has different definitions. Some health professionals use insurance weight charts, some use the 'rule of five', and others use the Suggested Weights for Adults from the US Department of Agriculture and US Department of Health and Human Services. You could also define ideal body weight as the weight at which you feel best.

To use the 'rule of five' (for women), start with 100 pounds for 5 feet of height. Add 5 pounds for every inch over 5 feet you are. Keep in mind a 10 per cent variance to account for body build and so on.

Monitoring Your Weight Gain

Remember that your *pattern* of weight gain is just as important as the *amount* of weight you gain. Your weight gain should be gradual and should roughly follow the Pregnancy Weight Gain chart on the left. You should gain approximately 900 g to 1.75 kg (2 to 4 pounds) during the first trimester and close to 450 g (a pound) per week during the second and third trimesters, when the baby grows the most. If your goal is more or less than average, adapt these numbers accordingly.

If you are eating healthy foods with just a few splurges, your weight gain will follow the right pattern for you. Remember that women have fluctuating weights, which vary even more during pregnancy. A few tips for weighing yourself are listed below.

▶ **Always weigh yourself at the same time of day and under the same conditions.**

For example, you might weigh yourself first thing in the morning after you use the bathroom, wearing the same nightgown.

▶ **Weigh yourself weekly, not daily.**

Weighing yourself daily could drive you nuts! Since your weight depends on what you've had to eat and drink, the amount of sodium you've consumed, and your bowel habits, you could show a 1.3-kg (3-pound) 'weight gain' on Monday and a 1.75-kg (4-pound) 'weight loss' on Wednesday.

▶ **Compare only weights from the same scale.**

If your clinic's scales shows a 1.75-kg (4-pound) weight gain compared to your home scale, don't panic! Scales are often different, so compare only weights from the same scales.

Gaining Too Fast or Too Much

Most women fear gaining too much, because they think the weight will be difficult to take off. Also, gaining too much weight can cause excessive infant size and increased risk of a caesarean section. Regardless of how much you gain, pregnancy is never the time to try to lose weight. If you have reached your goal of a 13.6-kg (30-pound) weight gain by week thirty-five, don't think you should not gain any more for the remaining five weeks!

Here are several explanations for gaining too much weight or gaining weight too fast:

- You may be overeating or eating too many high-fat, high-calorie foods. Are you trying to eat for two? See the quiz below to evaluate the extras in your diet.
- You may be carrying multiple foetuses. If you don't feel that your weight gain is related to eating, consult your doctor or midwife about the possibility of multiple births.
- Inaccurate weighing or weighing after eating or drinking. (Weighing after drinking a litre [1³/₄ pints] of water, for example, will add 900 g [2 pounds] to your weight!)
- Pre-eclampsia/high blood pressure. If you gain 1.5 kg (3 or more pounds) per week in the second or third trimester of pregnancy and also experience swelling of feet and/or hands, severe headaches, or vision problems, contact your doctor or midwife immediately! These could be the first signs of pre-eclampsia, a potentially serious problem. (See page 123.)

Will You Gain Too Much Weight?

1. Do you eat sweets four times a week or more?
2. Do you snack on foods like crisps, nuts, nachos, or chips four times a week or more?
3. Do you use a lot of margarine, salad dressing, soured cream, or cheese?
4. When you cook, do you pour more than 1 teaspoon of oil per serving into the pan?
5. Do you regularly eat the skin on chicken, fat on steak, and so on?
6. Do you eat typical fast food or fried food more than once a week?
7. Do you often eat when you're bored, depressed, angry, or happy – but not hungry?
8. Do you usually eat while doing something else, such as reading or watching TV?
9. Do you eat snacks like ice cream and cheese?

If you answered 'yes' to three or more of the above questions, you have a good chance of gaining too much weight (or too much fat) during your pregnancy. Keeping an eye on fat intake will help you now – and later, when you are trying to lose your 'baby fat'.

How to Avoid Gaining Too Much Weight

Now that the recommended weight gain is higher than it was a few years ago, you will definitely look pregnant! However, three factors control your weight gain and how it looks on you: your genes, your activity level, and your diet.

The distribution of pregnancy weight varies among women. You will hear myths about your weight gain. Some people will tell you that if you're having a boy, the weight will be all in your abdomen. And if your weight gain is spread out all over, many will predict a girl. The truth is, your genes control where the weight goes.

If you start a low-impact exercise programme approved by your doctor or midwife (such as swimming or walking) or continue an established exercise programme, you will be well toned and will look and feel better. Being in good overall physical shape will help you feel good about your expanding waistline. Having more lean muscle tissue will also help you lose weight after you have your baby.

One mother of two says: 'I lost all my weight within a few months after having Brian. I swam regularly right up to delivery. However, with Emily, I was very sick with bronchitis the last six weeks of pregnancy and spent a lot of time in bed. Overall, I was much less active when I was pregnant with Emily, and it took me much longer to take the weight off after Emily was born.'

Of course, your diet may need critical analysis. If you follow the Eating Expectantly Eating Plan (see Chapter Three), you shouldn't have any problem with excess weight gain. The quiz on page 23 may shed some light on your eating habits.

Not Gaining Enough

There are as many reasons for not gaining enough weight as there are for gaining too much. Though not gaining enough weight may seem like a blessing, the lack can cause major problems for your baby. Women who don't gain enough are more likely to deliver premature babies, and their babies are likely to be smaller. Newborn death is more related to prematurity and low birth weight than to any other cause.[9] So, if you are having problems gaining enough weight, be sure to find the reason below and do something about it.

- You have fast metabolism. Women who were underweight before pregnancy may simply burn calories more quickly. You may need help from a registered dietitian, who can closely analyze your diet for ways to increase calories.
- You can't eat much because of nausea, heartburn, stress, or other problems. First, you need to get to the root of the problem. Nausea usually goes away after the first trimester. The other problems may have simple solutions. Psychosocial stress has been known to decrease weight gain, and you may need help from a counsellor or social worker. Ask your midwife for assistance.
- You go a mile a minute. Some mothers-to-be have very active lifestyles and don't slow down for pregnancy. This could result in burning too many calories or not taking the time to eat

enough. Either scenario leaves fewer calories for baby to grow on. If your lifestyle is interfering with your weight gain, you may need to look at reducing your activities or exercise and/or increasing your calories.

• Psychological factors are interfering. If you have ever had a weight problem or an eating disorder, you might find gaining weight psychologically difficult. Your overall psychosocial well-being may also have an effect on your weight status. Depression, anxiety, low self-esteem, and lack of social support may all affect your weight gain.[10] You may need help from your midwife or a psychotherapist.

• You smoke. Smoking is associated with reduced weight gain, sudden infant death syndrome (SIDS), foetal death, and placenta previa (an abnormal placement of the placenta that may cause complications during delivery).[11] Do your best to quit or cut down.

What to Do If You Aren't Gaining Enough Weight

▶ **Make sure your diet is similar to the Eating Expectantly Eating Plan on page 53.**

▶ **Slow down!**

▶ **Increase the amount of food you eat.**

If you are having trouble eating more, increase fat intake – the easiest way to increase calories without increasing bulk. To increase fat intake, the best foods to add are those rich in unsaturated fats, such as vegetable oils, salad dressings, wheatgerm, nuts, seeds, avocado, peanut butter, and margarine with liquid oil or water as the first ingredient.

▶ **Don't forget the snacks.**

If you're eating only three meals a day, you're probably not eating enough. Most pregnant women need a few additional snacks to fit in all the nutrients and calories they need. (See page 247 for snack ideas for high-energy mums.)

▶ **Increase what I call 'healthy splurges' – foods that have some nutritive value, but have extra calories, too – such as milk shakes, frozen yogurt, breads made with fruits or vegetables (like banana bread or courgette bread), sweet potato or pumpkin pie, puddings and egg custard.**

To add calories, you may also want to add a food supplement to your milk.

All about Fat

Watching the types and amounts of fat you eat is important – for the short and long term – for several reasons:

• Gram per gram, fat has more than twice as many calories as carbohydrate or protein.

• Some types of fat are absolutely essential for humans because the body cannot make them. Eicosapenaenoic acid (EPA) and docosahexanenoic acid (DHA), two omega-3 oils found in fish, are important for the building of foetal brain tissue (which is 60 per cent fat) and eye tissue. The body can convert alpha-linolenic acid found in polyunsaturated vegetable oils into EPA and DHA, but not very efficiently. Sources of alpha-linolenic acid include flaxseed and linseed oil, canola oil, soybean oil and soy products, walnut oil and walnuts, and wheatgerm oil.

Another essential fat that can't be made in your body is linoleic acid (omega-6). All vegetable oils contain linoleic acid, but safflower oil is richest. Most people's diets contain too much omega-6 and not enough omega-3. Omega-6 and omega-3 oils form biologically active compounds that affect body functions such as blood pressure, blood clotting, and immune response, so the right balance could make a profound difference in overall health. To get enough of these essential fats in your diet, try to have a balance of oils rich in omega-6 and omega-3. Eating fish (especially fatty fish) a few times per week can help ensure adequate omega-3 intake. (See page 217 for 'The Facts on Fish.')

- Fat calories are stored easier than calories from other sources. The more fat you eat, the more fat you wear.
- A high-fat intake is implicated in heart disease and certain types of cancer, especially breast, prostate, and colon cancer.[12]
- A high-fat diet from eating fried foods can aggravate the nausea of early

pregnancy and heartburn later in pregnancy.
- Types of fat called trans-fatty acids (also called trans fat) are made when liquid oils are hydrogenated for storage or cooking – for example, when oil is made into shortening or stick margarine. These types of fat appear worse than saturated fat regarding heart disease and may have widespread implications for other diseases. Research also shows that trans fat gets into the foetal bloodstream in proportion to the mother's consumption; trans fat could restrict birth weight.[13] Trans fat is mostly found in margarine, shortening, and products made from these, such as bakery goods, commercially fried foods, and snack foods. You may want to avoid margarine or use as little as possible and keep processed, high-fat foods to a minimum. Look at the label of several margarines and choose a tub product that has liquid oil as the first ingredient. Currently, the amount of trans fat is not listed on food labels. It has been proposed that the amount of trans fat per serving be added to the amount of saturated fat per serving, so that the resulting amount and per cent of Daily Value (%DV) per serving on Nutrition Facts panels will be based on the sum of both types of fat.

Most health organizations recommend that we eat 30 per cent or less of our calories from fat. A specific guideline for pregnancy hasn't been established, but somewhere around 30 per cent fat is a prudent recommendation.

Sonja Connor, M.S., R.D., research associate professor in the Department of Medicine at Oregon Health Science Center in the US, says that a case can be made for watching fat intake during pregnancy, but she cautions intake below 20 per cent, saying, 'You may have trouble gaining weight and not laying down the fat you need to support lactation.' If you are having difficulty gaining weight, you may need to increase your fat intake, but try to get the extra fat from vegetable sources such as avocado, nuts, peanut butter, and vegetable oils.

The average pregnant woman needs 2,200 to 2,400 calories, and 30 per cent of those calories would be about 70 to 90 grams of fat. This may sound like a lot. Are you savvy about fat? Look at the following diet and guess how much fat it contains.

How Much Fat?

Breakfast
Cereal with 1 teacup semi-skimmed milk
2 slices toast with 2 teaspoons margarine
Fresh fruit
Snack
25 g (1 oz) cheese
10 wheat biscuits
Lunch
Deluxe cheeseburger
Chips
Side salad with 2 tablespoons dressing
Snack
2 tablespoons peanut butter on Melba toast
1½ teacups semi-skimmed milk

Dinner
175 g (6 oz) fish sautéed in safflower oil
Baked potato with 2 tablespoons soured cream and 2 teaspoons margarine
Fresh, steamed spinach
Tomatoes and cucumbers with 2 tablespoons vinaigrette dressing
Snack
Ice cream
Chocolate-chip cookie

Believe it or not, the above menu has 160 grams of fat, or double the amount recommended. Let's change a few things and see how the fat adds up in our modified menu.

Breakfast
Cereal with 1 teacup skimmed milk
2 slices toast with 1 teaspoon margarine and 2 teaspoons fruit spread
Banana
Snack
25 g (1 oz) low-fat cheese
8 wheat biscuits
Lunch
Grilled chicken sandwich
Side salad with pasta salad and light vinaigrette dressing
Peaches and pineapple
1 teacup semi-skimmed milk
Snack
2 tablespoons peanut butter
½ bagel
Vegetable juice
Dinner
175 g (6 oz) fish baked with a crumb topping of Parmesan cheese and 1 teaspoon margarine
Boiled new potatoes with 2 teaspoons margarine

Steamed fresh spinach
Melon balls
Skimmed milk
Snack
Frozen yogurt
Digestive biscuits

We've cut the fat in half with just a few changes! The menu now has under 80 grams of fat, a much better number. You can check the vitamin and mineral aspects of your diet by taking the nutrition quiz on page 62.

Changing Your Mindset for Pregnancy

Up to now you've been the perfect model of health. You don't eat eggs, you work out five times a week, and you haven't eaten red meat in years. Now you're craving a steak, don't feel like exercising (or doing much of anything, for that matter), and eggs seem to go down really well. What's a woman to do? First, let's set a few things straight.

The average Western diet does contain too much protein, but eating lean red meat in moderation is fine. You just need to choose lean cuts like top side, and flank steak. Red meat is rich in iron, and small amounts of red meat can help your body absorb iron from non-meat sources. It is also a good source of zinc, an important nutrient during pregnancy.

Eggs are a great source of protein, and eating them in moderation is not a problem for most people. Even the American Heart Association allows three to four egg yolks a week in its Eating Plan for Healthy Americans.[14] Sometimes eggs are easier to get down, so don't feel guilty about eating extra eggs. Just take it easy on the bacon, sausage, biscuits, hash browns, cheese, and so on.

Your body is going through a tremendous amount of change (no kidding!), and not feeling quite as energetic as you are used to is normal. You may also feel uncomfortable about the size or look of your 'body with baby', which may make you squeamish about getting into an exercise outfit or swimsuit. Try to get some exercise, even if it's just walking around the neighbourhood. Exercise will help maintain muscle tone and will make you feel good mentally and physically. (See Chapter Ten for more on exercise.) And remember that pregnancy doesn't last forever, even though sometimes it feels as if it might!

The Essential Guide to Vitamins and Minerals

The body needs many different nutrients every day. Every vitamin and mineral plays a small but important role in the making of a healthy baby.

New Terminology: Dietary Reference Intakes

Since 1943, the Recommended Daily Allowance (RDA) has been the standard for suggested nutrient intake. However, expanded knowledge about nutrient needs made it necessary for the US Food and Nutrition Board to coin a new term, Dietary Reference Intake (DRI). Dietary Reference Intake is based on four different ways of estimating nutrient needs. If you'd like to learn more about the development of and rationale behind DRIs, visit the US Food and Nutrition Board's website at www.nas.edu/iom/fnb.

The Energy-Releasing Nutrients

You have probably heard people say, 'Vitamins give me more energy.' Actually, vitamins have no calories, but you need them to be able to use the energy in your food. Because of this, the nutrients listed below are needed in amounts relative to the amount and type of food you eat.

Thiamin (Vitamin B₁)

DRI for pregnancy: 1.4 milligrams; for breastfeeding: 1.5 milligrams.

Functions: Releases energy from carbohydrate. Used in appetite and nervous-system function.

Sources: Brewer's yeast, enriched cereals and breads, pork, sunflower seeds, oatmeal, wheatgerm, dried beans, and peas.

Note: Thiamin is unstable in heat and light. Vegetables high in thiamin and other water-soluble vitamins should be cooked minimally, with as little water as possible.

Riboflavin (Vitamin B₂)

DRI for pregnancy: 1.4 milligrams; for breastfeeding: 1.6 milligrams.

Functions: Helps release energy from all foods. Maintains normal vision and skin health.

Sources: Fortified cereals, milk, yogurt, and cheese.

Niacin (Vitamin B₃)

DRI for pregnancy: 1.8 milligrams; for breastfeeding: 1.7 milligrams.

Functions: Helps release energy from food. Supports health of skin, nervous system, and digestive system.

Sources: Fortified cereals, poultry, fish, meat, legumes, and nuts.

Pantothenic Acid

DRI for pregnancy: 6 milligrams; for breastfeeding: 7 milligrams.

Functions: Helps release energy from food. Involved in antibody production.

Sources: Widespread in many foods. Salmon, trout, and avocado are good sources.

Biotin

DRI for pregnancy: 30 micrograms; for breastfeeding: 35 micrograms.

Functions: Helps release energy from food. Assists in fat synthesis and carbohydrate storage.

Sources: Widespread in many foods. Oatmeal, hazelnuts, and peanuts are good sources.

The Building Nutrients

These nutrients are responsible for helping build bone, muscle tissue, hormones, and other tissues.

Calcium

DRI for pregnancy and breastfeeding: 1,000 milligrams. The US National Institutes of Health Consensus Conference on Optimal Calcium Intake recommends an intake of 1,200 to 1,500 milligrams of calcium daily for pregnant and nursing women.[15]

Functions: Principal ingredient in bones and teeth; vital in muscle contraction, nerve function, blood clotting, blood pressure, and immune defence. Research shows a possible relationship between adequate calcium in the diet and reduced risk of hypertension and colon cancer.[16] Adequate calcium over the lifespan protects against osteoporosis.

Sources: Milk and milk products, small fish with bones, blackstrap molasses, calcium-fortified tofu, broccoli, greens, legumes, some seaweed, and sea vegetables.

Choline

A DRI has been established recently for choline. DRI for pregnancy: 450 milligrams; for breastfeeding: 550 milligrams.

Functions: As a component of lecithin, choline is important in the structure of all cell membranes, lipoproteins, and pulmonary surfactant.

Sources: Eggs, soyabeans, cauliflower, and lettuce.

Vitamin B$_{12}$ (Cobalamin)

DRI for pregnancy: 2.6 micrograms; for breastfeeding: 2.8 micrograms.

Functions: Helps in new red blood cell production; helps maintain health of nerve cells.

Sources: Muscle meats, fish, eggs, milk and milk products, and fortified foods.

Note: Only foods of animal origin and certain fortified foods contain Vitamin B$_{12}$. Check food labels to see whether B$_{12}$ is added. (See page 92 for more information.)

Phosphorus

DRI for pregnancy and breastfeeding: 700 milligrams.

Calcium and phosphorus make up three-quarters of the total weight of minerals found in the body. Unlike calcium, a deficiency of phosphorus is rare.

Functions: Used in building bones and teeth. Needed in every cell membrane, in genetic material, as part of energy production, and in the body's buffering system.

Sources: Primary sources of phosphorus in the Western diet are animal protein and carbonated sodas.

Note: Excess phosphorus may draw calcium out of the body.

Magnesium

DRI for pregnancy: 350 milligrams; for breastfeeding: 310 milligrams.

Functions: Used in bone mineralization, protein building, enzyme action, muscle contraction, transmission of nerve impulses, and maintenance of teeth. Also helps in the regulation of blood sugar and insulin. Low intakes of magnesium have been implicated in increased risk of heart disease.

Sources: Nuts, legumes, whole grains, dark green vegetables, and seafood.

Vitamin A

DRI for pregnancy: 800 retinol equivalents; for breastfeeding, first six months: 1,300 retinol equivalents, for second six months: 1,200 retinol equivalents. One retinol equivalent is equal to 1 microgram of vitamin A or 6 micrograms of beta-carotene. The body converts beta-carotene into vitamin A.

Functions: Helps in cell growth and development and in formation of bones and teeth. Needed for healthy skin, mucous membranes, cornea of the eye, and reproductive health. Diets rich in beta-carotene, an antioxidant, have been shown to be related to decreased risk of heart disease and cancer.

Sources: Fortified milk, cheese, and eggs.

Warning: Excess vitamin A is very toxic to the foetus, so if you are taking an individual supplement of vitamin A, a high-potency multivitamin containing several times the DRI for vitamin A, or medication containing vitamin A (such as Retin-A), STOP IMMEDIATELY and consult your doctor. Recent research shows that women who took a supplement of just four times the DRI for vitamin A were nearly five times more likely to have a baby with a birth defect.[17] You should also avoid all types of liver and fish liver oils while you are pregnant, because liver is a very concentrated source of vitamin A.

Beta-Carotene

The body converts beta-carotene to vitamin A as needed, so don't worry about consuming too much beta-carotene. However, people who have consumed large amounts of carrots or carrot juice have had their skin turn orange! The skin returns to normal after the person resumes a moderate diet.

Sources: Spinach and other dark leafy greens; broccoli; deep-orange fruits like apricots, peaches, and cantaloupe melon; and orange vegetables like squash, carrots, sweet potatoes, and pumpkin.

Vitamin K

DRI for pregnancy and breastfeeding: 65 micrograms.

Vitamin K is made in the digestive tract. Infants are given a dose at birth before their own vitamin K production starts.

Functions: Needed in the synthesis of blood-clotting proteins.

Sources: Seaweed (dulse and rockweed), green tea, soyabean oil, turnip greens, and lettuce.

Vitamin D

DRI for pregnancy and breastfeeding: 5 micrograms or 400 International Units (IU).

Functions: Used in bone mineralization through control of calcium and phosphorus in the body.

Sources: Sunshine, fortified milk, fortified cereals, and egg yolks.

Note: The best source of vitamin D is sunlight! Your skin produces its own vitamin D when exposed to sufficient sunlight. Women who develop deficiencies generally avoid dairy products, have very dark skin, or usually protect their skin from the sun with clothes or sunscreen. Women who live in northern latitudes (such as Boston, Massachusetts) or possibly southern latitudes (such as Christchurch, New Zealand) are also at risk for vitamin D deficiency because those areas don't get sufficient sunshine in the winter.[18] If any of the above risk factors apply to you, you should eat more foods fortified with vitamin D, spend more time in the sun, or ask your doctor or midwife about taking a supplement. (Use caution in supplementing vitamin D on your own; it is toxic in large doses.)

Exposing your hands and face to sunshine ten to fifteen minutes per day, two to three times per week in the summer is enough to produce adequate vitamin D levels. (Sunscreen and air pollution can block vitamin D synthesis.) If you do not get this much unprotected exposure or you have dark skin, make sure you have a dietary source of vitamin D. The DRI for vitamin D can be obtained from 500 ml (17 fl oz) of milk.

Another good reason to make sure your body makes enough vitamin D: Studies show that reduced circulating vitamin D may lead to increased risk for breast, colon, and prostate cancer.[19]

Vitamin B_6 (Pyridoxine)

DRI for pregnancy: 1.9 milligrams; for breastfeeding: 2.0 milligrams.

Functions: Used in amino acid and fatty acid metabolism; helps make red blood cells. Vitamin B_6 is needed in amounts proportional to the amount of protein in the diet.

Sources: Green and leafy vegetables, meats, fish, poultry, shellfish, legumes, fruits, and whole grains.

Note: Women – pregnant or not – don't seem to have enough vitamin B_6 in their diets. Some women who take birth control pills may have a slightly increased need for vitamin B_6. Deficiency can cause anaemia, irritability, and abnormal brain wave pattern.

Vitamin B_6 and Morning Sickness: Vitamin B_6 appears to be useful in treating morning sickness. However, large amounts of B_6 can be neurotoxic, so please discuss B_6 supplements with your doctor before self-prescribing.

Folic Acid (Folacin)

DRI for pregnancy: 600 micrograms; for breastfeeding: 500 micrograms.

Functions: Needed for all new cell production and use of amino acids. Also needed for some enzymes.

Sources: Spinach, leafy green vegetables, black-eyed peas, lentils, red kidney beans, broccoli, Brussels sprouts, beets, okra, green peas, asparagus, legumes, orange and grapefruit juice, and fortified cereals.

Note: The need for folic acid more than doubles during pregnancy due to vast increases in the number of new cells being made. Folic acid can be easily destroyed in cooking. Certain medications, such as oral contraceptives, anticonvulsants, aspirin, chemotherapy drugs, and antacids, can affect your folic acid status. Alcohol and smoking can also increase the need for folic acid.[20] If you take any of the above medications, smoke, or drink regularly, or if you did just prior to pregnancy, your need for folic acid is probably greater than average. You will need to choose your diet carefully and may want to discuss folacin supplementation with your doctor.

Folacin and Birth Defects: A landmark study done in several countries showed that folacin supplementation around the time of conception could prevent about 70 per cent of recurrent neural tube defects. It is thought that folacin supplementation can also prevent first-time occurrences. The US Institute of Medicine recommends that all women of childbearing potential consume 400 micrograms of folic acid per day from fortified foods or a supplement in addition to the folic acid found in a healthy diet. (An intake of 600 micrograms is recommended in pregnancy.)[21]

Iron

DRI for pregnancy: 30 milligrams; for breastfeeding: 15 milligrams.

Functions: Plays a very important role in pregnancy. Part of the blood protein haemoglobin, which carries oxygen in the body. Part of muscle protein. Necessary for the use of energy in the body.

Sources: Clams, fortified cereals, tofu, lentils, eggs, chicken, legumes, and dried fruit.

Note: Iron-deficiency anaemia is still a public health problem in the US. Pregnant women with iron-deficiency anaemia are more likely to have a premature or low-birth-weight baby. In the US 1985 Continuing Surveys of Food Intakes of Individuals (CSFII), only 4 percent of women met or exceeded the DRI for iron.[22]

Zinc

DRI for pregnancy: 15 milligrams; for breastfeeding, first six months: 19 milligrams, for second six months: 16 milligrams.

Functions: Promotes normal growth of tissues and bones; needed for the normal development of a foetus; involved in making genetic material, in immune reactions, in taste and smell, and in wound healing. Zinc is also required for sperm production.

Sources: Oysters, turkey, lean pork, wheatgerm, whole grains, lima beans, and almonds.

Note: Zinc deficiency during pregnancy can cause low birth weight, increased pregnancy complications, and premature births. A zinc deficiency during foetal brain development could cause foetal brain injury.[23]

Vitamin C (Ascorbic Acid)

DRI for pregnancy: 70 milligrams; for breastfeeding, first six months: 95 milligrams; for second six months: 90 milligrams.

Functions: Needed for thyroid hormone, collagen synthesis, and production of amino acids. Strengthens resistance to infection, helps absorption of iron, and acts as an antioxidant, meaning it breaks down oxidants, or free radicals, which can be destructive to cell membranes.

Sources: Kiwifruit, mango, papaya, citrus fruits, melons, peppers, berries, leafy green vegetables, tomatoes, broccoli, cauliflower, and cabbage.

The Support Nutrients

These nutrients help all the other nutrients with their functions.

Vitamin E (Tocopherol)

DRI for pregnancy: 10 milligrams; for breast-feeding, first six months: 12 milligrams, for second six months: 11 milligrams (all based on alpha-tocopherol equivalents).

Functions: Strong antioxidant. Works together with other antioxidants, vitamin C, and beta-carotene. There is some evidence that vitamin E intake above the DRI may be associated with decreased risk of heart disease and certain cancers. Research continues. If you followed a low-fat diet or took cholesterol-lowering drugs before your pregnancy, your body may be partially depleted of vitamin E.

Sources: Wheatgerm and wheatgerm oil, sunflower oil, safflower oil, almond oil and almonds, hazelnuts, and mayonnaise and salad dressings made with the above oils.

Sodium

There is no DRI for sodium; estimated minimum requirement for pregnancy: 570 milligrams; for breastfeeding: 635 milligrams.

Functions: Maintains normal fluid balance. Needed for nerve impulse transmission.

Note: Historically, women lowered their salt and sodium intake during pregnancy to reduce water retention and sometimes to prevent pre-eclampsia. Now, moderation rather than restriction is the key for pregnant women.

Potassium

There is no DRI for potassium; estimated minimum requirement for pregnancy: 2,000 milligrams; for breastfeeding: 2,500 milligrams.

Functions: Maintains fluid balance and helps maintain normal blood pressure. Helps with nerve impulses and muscle contractions.

Sources: Bananas, oranges and orange juice, watermelon, cantaloupe melon, vegetables, meats, milk, grains, and legumes.

Note: A high potassium intake has been linked to a reduced incidence of high blood pressure in certain populations.[24] In the US 1985 CSFII, women's potassium intakes were well below the estimated safe and adequate daily dietary intake.[25]

Other Trace Elements

Zinc and iron are considered trace elements, but they are so important during pregnancy that I included them in the section above. Other trace elements are copper, iodine, selenium, fluoride, manganese, chromium, and molybdenum. According to the US Subcommittee on Dietary Intake and Nutrient Supplements, routine supplementation of trace elements (with the exception of iron) does not seem to be necessary in pregnancy.

Copper

The estimated DRI for adults is 1.5 to 3 milligrams.

Functions: Helps in red blood cell production; is found in nerve coverings and connective tissue. Also assists in energy production and in respiration. Copper deficiency during pregnancy is unknown.

Sources: Whole grains, shellfish, kidney, raisins, nuts, peas, and beans.

Iodine

DRI for pregnancy: 175 micrograms; for breastfeeding: 200 micrograms.

Functions: An essential component of the thyroid hormone thyroxine, which is responsible for regulating the basal metabolic rate (the amount of energy the body needs at rest). Iodine deficiency during pregnancy can cause foetal disorders such as stillbirth, birth defects, and neurological impairment.

Sources: Seafood, iodized salt, and food grown in ocean areas that contain iodine-rich soil.

Selenium

DRI for pregnancy: 65 micrograms; for breastfeeding: 75 micrograms.

Functions: As an antioxidant, selenium works to protect body compounds from oxidation. Research links selenium and other antioxidants with reduced cancer risk.

Sources: Seafood, meats, and grains.

Fluoride

The estimated safe and adequate daily dietary intake for adults is 1.5 to 4 milligrams.

Functions: Bonds calcium and phosphorus in bones and teeth; prevents cavities in teeth.

Sources: Water that naturally contains fluoride or water that has fluoride added. If you are not sure whether your water contains fluoride, you might want to have it tested.

'The bottom-line message: The emphasis on optimal diet is of the greatest importance to all women of the childbearing age at all times – not only when pregnancy has been confirmed.'

– *Michael Hambidge, M.D., Sc.D., Director of the Center for Human Nutrition, University of Colorado Health Sciences Center, US*

Manganese

The estimated safe and adequate daily dietary intake for adults is 2 to 5 milligrams.

Functions: Part of enzymes that are active in many cell processes and a component of an important antioxidant.

Sources: Whole grains, beans, peas, and nuts.

Chromium

The estimated safe and adequate daily dietary intake for adults is 50 to 200 micrograms.

Functions: Associated with insulin; needed for the release of energy from glucose. Inability to use glucose results in diabetes-like deficiency symptoms. There is some concern that increased refinement of foods such as whole grains could lead to decreased intake of this trace mineral.

Sources: Whole grains, meat, mushrooms, asparagus, and brewer's yeast.

Molybdenum

The estimated safe and adequate daily dietary intake for adults is 75 to 250 micrograms.

Functions: A component of enzymes used in many body processes.

Sources: Legumes, cereals, and offal.

Nutrient Content of Protein Foods

Food	Fat (grams)	Protein (% DRI)	Thiamin (% DRI)	Iron (% DRI)	Zinc (% DRI)	Vitamin B$_6$ (% DRI)	Vitamin B$_{12}$ (% DRI)	Niacin (% DRI)
Beef sirloin, fat trimmed off 90 g (3.5 oz)	10	40	7	9	35	19	91	19
Beef braising steak, trimmed to 3mm (⅛ in) fat 90 g (3.5 oz)	19	40	3	9	40	13	98	15
Minced beef, extra lean 90 g (3.5 oz)	13	40	3	8	36	14	83	28
Leg of lamb, lean 90 g (3.5 oz)	6	40	6	6	28	8	88	30
Pork loin, lean 90 g (3.5 oz)	7	44	54	2	13	18	23	25
Chicken breast 90 g (3.5 oz)	3	44	3	3	6	27	11	65
Salmon 90 g (3.5 oz)	7	34	6	1	3	25	103	35
Tuna 90 g (3.5 oz)	1	36	1	4	2	15	98	62
Prawns 90 g (3.5 oz)	1	29	1	9	9	6	48	12
Clams, steamed 90 g (3.5 oz)	2	36	9	79	15	5	3200	16
Tofu, firm 90 g (3.5 oz)	2	10	6	3	3	0.5	0	1
Pinto beans 90 g (3.5 oz)	1	23	22	15	12	14	0	4

Source: U.S. Department of Agriculture. USDA Nutrient Database for Standard Reference, Release 13, 1999.

Of Special Concern

Studies of pregnant women's diets have shown that intakes of folic acid, iron, calcium, zinc, magnesium, and vitamins B$_6$, D, and E were below the DRIs. Check the preceding pages to see if you have sources of these nutrients in your diet.

Selected Nutrients in Various Cuts of Meat

All animal proteins are not equal; they provide varying amounts of zinc, iron, and vitamins B$_6$ and B$_{12}$. The graph above shows why you should eat a variety of meats.

Vitamin Supplements: You May Need Them

The general need for vitamin/mineral supplements has been debated for years, and so has their use during pregnancy.

Prenatal vitamins have been prescribed across the board for most pregnant women. However, a US National Academy of Sciences subcommittee recommends in its report *Nutrition during Pregnancy* that prenatal vitamin supplements should be prescribed on an individual basis, based on each woman's current nutritional status.[26]

The reason for the concern is that large doses of certain nutrients – including iron, zinc, selenium, and vitamins A, B_6, C, and D – can be toxic to the foetus. Moreover, an increase in the amount of one nutrient may negatively affect how other nutrients are absorbed and used.[27]

Because of the evidence about folic acid and neural tube defects, several organizations have come out in favour of taking either a folic acid supplement or a multivitamin supplement containing folic acid before conception. For example, the March of Dimes Foundation in the US recommends that all women capable of becoming pregnant take a daily multivitamin supplement that contains 400 micrograms of folic acid. The US Institute of Medicine recommends women consume 400 micrograms of folic acid from fortified foods or a supplement in addition to the folic acid found in a healthy diet. A US federal regulation mandates that any grain products calling themselves fortified must be fortified with folic acid.

Even if you eat fortified grains, you must still eat other foods containing folic acid to meet the recommended intake.

Since up to 60 per cent of pregnancies may be unplanned, it makes sense to have the proper mix of nutrients in your body before conception to prevent birth defects.

If You Take Supplements

Here are some words of advice about taking vitamin supplements:

▶ **DO NOT TAKE INDIVIDUAL SUPPLEMENTS, except for calcium or vitamin C.**

Large amounts of certain vitamins can be toxic to the foetus, causing birth defects, or can create imbalances, with certain nutrients competing with other nutrients for absorption. Recent research shows that women who took more than 10,000 IU of vitamin A – just four times the DRI – had five times the risk of birth defects compared to women who consumed 5,000 IU or less.[28]

▶ **Three months before you are pregnant and during the first months of pregnancy, it is important to take a multivitamin/mineral supplement that contains 400 micrograms of folic acid and no more than 100 per cent of the DRI for all nutrients. It may also be advisable for men to take a multivitamin/mineral supplement three months prior to conception.**

You can find this information on the label. When you confirm your pregnancy, your doctor might suggest that you take a prenatal vitamin. Remember that a vitamin/mineral supplement is no substitute for a healthy diet!

▶ **Remember that vitamin supplements are not the only sources of substantial amounts of vitamins.**

Fortified cereals can also provide 100 per cent of the DRI for many nutrients. If you were to take a multivitamin in addition to several servings of fortified food, you could potentially get too many vitamins, and the excess could be toxic.

▶ **If your doctor or midwife suggests a supplement that is nauseating you, consider taking the supplement with a light snack before you go to bed.**

Calcium Supplements

Calcium is vital during pregnancy for your baby's health and especially for your future bone health. Research also shows some correlation between increased calcium in the diet and reduced incidence of high blood pressure during pregnancy.[29]

Yet many women, both pregnant and not, do not have enough calcium in their diet. Women often start thinking about osteoporosis around the time of menopause, but they should actually consider their bone health all their lives. Bone continues to grow until the age of twenty-five and gradually starts losing mass after thirty-five. (See page 66 for information on how to sneak calcium into your diet.)

Recent research shows another good reason to have enough calcium in your diet: As your bones lose calcium to make up for calcium missing from your diet, lead stored in your bones is released. You are exposed to small amounts of lead over a lifetime from drinking water and other sources, and it is stored in your bones. During times when bones lose calcium (during pregnancy and lactation and after menopause, in women), lead is released into the bloodstream.

Adequate dietary calcium is essential in preventing, or at least minimizing, the turnover of bone. If you have had substantial lead exposure (by living in a house with lead pipes or eating leaded paint chips as a child), adequate calcium is even more important to prevent lead poisoning of yourself and your unborn child.[30]

The US National Institutes of Health recommend 1,200 to 1,500 milligrams of calcium per day for pregnant and breast-feeding women. They suggest you try to get your calcium from food first. If you can't, then take a supplement.

If you are currently taking a calcium or iron supplement, you should consider a few things about the way you take them:

Type of Calcium

Calcium is best absorbed from calcium citrate and calcium carbonate. Calcium carbonate is the most concentrated and economical form of calcium. Many women take Tums because it contains calcium carbonate. If you take too much calcium carbonate at one time, it can cause 'rebound hyperacidity' – excess stomach acid. If this becomes a problem, consider taking the calcium supplement in several doses during the day, since it is absorbed better that way. Avoid oyster shell calcium and dolomite due to possible lead and heavy metal contamination.

What You Take with It

Calcium is best absorbed when taken with food; iron is best absorbed on an empty stomach. If you take an iron supplement along with calcium citrate or calcium phosphate on an empty stomach, the amount of iron you absorb may be decreased.[31]

The Solution

If you take both iron and calcium, take them at different times. Take your iron supplement on an empty stomach or with a light snack that does not include a dairy product. Take your calcium supplement with a light snack. Registered US pharmacist Nellie Whaley suggests that if you take both calcium and iron, take the calcium at least two hours after or one hour before you take the iron.

Some women find that iron or prenatal vitamin supplements nauseate them. Taking supplements right before bedtime or with a snack usually helps. Whenever you decide to take your supplements, make it a ritual; calcium or iron left in the bottle won't bring you any benefit!

▼

Keeping Your Baby's Environment Safe

The 'don'ts' – you knew they were coming. An obstetrician who specializes in high-risk pregnancies once told me, 'You have only one chance to give your baby what it needs. Why not do everything you can to help your baby along? It's only nine months.' Giving advice is easy, but following it may not be so easy. If you are having problems with your health habits, talk to your doctor.

Smoking

The first trimester – and before pregnancy if possible – is a good time to kick some bad habits and pick up some good ones. Kiss your cigarettes good-bye, because babies of smokers weigh an average of 225 grams

(½ pound) less than those of non-smokers. Research shows that quitting smoking is the single most important thing you can do to improve the growth and long-term health of your baby.

Other adverse affects of smoking while pregnant include higher risk of pre-term delivery, early infant death, and possible problems with long-term growth, intellectual performance, and behavioural development. Babies of mothers who smoked during pregnancy were found to have a greater risk of obstructive sleep apnea, a disorder that causes infants to stop breathing while sleeping.[32] Smoking while you are pregnant may also affect your baby's neurological development.[33] Recent research has shown that the chemicals to which a foetus is exposed when a mother smokes can affect the brain in various ways. Girls are more likely to smoke and are five times more likely to be addicted to drugs in adolescence. Boys are more likely to have conduct disorders as adolescents and to be involved in criminal behaviour as adults.[34] And after your baby is born, he or she will also suffer the ill effects of secondhand smoke: higher risk of lower respiratory infections, middle ear infections, sudden infant death syndrome, and asthma.[35]

Smokers may need extra nutrients, such as vitamins B_{12} and C, amino acids, folic acid, and zinc, so a multivitamin/mineral supplement may be necessary.[36]

Quitting smoking has many benefits – but it may be easier said than done. For help, call the National Helpline for Smoking Cessation on 0800 169 0169.

Lead Exposure

Although lead isn't something you consume consciously, you may receive a regular dose of it from your drinking water. According to the US Environmental Protection Agency (EPA), as many as forty million people in the US may have too much lead in their drinking water. Pregnant women and children run the highest risk of problems from lead exposure because of increased absorption. Lead exposure can cause increased rates of miscarriage and stillbirth and may lead to such long-term effects as learning disability, brain damage, hyperactivity, high blood pressure, and kidney disease.[37] You may have too much lead exposure if:

- Your home was built in the last five years. The use of copper pipes with lead solder is widespread. As time passes, mineral deposits form a coating on the inside of the pipes that insulates the water from the solder. But during the first five years (before the coating forms), water is in direct contact with the lead.
- Your home was built before 1930. These homes often used lead pipes instead of copper ones. Also, water companies installed lead pipes underground to bring water to homes built during the first part of the century.
- You have 'soft' or acidic water. Soft or acidic water can strip away the mineral coating on water pipes and thus expose lead solder. Soft water is not dangerous if no lead was used either in your pipes or in the service pipes carrying water to your home.

- Your home has taps or fittings made of brass, which contains some lead.

To be safe, you should have your water tested. Contact your local Environmental Health Department. Avoid do-it-yourself tests – they are often inaccurate. Beware of scam artists who provide free lead testing and then sell you a treatment system you don't really need. The EPA action level for lead is fifteen parts per billion. You should take action to decrease the lead in your water if it has fifteen parts per billion in the 'first draw' or five parts per billion after you have let the water run for a minute or more.[38]

To decrease the lead in your water until you can do further testing or treatment, run cold water for several minutes before using for drinking or cooking. (Instead of wasting the water, consider saving it to water plants or wash windows.) If you usually use hot water to make coffee, tea, or for cooking, use cold water instead.

Inexpensive carafe water filters are now available, manufactured by Brita and Kenwood. Filtered water is also available for purchase in most grocery shops. Keep in mind that water filters may filter out fluoride; if yours does, check with your dentist to see if you should have supplemental fluoride.

Other possible sources of lead exposure include leaded crystal, pottery with leaded glaze, and lead-based paint that is chipping or being removed. Paint applied before 1978 contains lead.

Stripping lead paint from your home should be done only by a professional who is certified or licensed in lead safety. If not removed properly, fine lead particles can circulate throughout the home and cause even more problems.

Hot, acidic drinks like coffee can cause lead to leach from lead-glazed mugs. Similarly, fruit juice and acidic foods can cause lead to leach from leaded crystal. If you eat tinned foods regularly, be aware that the tins may contain lead solder.[39]

For More Information, Contact:
US National Lead Information Center
www.epa.gov/lead/nlic.htm

US National Sanitation Foundation International
P.O. Box 130140
Ann Arbor, MI 48113-0140
www.nsf.org
This nonprofit organization certifies and sets standards for water filtration systems.

US Coalition to End Childhood Lead Poisoning
www.leadsafe.org
This nonprofit group offers an educational website and encourages legislative action.

In the UK the Drinking Water Inspectorate is responsible for assessing the quality of the drinking water supplied by the water companies.

Illness during Pregnancy

Though no one plans to get sick or to be exposed to illness during pregnancy, knowing the facts can help. Some illnesses can affect your risk of miscarriage or low birth weight, and some can cause birth defects.

Immunization against the diseases listed below is often recommended before pregnancy. Ask your doctor or health visitor for information.

Chickenpox (varicella): Can cause birth defects and low birth weight.

Hepatitis B: Can cause low birth weight.

Rubella (German measles): Can cause birth defects and low birth weight.

Practising good hygiene, such as frequent hand washing, can prevent the spread of infectious diseases like the ones below.

Cytomegalovirus (CMV): Can cause birth defects, low birth weight, and developmental disorders.

Human immunodeficiency virus (HIV): Can cause low birth weight and cancer.

Human parvovirus B19: Can cause miscarriage.

Toxoplasmosis: Can cause miscarriage, birth defects, and developmental disorders. This parasite is passed in cat faeces and can also be transmitted by uncooked and undercooked meats and unwashed fruits and vegetables.

Women with immunity through vaccinations or earlier exposures are not generally at risk from hepatitis B, human parvovirus B19, German measles, or chickenpox. But pregnant women without prior immunity should avoid contact with infected children or adults.

Warning: Alcohol Can Cause Birth Defects

'Think before you drink' is a slogan that the US March of Dimes has used to remind women of the risk of drinking alcohol when pregnant. Foetal Alcohol Syndrome (FAS) and a variation, Foetal Alcohol Effect (FAE), can scar children whose mothers drink during pregnancy. FAS occurs in as many as three out of every thousand births, making it a leading cause of mental retardation. FAS can also cause permanent damage to growth and the central nervous system.[40] Mild cases of FAE can cause irritability, impulsiveness, and learning disabilities and may go undiagnosed for years. Many kids affected by FAE end up dropping out of school.

Alcohol is now recognized as a potent teratogen (a substance capable of causing birth defects) that can cause growth retardation (both in the womb and after birth) and facial abnormalities. Chronic alcohol abuse has been defined as more than two drinks per day. One drink per day has been shown to decrease birth weight.[42] Since alcohol freely crosses the placenta, the foetus's blood alcohol level is equal to the mother's. So one drink in a day might not be risky, but a drinking binge on a critical day of development could damage the foetus.

According to the US Public Health Service, as many as 86 per cent of women drink once during pregnancy; women with a higher level of education appear to drink more. In the past twenty years, there has been a fourfold increase in FAS in the United States.[43]

The good news is that if you are a drinker, whenever you stop, you increase your chances of having a healthy baby. Women who stopped drinking before their seventh month of pregnancy had healthy babies with no symptoms of FAS.[44]

What about an occasional drink? Research concerning low levels of alcohol consumption is limited and inconsistent. 'Because there is no level of drinking that is known to be safe, it is best to completely avoid alcohol during pregnancy,' says March of Dimes Medical Director Richard B. Johnston, M.D. If you have other concerns about alcohol, discuss them with your doctor.

Caffeine

You may be one of those people who 'aren't worth a darn' before their first cup of coffee. The bulk of the research about caffeine and pregnancy shows that moderate consumption (one cup of coffee per day, for example) is probably safe, yet there is some conflicting research. Heavy caffeine consumption of 300 milligrams per day has been shown to cause small reductions in birth weight, which could be detrimental to low-birth-weight or premature babies. Several studies have also suggested an association between caffeine and miscarriage.[45]

The US Food and Drug Administration continues to advise pregnant women to consume caffeine in moderation. Caffeine stimulates the central nervous system, is addictive, acts as a diuretic, and interferes with mineral absorption. The best advice: Instead of relying on caffeine, get more sleep and take a brisk afternoon walk for a pick-me-

Caffeine Content of Your Favourite Beverages and Foods			
Beverage or Food	**Caffeine (milligrams)**	**Beverage or Food**	**Caffeine (milligrams)**
Soft Drinks 375 ml (12 fl oz)		**Tea***	
Mountain Dew	55	250 ml (8 fl oz) black (Ceylon, Darjeeling, English Breakfast, Earl Grey)	25–110
Coke, Cherry Coke, Diet Coke	31		
Tab	31		
Pepsi	37	250 ml (8 fl oz) green	8–16
Diet Pepsi	36	250 ml (8 fl oz) herbal	0
Sprite, 7-Up (regular or diet)	0	Instant (1 teaspoon)	31
Any decaffeinated sodas	0	4.75 ml (8 fl oz) Snapple	48
Coffee		**Cocoa Drinks**	
Brewed 250 ml (8 fl oz)	135	Chocolate powder in milk (2–3 heaping teaspoons)	8
Instant 250 ml (8 fl oz)	95	Hot cocoa 25 g (1 oz) powder	5
Instant, decaffeinated (1 rounded teaspoon)	2	**Foods**	
Starbucks espresso 25 ml (1 fl oz)	90	25 g (1 oz) milk chocolate	11
Starbucks filter 250 ml (8 fl oz)	200	¼ cup chocolate chips (semisweet)	26

*Caffeine content varies with tea type, leaf size, and steeping time.

Sources: *Food Values of Portions Commonly Used*, 17th edition, by Jean Pennington; General Foods; Starbucks; Center for Science in the Public Interest, *Caffeine Content of Food and Drugs*.

up. If you must have some caffeine, switch to lower-caffeine products and consume as little as possible.

Herbal Preparations and Teas

Many people turn to herbal teas to cut their caffeine intake. However, you should stay away from teas containing coltsfoot, sassafras, calamus, or comfrey, all of which are carcinogenic.[46] Many herbal preparations, whether sold as teas or quasi medications, can act as drugs because they contain natural active chemicals. Some of these chemicals can be harmful to a foetus. Dr. Varro Tyler, Professor of Pharmacognosy at Purdue University, US and author of *The Honest Herbal,* advises, 'It is best to avoid herbal supplements during pregnancy unless you have expert knowledge about herbs or you are under the care of a doctor who does. Because they aren't approved as drugs, herbs don't undergo long-term toxicity testing.'

Remember that many of the drugs we use today first came from herbs, flowers, and trees. Exceptions are teas accepted as harmless, such as peppermint and chamomile. You should be safe if you stay with name-brand herbal and decaffeinated teas.

Drugs

All drugs, legal and illegal – even those as seemingly harmless as aspirin – have the potential to seriously harm your baby. So, let your midwife know if you are regularly taking any kind of drug. Also, ask what is safe to take for a cold, flu, or bad headache. Avoiding all medications is best when you're pregnant, especially during the first trimester. However, if you must take something, have your doctor approve it first.

When you are pregnant, you'll still be susceptible to headaches, colds, flu, and other problems for which you might ordinarily take medication. You may be on vacation and suddenly have a bad case of hay fever. For these times, have a list of over-the-counter medications approved by your doctor.

Cocaine

It has been estimated that over half the people addicted to crack cocaine are women.[47] Three studies done in US urban areas showed that between 10 and 17 per cent of women registered for prenatal care showed evidence of cocaine use.[48]

Cocaine addiction is, of course, harmful to the mother, but it can also have lifelong effects on a baby. Cocaine may take up to six days to leave the foetal blood supply. This increased exposure to the drug can result in premature separation of the placenta, foetal growth retardation, premature delivery, and decreased birth weight, length, and head circumference. Cocaine may also cause miscarriages, birth defects, and increased neurological and behavioural problems that may last a lifetime.[49]

If you are addicted to cocaine or any other drug, seek help through your doctor. If you'd like to read more about drugs and pregnancy, I recommend an excellent handbook titled *Drugs, Vitamins, and Minerals in Pregnancy* by Ann Karen Henry, Pharm. D., and Jil Feldhausen, M.S., R.D., Fisher Books, 1989.

▼

Travelling during Pregnancy

Chances are that during the nine months of pregnancy, you will travel somewhere. Travelling while pregnant may be 'business as usual', but it could also be challenging. Travelling can affect your exercise schedule and the types and amounts of food that you eat.

In the Plane

▶ **Find out whether a meal will be served.**

If you'd like a bit more control over your food on the flight, call the airline at least twenty-four hours before your flight to request a special meal. Some options are low-fat, vegetarian, diabetic, and seafood.

▶ **If you have a stopover between flights, use the time to exercise.**

Walk to your gate instead of using moving sidewalks or a bus.

▶ **Bring your own supply of snacks.**

Unless you are flying cross-country or overseas nonstop, you probably won't have a complete meal. And on a plane, even 'meals' can be skimpy. You will need snacks! Bring along fresh or dried fruit, wholegrain or digestive biscuits, granola bars, nuts, and other non-perishable snacks.

▶ **Request an aisle seat so you can get up to walk and stretch or go to the toilet.**

Bulkhead seats in the first row of each section offer more leg room.

▶ **If your flight is a long one, drink plenty of fluids before and during the flight.**

Flying can dehydrate you. During long flights, avoid carbonated beverages; they can increase gas.

▶ **Get up and walk around several times during the flight.**

Or, you may want to go to the back of the plane and just stand or stretch for a while. While sitting down, you can do isometric exercises, which can improve circulation.

▶ **Avoid taking heavy carry-on luggage unless someone else can carry it for you.**

The weight can increase back pain.

In the Car

▶ **Bring along a small coolbag in which you can keep yogurt, cheese, veggies, milk, fruit, and other snacks.**

You can even bring the makings of a sandwich, which can save you money on restaurant food. If you forget a coolbag, you can always stop at a supermarket along the way and pick up fresh or dried fruit and ready-to-eat raw vegetables.

▶ **Instead of eating regular-size meals when you stop, order appetizers or eat just half a portion.**

Sitting in the car for extended periods of time may induce 'boredom eating', yet you won't need as many calories while just sitting. Try to limit snacking to when you are actually hungry.

▶ **Drink plenty of fluids.**

If you are travelling to a higher altitude, your fluid needs will increase. Lack of activity can slow down your digestion and increase constipation. 'Pit stops' will allow you to get out and stretch, which can prevent back pain and increase circulation.

▶ **Plan 'adventure stops'.**

Try to include enough time in your itinerary to make extended stops to see things of interest. Use the stops as your exercise time to walk and stretch.

At Your Destination

▶ **If you are planning to stay at a hotel, try to get a room with a minifridge or kitchenette.**

This will allow you to keep your own snack foods as well as high-fibre cereals for breakfast or snacks.

▶ **Try to make wise food choices when eating out.**

When people eat most meals out, diets tend to be lower in fibre, calcium, vitamin C, and folacin and higher in fat and sodium.[50] (See page 237 for advice on eating out.)

▶ **If you are planning to stay with friends or relatives, bring along a few of the foods you usually eat, such as high-fibre cereal, milk, and extra fresh or dried fruit.**

This way your diet won't be lacking, and you won't have to ask your host to buy special foods for you.

▶ **Make sure you pack non-perishable snacks in your bag for those hectic tourist schedules.**

Good snacks include cheese biscuits, boxes of raisins, wheat biscuits, fibre bars, apples, bananas, and individual bags of pretzels. Don't forget the drinks! Juice boxes pack well.

▶ **If you are travelling to a foreign country, talk to your doctor before making reservations.**

Vaccinations may be required that you can't take while pregnant. Or, you may need to eat very carefully to avoid bacterial poisoning. You may want to take some non-perishable foods with you to snack on if familiar foods aren't available where you are going, or if food safety may be an issue.

▼

The Positives of Pregnancy

Although most people are familiar with only the negatives of pregnancy, pregnancy also has many positive aspects. For example, some women feel at their best when pregnant. And some women with chronic medical problems go into remission or experience decreased symptoms. By concentrating on the good things that occur during these nine months, life will be much more pleasant. Here are just a few of the good things about being pregnant. Try to think of them often!

• Your hair becomes thick and shiny.
• You radiate a warm, healthy glow.
• People open the door for you.
• Finally, you have a larger bra size!
• You can gain weight without guilt!
• You don't have to tuck in your blouse.
• You now have an excuse for being tired.
• You feel great all over.
• You feel good about taking care of yourself.
• You have a great reason for starting a walking programme and for eating right.
• You are the designated driver for the next nine months.
• Your partner brings you meals in bed.
• You're too tired for housework – a good excuse to get a cleaner!
• Finally, you have a long holiday to look forward to (maternity leave).
• Your kids learn how to help around the house.
• The love for your yet-to-be-born baby abounds.
• You don't have to worry about forgetting your birth control pill.
• You can wear one-size-fits-all clothes.
• You will become a member of Club Mother.
• You are part of a miracle.
• You have a special new friend living close by.
• This is an experience you'll have only once or a few times in your life. Enjoy it!

CHAPTER THREE

The First Trimester

What you will find in this chapter:

- *How Baby Is Growing*
- *Weight Gain and Energy Needs*
- *Protein Needs*
- *Other Nutrient Needs*
- *Focus on Fibre*
- *The Eating Expectantly Eating Plan*
- *Morning Sickness*
- *Other First-Trimester Challenges*
- *Food Planning for the First Trimester*

This chapter answers such questions as:

- *How much weight should I gain?*
- *I've read that I should eat 100 grams of protein; how much is that?*
- *How much protein is in an egg?*
- *How else can I get protein in my diet if I don't feel like eating meat?*
- *What can I do about morning sickness?*
- *How can I avoid constipation?*

How Baby Is Growing

During the first three months of pregnancy, good nutrition is vital for your baby's development. Babies born to poorly nourished mothers are more susceptible to birth defects and to infections in early childhood. Read on to learn about the many miraculous events taking place within your body during the first trimester.

At the End of One Week

For the first seven days after the sperm fertilizes the egg, the group of cells, or zygote, is travelling down the fallopian tube toward the uterus. Although the zygote is no larger than the tiniest speck of sand, it carries all the genetic material (DNA) necessary for development. During the first week, the cells are rapidly dividing into what will become organs, skin, hair, bones, and muscle. Even though the DNA and cells 'know' the sex of the baby, genital formation has not taken place yet, so we refer to the baby as 'it'.

The zygote implants in the uterine wall seven to eight days after fertilization; then it is known as an embryo. The mass of cells that includes both the embryo and what will become the placenta is only about the size of a blueberry.

At the End of Four Weeks (One Month)

By this time, you may be confirming your pregnancy and experiencing some of the telltale signs. The embryo is no bigger than a grain of rice, and its heart is beating by the twenty-fifth day. Its digestive system, backbone, and spinal cord are all beginning to form. Tiny limb buds that will become arms and legs are appearing. The next four weeks will be vitally important as development occurs rapidly.

At the End of Eight Weeks (Two Months)

The embryo is now about the size of your big toe, or a little over 25 mm (1 inch) long. All the major organs and systems are formed, yet some are not completely developed. The embryo clearly looks human. Its long arm and leg bones are beginning to form and are visible under its thin skin. The embryo now has a face, and its brain has taken shape. The head makes up almost half of the embryo. The embryo weighs only 6 g (¼ ounces)!

At the End of Twelve Weeks (Three Months)

From the ninth week on, the unborn baby is called a foetus. The nails are developed, and the foetus can suck its fingers and curl its hands into a fist. The kidneys are beginning to produce urine, and tooth buds for all the baby teeth are appearing. The foetus is only about as long as your middle finger (75 mm/3 inches) and weighs about 40 g (1½ ounces).

Although you may be just starting to buy maternity clothes or adjusting your belt to the next notch, most of your baby's organs and tissues are already formed.

Weight Gain and Energy Needs

Do you believe you have a special licence to eat for two because you're pregnant? Well, your licence is being revoked. You do need larger amounts of many nutrients during pregnancy, but you don't need to eat twice the food and calories, especially in the first trimester.

The Subcommittee on Nutritional Status and Weight Gain During Pregnancy of the US National Academy of Sciences recommends that you gain about 450 grams (1 pound) (or less) per month during the first trimester. That translates into 135 (or fewer) extra calories per day.[1] Uh oh, there go the visions of sundaes dancing in your head! Later in this chapter we'll talk about how to make your diet a winner without gaining too much weight.

Protein Needs

Protein is essential during pregnancy because your body uses it to build each new cell for your baby. Protein is also needed for the placenta – the lifeline that brings nourishment from you to your baby. Protein helps make new blood cells and muscle tissue that supports your baby. To top it all off, protein is used to make all the hormones that wreak havoc in your body when you're pregnant.

In the first trimester, your protein needs don't increase very much – only about 1⅓ grams extra each day, or the equivalent of 4 grams (⅙ ounce) of meat. The Daily Reference Intake (DRI) for protein throughout pregnancy is 10 grams higher than non-pregnancy needs, or 60 grams per day.[2] The additional protein you need is equal to 40 g (1½ ounces) of animal protein, 150 grams (5 ounces) of legumes, 1½ eggs, or 30 grams (1¼ ounces) of cheese.

Several factors influence your body's protein needs. To enable your body to use the protein you eat for building tissues and cells, you must eat enough calories (energy). This is because your body's first priority is supplying energy. If you eat enough protein but not enough calories, your body will use the protein for energy instead of for tissue building and other protein-dependent functions. Let's say you eat 275 grams (10 ounces) of fish and chicken every day. You don't have much of an appetite, so this fills you up and you don't eat much else, making your calorie intake from fats and carbohydrates inadequate. Because your body must use the protein for energy, your body will lack the protein it needs for other important purposes.

Also, you won't have enough glucose (blood sugar) to supply your brain with energy, so your body will start breaking down fat into fragments called ketones. The presence of ketones is a sign that your body can't complete the metabolic process. Large amounts of ketones can be harmful to your body. Avoid the production of ketones by having enough calories and carbohydrates in your diet.

Consuming a certain *quantity* of protein is not the only goal. The *quality* of protein also affects how your body uses it. Protein needs are calculated by determining the need for high biological value, or high-quality, protein. High-quality protein can be turned into body tissues. These proteins include

Protein Content of Food Groups

Food	Serving Sizes	Protein per Serving (grams)
Legumes	50 g (2 oz)	7–11
Dairy products	250 ml (8 fl oz) milk/ 25 g (1 oz) cheese	6–8
Meat, poultry, fish	25 g (1 oz)	6–8
Bread/cereal	1 slice/25 g (1 oz)	2–4
Vegetables	100 g (4 oz)	2–3
Fruits/juices	1 medium/125 ml (4 fl oz)	0–1
Fat, oil	Any amount	0

eggs, meat, chicken, milk, and fish. For all the bad press the egg has gotten over the years, it is well respected where protein is concerned. Egg protein is of the highest quality and is often used as a standard to which other proteins are compared.

If you do not eat animal products, your body will need greater quantities of lower-quality plant proteins to meet protein needs. Vegetarians, don't despair! You can meet your protein needs without eating meat, but you must look carefully at your intake of certain nutrients. (See page 94 for more information on vegetarian protein sources.)

As a rule, Westerners eat about twice as much protein as they really need. Pregnant women are no different, eating an average of 75 to 110 grams per day – well above the 60 grams per day recommended by the US Food and Nutrition Board. However, some doctors and birthing programmes recommend up to 100 grams of protein, especially for high-risk pregnancies. A daily diet that contains approximately 100 grams of protein might include four servings of dairy product, 175 grams (6 ounces) of animal protein (or the equivalent), four vegetables, four fruits, and eight servings of starch or bread.

Most women who eat a typical western diet don't have a problem meeting protein needs. In fact, the US National Academy of Sciences advises pregnant women not to use specially formulated high-protein supplements, protein powders, or high-protein beverages because some evidence suggests that these products might be harmful.[3]

Why You May Need to Work to Meet Your Protein Needs

You might not be able to meet your protein needs if you:

- don't drink milk or eat dairy products and also don't eat many other protein sources.
- have nausea or vomiting that prevents you from eating much of anything.
- just don't have the desire to eat meat.

If you eat or drink the recommended four servings of dairy products each day, you will be meeting half your protein needs. If you don't, you'll need to increase protein from other sources.

If you just don't feel like eating meat, you are not alone. Most pregnant women have some food aversion; your stomach may turn at the thought of eating what used to be your favourite food.

If your favourite high-protein foods turn your stomach, you can eat more dairy products, which are also good sources of protein, or you can turn to other sources. Many of the women I've talked to could tolerate eggs and cheese even if they couldn't eat meat. You may also tolerate many vegetarian protein sources. See page 65 for a list of protein sources and experiment to find what works for you.

If you can't eat much of anything due to first-trimester morning sickness, eat what you can. (See Chapter Thirteen for first-trimester recipes.) If the condition persists to the point where you are losing weight, alert your health-care provider, who may treat your nausea more aggressively or refer you to a registered dietitian for individual counselling.

Other Nutrient Needs

All vitamins and minerals play specific, essential roles during pregnancy, so be sure to have adequate amounts in your diet for the whole nine months.

Water is one of the most important nutrients in the first trimester – especially if you are suffering from morning sickness. Dehydration can be very serious! Folic acid is not only important in neural development but is also critical for cell production and division, which occur in leaps and bounds during the first trimester. Manganese is needed for developing the organs used for hearing. Vitamin A is needed for developing tissues. A low intake of zinc early in pregnancy is related to a threefold increase in the risk of very pre-term delivery.[4] Phosphorus, calcium, and vitamin D work together to produce strong bones..

Focus on Fibre

Fibre is one of those things most people don't eat enough of, even though every day new studies cite its benefits.

The old saying 'An apple a day keeps the doctor away' may well refer to an apple's fibre content. Here's why:

- Fibre-rich whole grains may protect against cancer, especially breast cancer and gastrointestinal cancers.[5]
- Soluble fibre has been shown to reduce cholesterol, thus reducing the risk of heart disease. Trace minerals and antioxidants in whole grains may also help cut heart disease risk.
- Soluble fibre helps control blood glucose, which is particularly beneficial to people with diabetes.[6]
- Fibre fills you up, not out!
- Fibre keeps your bowels moving, which can help prevent constipation and haemorrhoids.

Fibre Tips

Following are a few simple ways to make sure you get enough fibre every day:

▶ **Follow the slogan 'Five a Day for Better Health'.**

You'll be on your way to having adequate dietary fibre if you eat five fruits and vegetables daily.

Snack Tip

The fig may be the world's most under-appreciated fruit! Not only do figs have the highest amount of dietary fibre of any common fruit, nut, or vegetable, they are also higher in potassium than bananas and are considered a good calcium source. Eat this sweet, healthy treat as a between-meal snack.

Stuffed Figs

Cut a large slice in a fresh or dried fig. Fill it with low-fat or fat-free cream cheese, or puréed cottage cheese in a blender until it's the consistency of cream cheese. Add a dash of cinnamon or nutmeg for more flavour.

▶ **Choose wholemeal bread, savoury biscuits, and pasta.**

The American Dietetic Association supports the recommendation of three servings of wholegrain products daily.[7] Look at food labels; 'wholegrain' or 'wholemeal flour' should be the first ingredient.

▶ **Eat brown rice or bulgur instead of white rice.**

▶ **Start your day with a high-fibre cereal.**

Choose cereals containing at least 5 grams of fibre per serving.

▶ **When baking, replace part of the white flour with wheat bran, wholemeal flour, or oatmeal.**

Fibre Content of Foods

Food	Serving Sizes	Dietary Fibre (grams*)
Fruits		
Figs	5	9
Apple, fresh with skin	1 medium	4
Blackberries, raw	125 g (4 oz)	4
Raspberries, fresh	125 g (4 oz)	4
Dates	5	4
Pear, fresh with skin	1	4
Prunes	5	3
Banana	1 medium	3
Orange, fresh	1	3
Nectarine, fresh	1	2
Raisins	50 g (2 oz)	2
Pineapple, fresh	2 slices	2
Most other fruits contain 1–3 grams of fibre per serving.		
Vegetables		
Artichoke	1 medium	16
Potato with skin	1 medium	5
Green peas	50 g (2 oz)	4
Spinach, cooked and drained	75 g (3 oz)	3
Broccoli, cooked and chopped	75 g (3 oz)	3
Sweet potato, baked in skin	1 medium	3
Rhubarb, cooked	125 g (4 oz)	3
Corn, tinned	75 g (3 oz)	2
Cereals, Grains, and Legumes		
Black beans	125 g (4 oz)	8
Baked beans, tinned	125 g (4 oz)	7
Wheatgerm or wheat bran, unprocessed	4 tbsp	6
Bulgur or quinoa	75 g (3 oz)	5
Corn tortillas	2	3
Bran muffin	1	2–3
Popcorn	3½ cups	2–3
Wholemeal bread	1 slice	2
Brown rice, instant cooked	75 g (3 oz)	2

*Numbers rounded to the nearest whole number.

Sources: Pennington, J. *Bowes and Church's Food Values of Portions Commonly Used*. 17th Edition. Philadelphia: Lippincott Williams and Wilkins, 1998.

▶ Snack on high-fibre foods such as bran muffins, dried fruit, fresh fruit, vegetables, and wholegrain savoury biscuits.

If your diet is normally low in fibre, increase the fibre in your diet gradually. Adding a lot of fibre to your meals all at once can result in bloating and gas. Also, remember to drink plenty of fluids while eating high-fibre foods as they can cause constipation.

If you follow the advice above, you will be sure to get the 20 to 35 grams of fibre currently recommended by the US National Cancer Institute.[8] But if you want to be really aware of the specific amounts of fibre found in foods, look at the chart on page 52.

▼

The Eating Expectantly Eating Plan

What's the best way to eat for a healthy pregnancy? The guide below will help you plan your meals and snacks so that you obtain the nutrients you and your baby need. It may be helpful to write down what you eat for a few days and compare it to the Eating Expectantly Eating Plan.

Eating Expectantly Eating Plan

8 or more servings of grains

1 serving is 1 slice any type bread; ½ small bagel, pitta bread or English muffin; 1 150-mm (6-inch) tortilla; 8 tbsp cooked rice or pasta; 8 tbsp cooked cereal, barley, bulgur; 25 grams (1 ounce) ready-to-eat cereal, 3–4 savoury biscuits, or 2 biscuits.

Note: 3 or more of your 8 daily grain servings should be wholegrain.

4 or more servings of calcium-rich foods

1 serving is 250 ml (8 fl oz) any type milk or yogurt, 40 g (1½ ounces) natural cheese, 50 g (2 ounces) processed cheese, or 250 ml (8 fl oz) calcium-fortified orange juice or soya milk.

4 or more servings of fruit

1 serving is 1 medium fresh fruit; ½ grapefruit, mango, or papaya; 8 tbsp tinned or cut fruit; 4 tbsp dried fruit; or 200 ml (6.5 fl oz) fruit juice.

4 or more servings of vegetables

1 serving is 8 tbsp cooked vegetables, 250 ml (8 fl oz) leafy vegetables, 1 small potato, or 200 ml (6.5 fl oz) tomato or vegetable juice.

Note: Be sure to eat at least one fruit or vegetable that is high in vitamin C and one that is dark green or orange every day.

3 servings of protein foods

1 serving is 50–75 g (2–3 ounces) (the size of a deck of cards) cooked lean meat; 2 eggs; 8 tbsp tuna; 8 tbsp legumes, tofu, or textured vegetable protein; or 2 tablespoons nuts or nut butter.

Note: Eat a variety of protein foods, including fish at least once a week. Eat an additional ½ protein serving for each serving of milk that you don't drink.

Fats and sweets: Eat sparingly.

Most fat and sugar is hidden in foods, so watch out for fried foods, full-fat dairy foods, soft drinks, and so on.

Sample Meal Plan

Breakfast

Raisin bran cereal with strawberries

Wholemeal bagel with light cream cheese

Milk

Snack

Vegetable juice

Wholegrain savoury biscuits

Low-fat cheese

Lunch

Lean roast beef sandwich on wheat bread

Raw carrots and broccoli with dip

Melon balls

Biscuits

Milk

Snack

Popcorn

Dinner

Grilled salmon steak

Grilled corn on the cob

Spinach salad with tomato and mushrooms

Wholegrain roll

Fresh orange

Milk

Snack

Peanut butter and digestive biscuits

Yogurt with dried fruit

▼

Morning Sickness

A touch of queasiness may be your first clue that you are pregnant. If you have morning sickness, you may need to figure out how to survive the day before you can even think about eating. Here's some information to help you through this trying time.

The Facts on Morning Sickness

- You are not alone. Morning sickness is the most common problem of pregnancy, occurring in as many as 90 per cent of pregnancies. A very small percentage of pregnant women have severe nausea and vomiting (hyperemesis gravidarum), which can lead to weight loss, dehydration, and hospitalization.
- Despite its name, morning sickness can (and often does) occur any time of the day or night.
- While nausea often subsides by the second trimester, for some women it doesn't. According to Miriam Erick, M.S., R.D., author of *No More Morning Sickness* and *Take Two Crackers and Call Me in the Morning*, the average duration of morning sickness is seventeen-and-a-half weeks. Some women have morning sickness throughout their pregnancies.
- Morning sickness may be a sign that your hormones are at a healthy level. Women with morning sickness have a lower risk of miscarriage – unless they suffer significant weight loss.

- While no one knows exactly what causes morning sickness, some have theorized that pregnancy hormones – specifically estrogen and human chorionic gonadotrophin (HCG) – are to blame. Heightened sense of smell has also been blamed as a potential cause.

Morning Sickness Survival Tips

If morning sickness is making you miserable, the following tips may help you feel better. The first five tips are summarized from Miriam Erick's *No More Morning Sickness: A Survival Guide for Pregnant Women* (Plume, 1993).

Note: If you experience severe nausea and vomiting, consult your doctor or midwife. Do not self-treat with medication, vitamins, or herbal supplements without your doctor's approval.

1. Track your environment.

Erick recommends keeping score of how you feel throughout the day to determine whether certain environments tend to make you sick. Are you more sensitive to smells? To noise? To light? Are you more likely to feel sick when you are tired or hungry? Do certain food tastes or textures make you feel better?

2. Take the sniff test.

Because a pregnant woman may have a heightened sense of smell, any odour could trigger nausea. It might be an unpleasant odour like your neighbour's cigarette smoke or the body odour of the person next to you on the train, or it might be a smell you nor- mally love, like garlic or your partner's cologne. Try to identify and avoid odours that make you turn green. Alternatively, experiment with smells that make you feel better. (Erick has found the smell of lemon to be helpful for many women.)

3. Change your environment.

If smells bother you, try to get rid of them. This might mean eating only cold foods for a while, eating outside, or having someone else do the cooking. If a colleague's cologne is the problem, ask him or her not to wear it for a while. If the drive to work makes you queasy, try walking, using public transit, or working at home.

4. Trust your intuition.

Sometimes it's most important just to keep something down – no matter what it is. Ask yourself: "What would make me feel better? Something sweet, salty, crunchy, sour, soft, bland, or wet?" Erick has found that the food that often does the trick is potato crisps. I once had a bout of morning sickness on the morning of a TV interview. What sounded good at the moment? Pretzels and a cola. It definitely wasn't the healthiest breakfast – but after eating it, I was able to get on with my day and eat healthier foods.

5. Drink enough fluids.

Dehydration, which can be fatal, is the biggest danger of morning sickness. Women with severe morning sickness are often hospitalized to be rehydrated intravenously. 'Fluids are the most necessary nutrients and the hardest to get in,' Erick says. Most pregnant women need 10 cups of fluids per day.

Some women find sparkling water appealing, while others get their fluids from fruits with high water content, like watermelon, cantaloupe melon, and grapes. Popsicles, slushy drinks, ginger ale, and lemonade may also be appealing.

6. Avoid having an empty stomach.

Eat small, frequent meals with snacks in between to keep your stomach from emptying out completely. This might mean eating a little something as often as every thirty minutes. Some women carry a box of savoury biscuits with them all day to keep nausea at bay.

7. Eat a substantial bedtime snack.

Eating a bedtime snack with protein, such as half a sandwich and milk or peanut butter and biscuits, may keep your blood sugar up during the night and prevent morning sickness.

8. Avoid greasy, spicy, and strong-smelling foods.

Such foods can aggravate nausea as well as heartburn. However, if this kind of food sounds really good to you, it's worth a try!

9. Eat a snack before breakfast.

Leave food beside your bed at night or have your partner bring you a snack in the morning before you get out of bed. (Now there's a fine habit to cultivate!)

10. Eat slowly and drink fluids between (not with) meals.

This strategy may help you keep your food down. Remember that fluids are vital to your health, so be sure to get them one way or another!

11. Eat cold foods or have your partner do the cooking.

The look of raw food or the smell of strong foods cooking may make you feel sick. Use the cooking time to take a walk or do some shopping. You might also want to eat outside when possible to get more fresh air.

12. Think differently.

Some alternative therapies may help morning sickness. Acupressure and Sea-Bands (for motion sickness) have been shown to ease nausea during pregnancy. The use of ginger, hypnosis, and vitamin B_6 has also helped some women. Vitamin B_6 can be toxic in large amounts, so consult your doctor before self-treating! Prescription drugs may also be a safe and effective treatment for your morning sickness.[9]

▼

Other First-Trimester Challenges

Frequent Urination

In those first few months, you might feel as though you're wearing a path in the carpet with all your trips to the bathroom. The increased frequency of urination may be an early hint that you're pregnant. Your baby, within the uterus, sits right above your bladder. As your uterus engorges with blood and your baby grows, the pressure on your bladder increases and the space for storing urine decreases.

What You Can Do:

▶ **DON'T decrease your total fluid intake!**

However, if you're getting up several times during the night to urinate, you might want to slightly decrease your intake of fluids during evening hours.

▶ **Sleep on your side.**

Lying on one side may help relieve pressure on your bladder.

▶ **Start doing pelvic floor exercises now and continue during and after your pregnancy.**

These exercises tone up the muscles that hold in urine. Have you ever sneezed or coughed and felt as though you nearly emptied your bladder? This can happen more frequently during pregnancy and again later in life. The weakened bladder control may be due to poor muscle tone in the area, along with added pressure from baby. Keeping these muscles toned during pregnancy can also help you get back in shape and heal more quickly after you have the baby. Ask your doctor or midwife for information.

Note: If urination is painful, contact your doctor.

Fatigue

You may feel as though you could sleep for the rest of your pregnancy. During the first trimester, when your hormones are playing tag and you're it, fatigue is common.

What You Can Do:

▶ **Accept your need for rest and slow down your lifestyle.**

▶ **Eat regular, balanced meals that are high in the essential nutrients.**

If you're not eating enough calories or not getting enough essential nutrients, your diet could be partly to blame for the fatigue. (See page 28 for more information on essential vitamins and minerals.) During the first trimester, your health-care provider will probably check the amount of iron in your blood. Iron-deficiency anaemia can cause fatigue and is fairly common in pregnancy due to the greatly increased need for this mineral. Consuming adequate amounts of dietary iron before and during pregnancy can prevent anaemia. (See pages 70–71 for good sources of iron.)

▶ **Exercise regularly.**

Even though you may not feel you have the energy to exercise, afterwards you'll be glad you did. (See Chapter Ten: Fitting Fitness In.)

Cravings and Aversions

We've all heard stories about the husband who runs to the shop in the middle of the night to get his wife chocolate-fudge ice cream. You may be experiencing something similar. No one is sure what causes cravings. Sometimes, a craving signals a dietary need. (No, we don't have a DRI for chocolate-fudge ice cream yet!) Some women crave non-food items like clay, starch, dirt, or ice. This particular type of craving, called pica, usually stems from an iron deficiency. Other cravings may be due to – you guessed it – those crazy, mixed-up hormones.

Cravings for sweets can be explained by drops in blood sugar, which can happen easily if you don't eat often enough. In this case, your body needs any carbohydrate food and you may, for example, turn the need into a craving for your favourite high-carbohydrate food, such as ice cream.

Cravings can often be healthy. I'm generally not a grapefruit eater, but when pregnant with my second child, I asked for grapefruit frequently. I also often wanted a stick-to-your-ribs food like a bean burrito or hamburger. This may have been due to the need for more calories or protein.

Aversions to certain foods are just as common as cravings, so don't be surprised if your favourite food now turns you off. Sometimes an aversion (to cigarettes or alcohol, for example) acts to protect your baby. Meat is often unappealing during pregnancy, while eggs, cheese, milk, and beans are often more easy to tolerate. (See Chapter Six for vegetarian eating tips.)

Whatever your particular fancy, rest assured it will probably change during your pregnancy and will be different during your next pregnancy!

What You Can Do:

▶ **To keep cravings in check, make sure to eat regular meals and snacks, including breakfast.**

▶ **If you *must* have something, then have it!**

If the craved food is less than nutritious, try to eat a small amount. Or, try to steer your craving toward a healthier alternative – such as a wholemeal raisin bagel instead of a doughnut.

Breast Changes

Breast enlargement and sensitivity are common early signs of pregnancy. In the first trimester the fat layer of your breast thickens, and the number of milk glands increases. The veins close to the surface enlarge due to your increased blood flow. Your nipples and areolas (the dark areas around your nipples) will enlarge and probably get darker.

What You Can Do:

▶ **Wear a good supportive bra, preferably one with flexible straps.**

If you plan to breast-feed, a nursing bra is a wise choice.

▶ **If you are large-busted, you might want to sleep in a lightweight bra.**

Teeth and Gum Changes

Hormones and increased blood flow affect many areas of your body, including your gums. They can soften and become more prone to infections.

What You Can Do:

▶ **Eat a balanced diet that contains plenty of vitamin C.**

Good nutrition is the first defence against gum disease.

▶ Don't neglect your teeth and gums during pregnancy.

Continue regular flossing, brushing, and professional cleaning. Have a dental checkup during your pregnancy. However, be sure your dentist knows that you are pregnant before your visit.

Note: If you are planning a pregnancy, visit your dentist first for a checkup and for any dental work that might be needed.

❓ Questions You May Have

Q: What if I skip meals – is that bad for the baby?

A: Yes, and for you, too! During pregnancy, your baby depends entirely on you for energy. When you don't eat, your baby may not get the energy and nutrients it needs and will then use your nutrient stores, which may leave you depleted. When you skip meals, you often eat much more food later to make up for it, and you may store those extra calories as fat. Try to avoid the feast-or-famine approach by taking the time to eat regular meals and snacks.

Q: I usually eat fast food for lunch every day. How can I eat more nutritiously?

A: I recommend planning ahead and taking the time to shop and cook. The time and effort will be well spent. Eating typical fast food is costly – both in money and to your health. Fast food provides lots of calories, but not many nutrients. To improve on a typical fast-food meal, have fruit with it. Good news: Fast food is improving, and eating nutritiously on the run is getting easier. (See page 309 for 'Meals in Minutes', and page 239 for 'Choosing Nutritious Fast Foods'.)

Q: What if I just can't eat much at all? My 'morning' sickness occurs all the time.

A: As noted earlier, extra calories aren't a priority in the first trimester. What is important is keeping your baby's environment safe, having an adequate intake of folic acid, and keeping well hydrated. Eat whatever you can to get through your nausea and make sure to drink plenty of fluids. The baby will draw on your stored nutrients if you aren't able to eat much. However, make your calories count. When you *are* able to eat, eat the most nutritious foods you can, and when your morning sickness has subsided, eat well to restock your body's nutrient stores.

▼

Food Planning for the First Trimester

During the first trimester, cooking and eating can be a big challenge. If you're looking for practical, realistic menus for your situation, browse the list overleaf and refer to Chapter Thirteen for menu details and delicious recipes.

Menus

- Don't Feel Like Eating
- Don't Feel Like Cooking
- Don't Feel Like Eating or Cooking
- Feel Like Staying in Bed, but Can't
- Feel Great
- Blender Breakfasts (or Snacks to Go)
- Snack Ideas
- High-Energy Snack Ideas

CHAPTER FOUR

The Second Trimester

What you will find in this chapter:

• *How Baby Is Growing*
• *Weight Gain and Energy Needs*
• *How's Your Diet?*
• *Protein Needs*
• *Other Nutrient Needs*
• *The Power of Soya*
• *Focus on Calcium*
• *Focus on Iron*
• *'Thrive on Five'*
• *Smart Snacking*
• *Second-Trimester Challenges*
• *Food Planning for the Second Trimester*

This chapter answers such questions as:

• *Doesn't my prenatal vitamin have enough calcium?*
• *Which foods are high in iron?*
• *What's a good snack?*
• *What about chocolate milk?*
• *Which has more calcium: milk or yogurt?*
• *When will I feel my baby move?*

You've made it through the first trimester – congratulations! The second trimester includes the thirteenth through to the twenty-sixth weeks and is usually when pregnant women feel their best. During this time you'll have lots of energy, especially if you're eating right and exercising. You'll mark the halfway point of your pregnancy and you'll feel your baby move!

How Baby Is Growing

The development of all the major organs and systems is either started or complete. From now on, the foetus will start to gain more weight. Your body is producing more blood in order to nourish your baby, so you need to be drinking plenty of fluids, preferably 10 cups per day of water, milk, juice, or soup. Anything with caffeine can cause you to lose your needed fluids.

At the End of Sixteen Weeks (Four Months)

Your baby is quite active, even though you might not feel it yet. Making facial expressions, swallowing, rotating feet, kicking, sleeping, waking, and even listening to you are all part of your baby's daily routine. Downy hair called lanugo is developing on the head. The foetus is now 150 to 175 mm (6 to 7 inches) long and weighs 175 to 225 g (6 to 7 ounces), the weight of a large apple.

At the End of Twenty Weeks (Five Months)

A growth spurt has occurred within the last month. The foetus now measures between 200 and 300 mm (8 and 12 inches) and weighs about 450 g (1 pound). Lanugo now covers the whole body, and the hair on the head is getting thicker.

Eyebrows and eyelashes are developing. You are beginning to sense your baby's movements as its muscles develop and it becomes stronger at turning and rolling.

At the End of Twenty-Four Weeks (Six Months)

Baby is now between 275 and 350 mm (11 and 14 inches) long and weighs between 674 and 750 grams (1½ and 1¾ pounds). The foetus looks like a wrinkled old man. Its skin is covered in vernix, a thick waxy coating that protects its skin while in the amniotic fluid. Baby opens and closes its eyes and can hear and respond to external noise and music. Its distinct fingerprints and footprints are formed. (Even identical twins have different fingerprints.) The alveoli in the lungs are just beginning to develop. If the baby were born at this time, it would need extremely specialized care.

Weight Gain and Energy Needs

During the last two trimesters of your pregnancy, your body needs about 300 more calories per day than it needed before you were pregnant. Eating at this rate will result in an 11.5- to 16-kilo (25- to 35-pound) weight gain – considered optimal for a healthy baby. However, many things will affect your energy needs, including pre-pregnant weight, activity level, and current weight. Some women are less active during the last half of pregnancy; others remain active and burn even more calories due to their increasing weight.

From now on, you should try to gain about 450 grams (1 pound) per week.[1] Remember that the extra calories and protein you are eating work towards creating a healthy environment for your baby to live in until birth. The extra nutrients are required for increased blood volume, placental growth, increased fat storage, increased breast tissue, and production of amniotic fluid. In addition, nutrients provide the building materials for your growing foetus.

In the next few weeks – usually between sixteen and twenty weeks gestation – you should feel a fluttering in your uterus; this is your baby moving! It's a very exciting feeling and also a reminder that during these special months you must take good care of yourself by eating right, exercising moderately, and trying to improve other lifestyle habits.

Now is a good time to take inventory of your diet and health habits. Complete the survey below to find out how your diet compares with the dietary needs of a mother-to-be.

How's Your Diet?

First write down in the spaces that follow everything you've eaten during the last day (or on a typical day). Then refer to the Eating Expectantly Eating Plan on page 53 to tally the number of servings of each food type you've eaten. Compare your totals for the day with those recommended.

Breakfast

_____

_____

_____

Snack

_____

_____

Lunch

_____

_____

_____

Snack

_____

_____

Dinner

_____

_____

_____

Snack

_____

_____

How Did You Do?

Your diet should contain at least:

8 or more servings of grains
Best choices: whole grains, wholemeal bread and cereal, sweet potatoes, winter squash, potatoes, dried beans, peas, corn, wheat biscuits, and popcorn.
Note: Don't forget that three servings should be whole grains.

4 or more servings of fruits
Best choices: papaya, mango, melon, berries, apricots, peaches, grapefruit, orange, and kiwifruit.

4 or more servings of vegetables
Best choices: broccoli, cauliflower, carrots, spinach, cabbage, leaf and cos lettuce, greens, peppers, and tomatoes.
Note: Don't forget to eat at least one vitamin-C-rich and one vitamin-A-rich fruit or vegetable every day!

4 or more servings of calcium-rich foods
Best choices: skimmed and semi-skimmed milk and yogurt, fat-free and low-fat cheeses, and tofu made with calcium.

3 servings of protein foods
Best choices: fish and shellfish, dried beans and legumes, tofu, poultry, lean beef, lamb, and pork. Be sure to eat a variety, and include fish at least once a week!

Fats and sweets: Eat sparingly.
Best choices: avocado, nuts, nut oils, seeds (especially flaxseed), canola and olive oil or products made with these oils.
Note: Remember that baked goods, fried foods, full-fat products, and desserts have

many hidden fats. Fat has twice as many calories as carbohydrate or protein.

8 to 10 cups of fluid

You should be drinking to thirst, or at least 8 cups of fluid per day, most of it from water.

Visit www.healthyfoodzone.com for more eating tips.

▼

Protein Needs

Protein is very important during the second trimester for the growing tissue of the foetus and placenta, your increasing blood volume, and your growing breast and uterine tissues.

All protein is not equal. Proteins are composed of amino acids, and for proteins to be used most efficiently, all the essential amino acids must be present in certain amounts and proportions. The term *complete protein* describes protein that contains all the essential amino acids (those your body can't produce) in the amounts needed to build proteins. *Incomplete proteins* lack one or more amino acids or contain small amounts of amino acids. This distinction is important for people who don't eat animal protein. In the past, nutritionists believed that we needed to combine incomplete proteins during the same meal. Now we know that eating a variety of different proteins throughout the day is adequate.[2]

Foods that contain complete protein include beef, poultry, fish, milk, eggs, and cheese. Foods considered incomplete-protein sources include beans, rice, grains, peanut butter, nuts, pasta, soya products, and some vegetables. (Fruit contains very small amounts of protein.) Various protein sources supply different nutrients, so eat a variety of foods, both those that contain complete protein and those that contain incomplete protein. (See the chart on page 65 to learn the protein content of many common foods.) Even if you are not vegetarian, I encourage you to eat non-animal protein sources, especially soya. Consider eating one or two meatless meals per week.

If you aren't much of a meat eater, eat smaller amounts of the higher-protein meats or eat more vegetable protein sources. (See Chapter Six: Vegetarian Eating for more information.)

▼

Other Nutrient Needs

Iron is important during the second trimester because the foetus starts to store iron for the future and you continue to need more iron for increased blood volume. Your body needs potassium for nerve impulse transmission. If you vomited a lot during the first trimester, your body may be depleted of potassium. Vitamin C is necessary to produce collagen, a binding substance used in muscle, blood vessels, and nerves. Chromium is a trace mineral used in the regulation of blood sugar, and inadequate intake may contribute to gestational diabetes, which often occurs during the second trimester.

Protein Content of Common Foods

The Dietary Reference Intake (DRI)* for pregnancy is 60 grams; for breastfeeding, 65 grams.

Food	Serving Sizes	Protein (grams[†])
Complete Protein Foods		
Turkey, light meat	75 g (3 oz)	26
Chicken breast	75 g (3 oz)	26
Beef, roast	75 g (3 oz)	25
Pork, centre loin	75 g (3 oz)	25
Tinned tuna, drained	75 g (3 oz)	22
Plaice	75 g (3 oz)	21
Beef, minced, extra lean	75 g (3 oz)	21
Prawns	75 g (3 oz)	18
Scallops	75 g (3 oz)	16
Ham	75 g (3 oz)	16
Cottage cheese	125 g (4 oz)	15
Eggs	2 large	12
Yogurt	250 ml (8 fl oz)	9–11
Milk, any type	250 ml (8 fl oz)	8
Cheddar cheese	25 g (1 oz)	7
Beef frankfurter, any type	1	6
Processed cheese, Kraft	25 g (1 oz)	5
Incomplete Protein Foods		
Tofu, firm	90 g (3½ oz)	20
Split-pea soup with ham	250 ml (8 fl oz)	20
Lentils, cooked	175 g (6 oz)	18
Miso or tempeh (soya products)	8 tbsp	16
Green peas	125 g (4 oz)	9
Peanut butter	2 tablespoons	8
Egg noodles	65 g (2½ oz)	8
Soya milk	250 ml (8 fl oz)	7
Nuts	25 g (1 oz)	6–7
Bulgur, cooked	150 g (6 oz)	6
Brown rice, cooked	150 g (6 oz)	5
White rice, cooked	150 g (6 oz)	4
Wholemeal bread	1 slice	3

*Formerly known as RDA

[†]Numbers are rounded to the nearest whole number.

Sources: Pennington, J. *Bowes and Church's Food Values of Portions Commonly Used,* 17th edition. Philadelphia: Lippincott Williams and Wilkins, 1998.

U.S. Department of Agriculture. USDA Nutrient Database for Standard Reference, Release 13, 1999.

Food and Nutrition Board. *Recommended Dietary Allowances.* Revised 1989. Washington, D.C.: National Academy Press, 1998.

The Power of Soya

Soya may just be the health food of the century. Several components of soya – protein, fibre, and phytochemicals (plant substances that are biologically active) – appear to have various benefits:

- Regular consumption of soya foods is linked to reduced risk of breast and rectal cancer.
- Soya protein seems to significantly lower serum cholesterol, low-density-lipoprotein (LDL) cholesterol, and triglycerides.[3] Soya-protein-based diets also significantly lowered cholesterol in children who had hereditary high cholesterol.[4] If high cholesterol runs in your family, eating soya regularly could help keep your cholesterol under control.
- Isoflavones, phytoestrogens found in soya foods, may affect how much calcium is lost from bones – an important consideration for those who have osteoporosis risk factors like family history of osteoporosis and fair skin.[5]

So how do you get soya into your diet? First, leave all preconceived ideas about tofu behind. Tofu is a bit like plain yogurt; it doesn't have much taste on its own. However, tofu will pick up any flavour you decide to give it. Textured vegetable protein (TVP) is dehydrated tofu and is a good substitute for hamburger in sloppy joes, chillies, and soups. Be creative and try some soya in your diet! (See Chapter Six: Vegetarian Eating and Chapter Fifteen: Menus and Recipes for the Third Trimester for more ideas.)

Focus on Calcium

Calcium is a vital mineral for your baby's bone development. Unfortunately, it's a mineral that adults often delete from their diets when they cut down on dairy products. Although the DRI is 1,000 milligrams,[6] a US National Institute of Health Consensus Conference on calcium intake recommended an intake range of 1,200 to 1,500 milligrams per day; 1 to 1.25 litres (1$\frac{3}{4}$–2 pints) of milk contain this amount. Milk and dairy products also provide such important nutrients as protein, magnesium, vitamin D, and riboflavin. If you don't use dairy products, you should consume calcium-fortified products like juices and high-calcium vegetables – and you'll have to eat a lot of them! You should try to get your calcium from food before considering supplements.

Twelve Ways to Sneak Calcium into Your Diet

If you don't like milk, the following foods contain good sources of calcium yet don't taste like milk. If you think creatively, you can sneak calcium into your diet in dozens of ways. Here are just a few ways to increase the calcium in your diet:

1. Make creamy soups (homemade or tinned) with milk or evaporated milk.

2. Use evaporated milk, which has twice the calcium, when preparing food like mashed potatoes, pudding, and cream sauces.

3. Eat dairy desserts such as pudding, frozen yogurt, milk shakes, and Berry Mousse Parfait (page 303).

4. Add reduced-fat or fat-free cheese to your mashed potatoes, vegetables, pasta, sandwiches, and sauces. Instead of meat, use low-fat cheese or tofu made with calcium in your lasagna or Spinach-Stuffed Shells (page 346).

5. Eat more corn tortillas! A meal of two bean tostadas contains almost 400 milligrams of calcium.

6. Add molasses to homemade quick breads, biscuits, and pancakes (or add it to your mix). Sesame seeds and tahini (sesame-seed paste) are also high in calcium and can be added to snack bars, cakes, vegetables, and dips. (See Favourite Snack Cake, page 351, and Quick and Healthier Pancakes, page 282.)

7. Add non-fat milk powder to prepared soups, prepared muffin and pancake mixes, milk shakes, and cream sauces.

8. Use plain yogurt as a base for salad dressing or veggie dip, or use fruit-flavoured yogurt as a sauce for fruit salad or as a dip for fresh fruit.

Calcium Content of Animal-Based Foods and Beverages

The DRI* for pregnancy and breastfeeding is 1,000 milligrams.

Food	Serving Sizes†	Calcium (milligrams)
McDonald's milk shake	1 small	350
Yogurt, fruit-flavoured, with non-fat dry milk	250 ml (8 fl oz)	314
Skimmed milk (1% fat)	250 ml (8 fl oz)	300
Full-fat milk	250 ml (8 fl oz)	291
Cheese pizza, thin crust	2 slices	290
Buttermilk, cultured	250 ml (8 fl oz)	285
Swiss cheese	25 g (1 oz)	272
Cheddar cheese	25 g (1 oz)	204
Salmon, tinned with bones	75 g (3 oz)	203
Cottage cheese (2% fat)	225 g (8 oz)	155
Processed cheese	25 g (1 oz)	150
Taco	2 small	140

*Formerly known as RDA

Sources: Pennington, J. *Bowes and Church's Food Values of Portions Commonly Used*, 17th edition. Philadelphia: Lippincott Williams and Wilkins, 1998.

U.S. Department of Agriculture. USDA Nutrient Database for Standard Reference, Release 13, 1999.

Manufacturers' labels.

Food and Nutrition Board. *Dietary Reference Intakes*, 1999.

9. Eat fish with small bones. Salmon Pâté (page 251) contains both salmon and fat-free cream cheese. (Make sure to leave the skin off the salmon.)

10. Prepare Broccoli Quiche (page 334) or egg custard, both of which contain milk. Eat more vegetables that are good sources of calcium.

11. Instead of buying plain orange juice, buy calcium-enriched orange juice.

12. Use silken tofu as a base for dips, puddings, and salad dressings; use firm tofu as a meat substitute in lasagna and 'meatloaf'. (See Tofu Loaf, page 347.) Check the label to make sure the tofu has calcium added.

Calcium Content of Vegetarian Foods and Beverages

The DRI* for pregnancy and breastfeeding is 1,000 milligrams.

Food†	Serving Sizes‡	Calcium (milligrams)
Agar (a product made from algae), dried	90 g (3½ oz)	625
Kale	175 g (6 oz)	358
Rhubarb, frozen, cooked	225 g (8 oz)	348
Blackstrap molasses	2 tablespoons	344
Orange juice, calcium-fortified	250 ml (8 fl oz)	300
Soya milk	250 ml (8 fl oz)	300
Spinach, frozen, boiled§	175 g (6 oz)	278
Firm tofu made with calcium sulfate (a processing agent)	100–125 g (4 oz)	200+ (varies)
Turnip greens, fresh, boiled	175 g (6 oz)	198
Kale, frozen, cooked	175 g (6 oz)	180
Okra	175 g (6 oz)	177
Sesame seeds	2 tablespoons	176
Kombu (a sea vegetable), raw	90 g (3½ oz)	168
Mustard greens, frozen, boiled	175 g (6 oz)	152
Wakame (a sea vegetable), raw	90 g (3½ oz)	150
Tortillas, corn	2	90
Nori (a product made from algae), raw	90 g (3½ oz)	58

*Formerly known as RDA

†Foods are cooked unless otherwise noted.

§Spinach contains oxalates, which can significantly cut down on calcium absorption.

Sources: Pennington, J. *Bowes and Church's Food Values of Portions Commonly Used*, 17th edition. Philadelphia: Lippincott Williams and Wilkins, 1998.

U.S. Department of Agriculture. USDA Nutrient Database for Standard Reference, Release 13, 1999.

Manufacturer's labels.

Food and Nutrition Board. *Dietary Reference Intakes*, 1999.

? Questions You May Have

Q: I can't tolerate milk! What can I do?

A: Many people of African or Asian origin have lactose intolerance, meaning they have trouble absorbing and digesting lactose, or milk sugar. The result is uncomfortable gas, stomachaches, and in some cases, diarrhoea.

If you have lactose intolerance, don't give up on dairy products! Research shows that as pregnancy progresses, especially in the third trimester, women who are lactose intolerant can break down much more lactose. This may be a compensatory effect, since the body needs large amounts of calcium in the third trimester.[7]

Lactase, the enzyme that is lacking in lactose-intolerant people, can be purchased in drops (to put into milk) or in pills (to take directly before drinking milk). Lactase is sold over the counter in chemists under the name of Lactaid.

Some lactose-intolerant people can tolerate milk with food, especially with food that contains fibre, such as milk over raisin bran at breakfast.[8] Cocoa may stimulate the body to produce more lactase, thereby increasing the tolerance of chocolate milk or hot cocoa.[9] I've found that some women tolerate whole milk better than skimmed or semi-skimmed milk. This may be because the fat slows digestion of the milk and thus improves lactose digestion. For those who can use the extra calories and energy, chocolate milk is an option for increasing calcium in the diet. Other low-lactose dairy options are yogurt, buttermilk and cheese.

If none of these solutions works for you, the last resort is to take a calcium supplement. (See page 38 for more about calcium supplements.)

Q: Doesn't my prenatal vitamin have enough calcium?

A: No, even though the pill is big. If it did contain all the calcium needed, you *really* wouldn't be able to swallow it! Most prenatal vitamins contain only a small percentage of the DRI for calcium. You must obtain the majority of calcium you need from your diet.

▼

Focus on Iron

Sometime between the twenty-fourth and twenty-eighth week, your doctor or midwife will probably test your blood again for iron-deficiency anaemia, a somewhat common problem during pregnancy. Because your blood volume increases up to 50 per cent, you need twice as much iron as you needed before you were pregnant. Knowing a few things about iron will help you prevent anaemia and improve your iron status if you are anaemic.

Iron is best absorbed from animal sources such as beef, eggs, and so on. If you are not a big meat eater, combine a small amount of animal protein with vegetable protein. This helps you absorb more iron from vegetable

Iron Content of Animal-Based Foods

The DRI* for pregnancy is 30 milligrams; for breastfeeding, 15 milligrams.

Food[†]	Serving Sizes	Iron (milligrams)[‡]
Clams	75 g (3 oz)	24
Oysters (also a great source of zinc)	75 g (3 oz)	8
Mussels	75 g (3 oz)	6
Chilli with meat[§]	225 g (8 oz)	2–5
Roast beef sandwich	1	4
Stuffed green pepper with beef and crumbs[§]	1	4
Spaghetti and meatballs with tomato sauce[§]	225 g (8 oz)	4
Prawns	75 g (3 oz)	3
Egg McMuffin	1	3
Green pepper steak[§]	275 g (10 oz)	3
Beef and vegetable stew[§]	225 g (8 oz)	3
Cheeseburger, Burger King	1	3
Lasagna with meat sauce	225 g (8 oz)	2–3
Bass, freshwater	75 g (3 oz)	2
Chicken breast	75 g (3 oz)	1

*Formerly known as RDA

†Foods are cooked, as applicable, unless otherwise noted.

‡Numbers are rounded to the nearest whole number.

§Also contains a significant amount of vitamin C, which helps absorption of iron.

Sources: Pennington, J. Bowes and Church's *Food Values of Portions Commonly Used*, 17th edition. Philadelphia: Lippincott Williams and Wilkins, 1998.

Food and Nutrition Board. *Recommended Dietary Allowances*. Revised 1989. Washington, D.C.: National Academy Press, 1998.

foods. For example, mix a small amount of ham with your pinto beans, or chop a hard-boiled egg into your cooked spinach or spinach salad.

You can also increase the amount of iron your body absorbs from food by eating a vitamin C food along with it. For example, have an orange, some melon, or berries for dessert after a meal, or have raw or cooked tomatoes, tomato juice, broccoli, cabbage, greens, cauliflower, or pepper as your veggie. Or, drink citrus juice, vegetable or tomato juice, or vitamin-C-fortified apple juice with your meal.

Factors that inhibit iron absorption are:

- Coffee
- Tea
- Calcium supplements
- Antacids
- Dairy products
- Soya protein
- Wheat bran
- Fibre

Factors that aid iron absorption are:

- Vitamin C. Vitamin C foods include tomato, greens, cabbage, citrus, peppers, pineapple, mango, and papaya.
- Cooking with an iron pan. The iron content of about 75 grams (3 ounces) of spaghetti sauce increases from 3 milligrams to 87 milligrams of iron when cooked in an unenameled iron pan.[11]

▼

'Thrive on Five'

The US National Cancer Institute uses the slogans 'Thrive on Five' and 'Five a Day for Better Health' to encourage Americans to eat more fruits and vegetables. Why? Fruits and vegetables are great sources of vitamins, minerals, and fibre. All plant foods also con-

Iron Content of Vegetarian Foods

The DRI* for pregnancy is 30 milligrams; for breastfeeding, 15 milligrams.

Food[†]	Serving Sizes	Iron (milligrams)[‡]
Quinoa	225 g (8 oz)	16
Tofu, firm	90 g (3½ oz)	13
Soya beans	225 g (8 oz)	9
Molasses	2 tablespoons	7
Black or haricot beans, tinned	225 g (8 oz)	5
Pinto beans, tinned	225 g (8 oz)	4
Chickpeas, tinned	225 g (8 oz)	3
Prune juice	250 ml (8 fl oz)	3
Spinach[§]	175 g (6 oz)	3
Potato[§]	1 medium	3
Peas, frozen, boiled	125 g (4 oz)	3
soya yogurt, natural	250 ml (8 fl oz)	3
Figs, dried	5 medium	2
Bulgur	175 g (6 oz)	2
Raisins	275 g (10 oz)	2
Pumpkin, tinned	125 g (4 oz)	2
Green beans or broccoli[§]	175 g (6 oz)	1
Tomato or vegetable juice[§]	250 ml (8 fl oz)	1

*Formerly known as RDA

†Foods are cooked, as applicable, unless otherwise noted.

‡Numbers are rounded to the nearest whole number.

§Also contains a significant amount of vitamin C, which helps absorption of iron.

Sources: Pennington, J. *Bowes and Church's Food Values of Portions Commonly Used*, 17th edition. Philadelphia: Lippincott Williams and Wilkins, 1998.

Food and Nutrition Board. *Recommended Dietary Allowances*. Revised 1989. Washington, D.C.: National Academy Press, 1998.

tain phytochemicals, biologically active substances that are widely believed to have many beneficial effects on health, such as prevention of cancer and heart disease.

The great thing about filling up on fruits and vegetables is that when you do so, you are less likely to eat crisps, biscuits, and other less-nutrient-dense foods. Try to eat a variety of fruits and vegetables from day to day.

Do you think that five fruits and vegetables per day sounds like a lot of food? Here are a few easy tips for adding fruits and vegetables to your meals:

Breakfast

▶ **Add mashed banana, dried fruit, or apple purée to pancake batter.**

Top pancakes and waffles with strawberries or other fresh fruit.

▶ **Whip up a fruit shake. (See pages 266–271 for recipes.)**

▶ **Add dried fruit, peaches, strawberries, blueberries, bananas, or other fresh fruit to your cereal.**

▶ **Eat a fruit or drink some juice before you have anything else.**

▶ **If you eat omelettes, add tomatoes, mushrooms, and red or green peppers.**

Lunch

▶ **Add apple, raisins, pineapple, mango, or mandarin orange slices to your chicken, tuna, or tossed salad.**

▶ **Have a salad or raw veggies before your meal.**

Use darker greens, such as cos or soft lettuce or spinach, for your salads.

▶ **Drink vegetable or tomato juice before or with your meal.**

▶ **Add soft lettuce, thinly sliced cucumber, finely shredded cabbage, or spinach and tomatoes to your sandwiches.**

▶ **Stuff leftover veggies or salad in a pitta pocket with cheese.**

▶ **To save time, buy ready-to-eat salads, carrots, broccoli, and so on. Talk about fast food!**

Dinner

▶ **Do a stir-fry for dinner. You can even buy the vegetables cleaned, chopped, and ready to go!**

▶ **Cheer up your spaghetti sauce with pepper, courgettes, carrots, or aubergine.**

Shred or chop these vegetables finely and they will cook quickly. If you have picky children at home, you can purée the cooked vegetables. Your kids will never know the veggies are there!

▶ **Use puréed roasted red pepper or another vegetable as the base for a sauce. (See page 348 for recipe.)**

▶ **Start dinner with a vegetable-based soup, such as minestrone or gazpacho. (See page 284 for recipe.)**

► Make a fruit salsa to accompany your grilled chicken or seafood. (See page 336 for recipe.)

► Make an appetizer of oven-fried courgette sticks or aubergine slices. (See page 258 for recipe.)

Dessert

► A mixed fresh fruit salad makes a great finish.

► Top angel food or pound cake with fresh or tinned fruit.

► Make a fruit shake with frozen strawberries, raspberries, and milk. (See page 271 for recipe.)

► Try a fruit sorbet.

► Have a frozen yogurt layered with fruit.

► Munch on a frozen banana or frozen grapes.

► Top off a grilled dinner with grilled fruit kebabs.

► Dip strawberries in a yogurt dip or chocolate sauce. (Everyone needs an occasional splurge!)

▼

Smart Snacking

When I ask my clients if they snack, they usually look embarrassed. You would think *snack* is a four-letter word. Most people think of snacking as eating foods they shouldn't or cheating. Actually, snacking can be healthy, and it's a must during pregnancy. Snacking helps you get all the nutrients you need when you can't eat much at a meal. It also gives you more energy during those times when baby seems to be sapping it all.

What Are the Best Snacks?

The best snacks are those that offer the most nutrition per calorie. Fruits and vegetables are tops; they offer lots of nutrition, virtually no fat, and few calories. Their fibre and fluid content are additional benefits.

The US Center for Science in the Public Interest, publisher of *Nutrition Action Healthletter,* recently published a list of the healthiest fruits, based on their nutrient and fibre content. Here are the top fifteen: papaya, cantaloupe melon, strawberries, oranges, tangerines, kiwifruit, mangos, apricots, persimmons, watermelon, raspberries, red or pink grapefruit, blackberries, dried apricots, and white grapefruit.[12] Don't despair if your favourite fruit isn't on this list; just try to include the above fruits more often to get the most nutrition.

The second category on our list of good snacks is other high-carbohydrate foods. These also provide energy, little fat, and contain fibre. Of course, they also taste good! Third on our list are dairy and protein food combinations. Try to eat a variety of snacks during the day. Here are some ideas to get you started:

Healthy Snacks

Fruits and Vegetables

• Dried or fresh fruit (Since dried fruits are concentrated, they are a great source of vitamins, minerals, and fibre. You can also keep them in your handbag or desk drawer.)

• Raw vegetables (You can buy them ready to eat and keep them in your refrigerator.)

• Leftover vegetables (Heat them up for a healthy snack.)

• Fruit or vegetable juice, fruit juice mixed with mineral water, or a fruit smoothie

High-Carbohydrate Foods

• Granola Bars (I like these if they are sweetened with fruit high in fibre.)

• Dehydrated bean soup in a cup

• Raisin bran or other high-fibre cereal

• Rice cakes

• Popcorn (Choose the one with the least fat, or pop your own.)

• Rye or wheat biscuits

• Digestive biscuits

• Fig Newtons

• No Oil Tortilla Chips, or other baked chips with salsa

Dairy Foods

• Milk

• Yogurt

• Low-fat cheese

At Last, Low-Fat Chips

As I write this, I'm snacking on tortilla chips that aren't fried – and they taste great! It is possible to do the impossible: Make tortilla chips, as well as black bean and pinto bean dips, salsas, and queso dips, without added fat! Twenty-five grams (one ounce) of chips also provides 80 milligrams of calcium. It is better to eat naturally low-fat chips than those made with Olestra (a fat substitute) while you are pregnant.

• Dip made with cottage cheese or fat-free cream cheese

• Milk shake made with fresh fruit (See pages 266–271 for yogurt shakes.)

High-Protein Snacks

Add protein foods for a big appetite. Eating a snack that contains protein before you go to bed at night can prevent low blood sugar in the morning.

• Peanut butter on savoury biscuits or with banana or apple

• Wholegrain cereal with milk

• Cheese and apple

• Tortilla rolled up with ham and cheese or with beans and cheese

• Yogurt with grape nuts or granola

• Cottage cheese and fruit

• Fat-free cheese on celery, carrots, and broccoli

• Tortilla chips and fat-free beans

See page 245 for lots more snack ideas!

Second-Trimester Challenges

Vaginal Discharge

Increased discharge is considered normal during pregnancy. It is usually whitish and is the result of an increased supply of blood and glucose to the vaginal walls and increased production of mucus by the endo-cervical glands. The acid level of your mucus changes during pregnancy, making you more susceptible to vaginal infections. If you have severe itching, irritation, or a foul odour, contact your doctor.

What You Can Do:

▶ **Continue to bathe daily.**

▶ **Wear cotton underwear.**

▶ **Avoid feminine deodorants, powders, and bubble baths.**

Constipation

Progesterone, a pregnancy hormone, slows down the movement of food in your intestine, causing more water and nutrients to be absorbed, and constipation is often the result. The pressure of the growing baby on your intestines and rectum can also cause this problem. An iron supplement can further worsen it.

What You Can Do:

▶ **Drink plenty of fluids – at least 8 to 10 glasses daily, mostly from water.**

▶ **Eat high-fibre foods. Eating at least five fruits and vegetables per day will keep constipation away! (See page 51, 'Focus on Fibre.')**

▶ **Exercise regularly.**

▶ **Avoid foods that cause constipation. Some people are constipated when they eat certain foods, such as cheese or bananas.**

▶ **Avoid caffeine, since it can cause a loss of even more fluid, which can make the stools hard.**

Haemorrhoids

Haemorrhoids are swollen or enlarged veins in the rectum. Hormones once again play a role in this problem, as does straining during a bowel movement. As the baby grows, greater pressure from the uterus displaces intestines, which can lead to constipation and then haemorrhoids.

What You Can Do:

▶ **Prevent constipation.**

▶ **Discuss haemorrhoids with your doctor or midwife.**

Your doctor may advise a stool softener or high-fibre laxative such as Fybogel or Isogel. If you do take a stool softener, keep in mind that it can take as long as three days to work.

Don't take more than one type of stool softener at the same time.

▶ **DON'T take over-the-counter laxatives, stool softeners, or haemorrhoid treatments without your health-care provider's approval.**

▶ **Taking warm baths and sitting on soft pillows can relieve the pressure.**

▶ **Avoid heavy lifting, pushing, and standing for long periods of time.**

Stress

We all live with stress. If you don't manage your stress, it can lead to chronic medical problems such as ulcers and heart disease. Pregnancy offers its own special stresses. Just wondering whether you are doing all the right things for your baby is a stress. You may be debating whether to work after you have the baby or preparing another child for your new arrival. You may be trying to figure out how you'll pay for all those baby things you'll need to buy. And pregnancy hormones can bring mood swings, causing you to cope less effectively with stress.

According to the US March of Dimes, some studies show that extreme stress can play a role in low birth weight.

What You Can Do:

▶ **Set realistic goals.**

You probably can't physically do what you did before pregnancy. You must put yourself first; take more time for rest, exercise, and planning and preparing healthy meals. Pare down your busy schedule if necessary.

▶ **Use relaxation techniques such as biofeedback and meditation.**

Many audio- and videotapes with relaxing music and scenery are available, and these can help you take a mental vacation. A daily walk can also relieve stress and help you put things in perspective.

▶ **Try to find support in your partner, friends, and colleagues or on the internet.**

Other new mothers or mothers-to-be will be especially empathetic. Remember that your partner will also be feeling stress and will probably need support, too. Below are some internet pregnancy resources that you may find helpful:

www.pregnancyguideonline.com
www.pregnancycalendar.com
www.fitpregnancy.com
www.epregnancy.com

Food Planning for the Second Trimester

Most women feel their best during the second trimester. Your appetite may be robust, and you may feel like spending more time in the kitchen. The menus listed below and detailed in Chapter Fourteen are a bit heavier than those I've recommended for the first trimester, and some of the recipes require more preparation.

Menus

- A Month of Breakfast Ideas
- Menus for a Hungry Appetite
- I Could Cook All Day
- Company's Coming!

CHAPTER FIVE

The Third Trimester

The third trimester is an important time for many reasons. It's the homestretch of your pregnancy, a time when you will be completing preparations for your baby's arrival. Likewise, your baby will be growing rapidly to prepare for its birth into the world.

How Baby Is Growing

Your baby is now rapidly filling your uterus. With less elbow room, the baby will be turning flips less often. You might, however, feel rhythmic movements. These are hiccups!

At the End of Twenty-Eight Weeks (Seven Months)

A baby born at this time is considered able to live outside the uterus, though its lungs are still not mature. Your baby did a lot of growing in the last month and should weigh between 1125 and 1350 grams (2½ and 3 pounds). It is 35 to 42 centimetres (14 to 17 inches) long. Baby is now storing calcium, and its bones are hardening. Many babies now find they fit better upside down and start to position themselves for birth. Your doctor can determine if your baby is positioned head down.

At the End of Thirty-Two Weeks (Eight Months)

All your baby needs to do now is develop lung surfactant (which enables the lungs to inflate and deflate properly) and store some fat. Baby is beginning to store minerals such as iron, calcium, and phosphorus. The kicks are strong and vigorous, and many women can feel a heel, fist, or elbow through their abdomen. Your baby now weighs between 2000 and

What you will find in this chapter:
• How Baby Is Growing
• Weight Gain and Energy Needs
• Other Nutrient Needs
• Focus on Vitamin B₆ and Zinc
• What about Sugar?
• Tips for Keeping Up Your Energy
• Third-Trimester Challenges
• Food Planning for the Third Trimester

This chapter answers such questions as:
• What if I have gained too much weight?
• I feel so tired; what can I do?
• What can I do for heartburn?
• I can't sleep; any advice?
• I have backaches and swollen ankles. Help!

2250 grams (4½ and 5 pounds) and is between 41 and 45 centimetres (16½ and 18 inches) long.

At the End of Thirty-Six Weeks (Nine Months)

Baby is now making great strides in growth and is gaining close to 225 grams (½ pound) per week. The bones in the head are soft and ready for delivery. Lanugo and vernix are disappearing. Fat deposits under the skin help fill out the body and eliminate the wrinkling of the skin. Baby will settle lower into your pelvis and may seem to slow its activity. However, you should still feel your baby move at least ten times in a twelve-hour period. If you don't, contact your doctor or midwife.

At the End of Forty Weeks (Ten Months)

Your baby is not considered full-term until thirty-eight weeks. At this time, the baby has a well-established sleeping pattern and individual styles of responses. The baby will continue to gain weight until the time of delivery. These last few weeks can be tiring as you wait for the arrival of your new little one.

▼

Weight Gain and Energy Needs

During the last trimester you will probably gain a large proportion of your total pregnancy weight. Just when you think you cannot gain any more weight or expand your belly any further, you do! Remember that as you prepare for the baby's arrival, you still need to eat well and make wise food choices.

You should continue to gain about 450 grams (a pound) a week during this time. Remember that if you are overweight or underweight, your weight gain should be adjusted accordingly. If you find that you have exceeded your goal weight already, discuss this with your health-care provider. He or she will still want you to continue gaining weight, but perhaps at a slower rate. Never try to lose weight while pregnant, no matter how much weight you have gained. Your baby needs you to eat adequately so that it can grow and develop enough to survive on its own in our world.

In the third trimester many women find that their get-up-and-go got up and went. Regular exercise (even a simple walk around the block) will improve your endurance and keep you from feeling like a couch potato. If you find that you are much less active now, you may not need the entire 300 extra calories I recommended earlier for the second and third trimesters. However, you still need all the added nutrients, so if you do cut down on food intake, you must make your food choices with even more care.

On the other hand, you may find that with your baby's arrival just around the corner, you have renewed energy! You may need to increase your calories. (See page 247 for high-energy snack ideas.)

As your due date gets closer, you might consider getting more of your calories from complex carbohydrates. Competitive athletes often load up on carbohydrates before a big event. Labour and delivery constitute such an event! Building up your store of carbohydrate may give you a bit more energy for labour.

Weighing In

Are you one of those weight-conscious women who weigh themselves daily? Don't! Although being aware of your weight is a good idea, during the third trimester you are more prone to water retention and fluctuations in weight gain. So when you panic, thinking you've gained a little weight in two days, the weight gain may simply be a result of water retention. Develop a healthy attitude about weight by weighing yourself just once a week at the same time of day under the same conditions. This will give you a truer idea of how your weight gain is progressing.

Note: If you do find that you have gained 900 or more grams (2 or more pounds) in two days; notice extreme swelling in your hands, face, or feet; or have headaches or vision trouble, notify your doctor. This may be a sign of pre-eclampsia. (See page 123 for more information.)

▼

Other Nutrient Needs

Your need for vitamins and minerals during the third trimester remains essentially the same as during the second trimester. Calcium is important during the third trimester for the laying down of calcium in the baby's bones. Brain development during the third trimester makes zinc a key nutrient. Zinc is critical throughout pregnancy, and a deficiency is related to premature delivery and many other problems. Vitamin B_6, essential for the use of protein, is necessary for the building of tissues, including brain and muscle tissue. B_6 is needed in proportion to the protein in your diet; the more protein you eat, the more B_6 you need. Also important for brain development are omega-3 fatty acids, primarily found in cold-water fish such as salmon and tuna. Try to eat fish at least once or twice a week.

Keep in mind that certain water-soluble vitamins such as thiamin, riboflavin, and niacin are required in amounts relative to your calorie intake. Thus, if you increase your calories, make sure your diet contains foods rich in these vitamins. Women who follow strict vegetarian diets (no animal protein) should take a vitamin B_{12} supplement of 2.6 micrograms per day.[1]

US research data shows that pregnant women's diets do not meet the Dietary Reference Intakes (DRIs) for vitamin B_6, vitamin D, vitamin E, folic acid, iron, zinc, calcium, and magnesium.[2] How does your diet stack up? Answer 'yes' or 'no' to the following questions.

1. I eat a variety of foods daily.
2. I eat an orange or dark green vegetable daily.
3. I eat a citrus fruit or another fruit or vegetable high in vitamin C daily.
4. I eat two to three servings of protein food daily.
5. I eat a variety of protein sources, including plant proteins.
6. I eat three servings of whole grains almost every day.

7. I eat six fruits and vegetables on most days.
8. I eat four servings of dairy products or high-calcium food daily.
9. I am gaining about 450 grams (1 pound) per week.
10. I avoid caffeine, alcohol, and drugs.

If you answered 'yes' to seven or more questions, you're doing pretty well. Fewer than that? Well, you know what you need to work on.

Focus on Vitamin B₆ and Zinc

Vitamin B_6 is necessary for many reactions in the body, namely building protein from amino acids and forming haemoglobin and neurotransmitters in the brain. Women usually don't have enough B_6 in their diets. Most recently, however, vitamin B_6 has made the news with the discovery that adequate amounts of B_6 help decrease blood levels of homocysteine, an amino acid that increases the risk of heart disease.

The more protein in your diet, the more B_6 you need. (Luckily, high-protein foods are good sources of vitamin B_6.) Also, women who take birth control pills seem to need more of the vitamin. If you have recently been taking birth control pills, try to have extra B_6 in your diet. Remember that vitamin B_6 is water-soluble and can be destroyed by cooking and processing.

Zinc performs many functions during preg-

Good Sources of B₆

The DRI* for pregnancy is 1.9 milligrams; for breastfeeding, 2.0 milligrams.

Food	Serving Sizes†	B₆ (milligrams)
Animal Sources		
Chicken, light meat	75 g (3 oz)	.51
Pork loin	75 g (3 oz)	.34
Ham	75 g (3 oz)	.34
Halibut	75 g (3 oz)	.34
Tuna, light	75 g (3 oz)	.29
Vegetable Sources		
Chickpeas, canned	225 g (8 oz)	1.14
Sweet potato, mashed	225 g (8 oz)	.80
Potato, baked with skin	1 medium	.70
Banana	1 medium	.66
Prune juice	250 ml (8 fl oz)	.56
Bran flakes	25 g (1 oz)	.50
Soya beans	225 g (8 oz)	.40
Lentils	225 g (8 oz)	.35
Brown rice, medium	175 g (6 oz)	.29
Wheat germ, toasted	4 tbsp	.28
Pinto beans	225 g (8 oz)	.275
Dates, dried	10	.16

*Formerly known as RDA

†Values represent cooked foods, as applicable.

Sources: Pennington, J. *Bowes and Church's Food Values of Portions Commonly Used*, 17th edition. Philadelphia: Lippincott Williams Wilkins, 1998.

Food and Nutrition Board. *Dietary Reference Intakes*, 1999.

nancy; it is necessary for conception, for every phase of growth, and for the immune system. Zinc even helps to ensure that your baby is not premature. Low zinc intake has been related to neural tube defects and other

Good Sources of Zinc

The DRI* for pregnancy is 15 milligrams; for breastfeeding, 19 milligrams.

Food	Serving Sizes†	Zinc, (milligrams)
Animal Sources		
Oysters, fried	75 g (3 oz)	74
Chuck arm pot roast	75 g (3 oz)	7.4
Crab, Alaskan	75 g (3 oz)	6.5
Prime rib	75 g (3 oz)	6.0
Veal roast, sirloin	75 g (3 oz)	4.0
Lamb chop, lean	75 g (3 oz)	2.8
Lobster	75 g (3 oz)	2.5
Pork roast, rump	75 g (3 oz)	2.4
Clams	75 g (3 oz)	2.3
Prawns	75 g (3 oz)	1.3
Vegetable Sources		
Wheat germ, toasted	4 tbsp	4.8
Chickpeas, tinned	225 g (8 oz)	2.5
Green peas, frozen	125 g (4 oz)	1.5
Bran flakes	25 g (1 oz)	1.5
Bran muffin	1 medium	1.5
Spinach	150 g (6 oz)	1.4

*Formerly known as RDA

†Values represent cooked foods, as applicable.

Sources: Pennington, J. *Bowes and Church's Food Values of Portions Commonly Used*, 17th edition. Philadelphia: Lippincott Williams and Wilkins, 1998.

Food and Nutrition Board. *Recommended Dietary Allowances*. Revised 1989. Washington, D.C.: National Academy Press, 1998.

birth defects. Unfortunately, zinc is a mineral that non-pregnant women often don't get enough of. High-fibre diets can interfere with absorption of zinc. Beef and shellfish are generally rich in zinc; vegetarian women need to eat plenty of zinc-rich legumes and whole grains.

▼

What about Sugar?

Sugar has received a lot of bad press over the years. Many myths are still circulating about sugar. Here are the facts:

- Sugar doesn't cause diabetes, though it does cause the body to produce more insulin in order to use the sugar. This happens with any carbohydrate food, but the effect is more pronounced with simple sugars.
- Sugar doesn't appear to cause hyperactivity. A review of twenty-three studies showed that sugar had no effects on either behaviour or cognitive performance. In fact, sugar has been shown to have a calming effect on newborns in pain.[3] The increased activity of children who have consumed sugar may often be caused by the accompanying caffeine, as in a cola. Another explanation may be that the settings in which children usually eat a lot of sugar, such as birthday parties and Hallowe'en outings, promote increased activity. However, individual reactions to any food are possible.
- Sugar does cause tooth decay, as do many other carbohydrate foods.
- Westerners have increased their calorie intake in recent years, and most of the extra calories come from added sugars. It is estimated that nearly one-quarter of their daily calories come from added sugar – mainly from soft drinks. Since high-sugar foods are often low-nutrient

foods, they can have a negative impact on the overall diet. *Dietary Guidelines for Americans 2000* recommends choosing foods and beverages that limit sugar intake.[4]

▼

Tips for Keeping Up Your Energy

You may have heard that the third trimester (especially the last month) is a real challenge. You feel as though you can't possibly get bigger. Getting out of your chair or bed (especially if you have a waterbed) is sometimes tough, and your energy level may need a boost. On the other hand, many women feel great and enjoy sudden bursts of energy (often called the nesting syndrome) when they want to get everything done. The following tips will help you feel your best during the last months of pregnancy.

▶ **Put up your feet from time to time.**

Some swelling in the feet and legs is considered normal during the last few months. Keep in mind that the extra 9 to 133.5 kilograms (20 to 30 pounds) you are now carrying are putting a lot of pressure on your legs, knees, and feet. Wear flat, supportive shoes; support hose may also be a good idea.

▶ **Take catnaps at lunch if you can,** *after* **you've eaten.**

I remember taking several naps on my boss's couch during lunch when I was pregnant.

Baby Pick-Me-Up: A High-Energy Drink
(2 servings)

1 frozen or 125 g (4 oz) tinned peach or nectarine (Freeze for 45 minutes or more.)

½ banana

175 g (6 oz) frozen strawberries

250 ml (8 fl oz) low-fat vanilla yogurt or 250 ml (8 fl oz) milk plus sweetener to taste

2 tablespoons non-fat dry milk

Combine all ingredients in blender. If you don't have frozen fruit, adding ice to desired consistency will increase the volume.

Nutrient analysis per serving:

274 calories
8 grams protein
6 grams fibre
2 grams fat

Percentage of DRI* for pregnancy:

46% vitamin C
23% vitamin B$_{12}$ and calcium
29% potassium

* Formerly known as RDA

▶ **Let the housework go!**

It's good practice for the first few months with baby. Start putting your feelings first and the housework second. Do only what has to be done (laundry, for example) or enlist the help of your partner or children.

▶ **Don't forget those in-between snacks – they help boost your energy.**

Keep a snack stash in your drawer: peanut-butter biscuits, raisins, dried figs, prunes, apricots, digestive biscuits, and granola bars.

▶ **Keep up with your exercise programme.**

Exercise is probably the last thing you want to do when you feel tired, but it really will help in the long run. I don't like to swim very much, but when I attended a water exercise class for pregnant women, I loved it. You feel weightless in the water – and that is a nice feeling! After a long workday, being in the water can be very refreshing.

▼

Third-Trimester Challenges

Backache

As pregnancy progresses and the uterus enlarges, spine curvature increases. Also, hormones cause the pelvic joints to loosen. You may notice that the way you walk is a bit different from before you were pregnant. This may be due to loosening of joints and an adjustment in posture to compensate for carrying a big load out front.

What You Can Do:

▶ **Practise good body mechanics and posture.**

▶ **Avoid bending over and lifting heavy objects (including children, if possible).**

Bend at the knees and keep your back straight.

▶ **Wear low-heeled shoes.**

▶ **Learn to do pelvic tilts; they will relieve pressure on your back and stretch and tone your muscles.**

Ask your midwife or antenatal clinic for instructions, or see page 189.

▶ **Bend your knees slightly when standing in place.**

Oedema (Swelling)

Many women experience ankle swelling in the last trimester because blood and fluid circulation (between the heart and the lower extremities) becomes more and more difficult. Let your doctor or midwife know if you have swelling in your hands or face; this could be a sign of pre-eclampsia.

What You Can Do:

▶ **Elevate your legs to the level of your hips as often as possible.**

▶ **Avoid standing for long periods of time.**

▶ **If you must sit for long periods, try to stand up, stretch, and move around a bit to improve circulation.**

▶ **Avoid anything that will restrict circulation: stockings with tight bands, tight slips or pants, tight knee-highs, and so on.**

▶ **Don't restrict fluid intake!**

Heartburn

As the baby grows, it compresses your stomach, leaving minimal space for food. The hormones that slow down your digestion also relax the sphincter muscle that keeps food in your stomach. These changes cause stomach acid to back up into your oesophagus, causing a burning sensation that feels as though it's around your heart.

What You Can Do:

▶ **Eat small, frequent meals.**

▶ **Stay away from gassy, spicy, and greasy foods.**

▶ **Don't overeat.**

▶ **Stand or walk around after eating, instead of lying down immediately after a meal.**

▶ **Keep your head slightly elevated when you're in bed.**

▶ **Cut down on caffeine; it causes heartburn for some women.**

▶ **Wear comfortable clothes.**

▶ **Talk with your doctor before using antacids; some contain sodium bicarbonate, which may interfere with absorption of some nutrients.**

Sleepless Nights

As your body gets larger, you may find that getting comfortable in bed is quite a chore. The baby kicking, heartburn, and anxiety about the arrival of the new person in your life can add to sleeplessness.

What You Can Do:

▶ **Try a bedtime ritual: warm bath, decaffeinated mint tea or warm milk, and soft jazz or easy-listening music.**

▶ **Support yourself with pillows.**

One new mother says, 'Our bed was a virtual oasis of pillows! I used two behind me to support my back, one between my knees to relieve back pressure, and one for my head.'

▶ **Practise the relaxation and breathing techniques that you learned in antenatal class.**

▶ **Continue regular exercise; it has a calming effect and can help with insomnia.**

Another new mother shares, 'My husband and I enjoyed a leisurely walk every evening after dinner. It gave us quiet time to talk and helped me sleep better at night. Of course we always had other things we could do, such as cleaning the house or paying bills, but we made our walk together a priority.'

▼

Food Planning for the Third Trimester

The main problems with eating during the last months of pregnancy are:

1. You get full quickly.

2. Fatigue may prevent you from wanting to cook.

3. Heartburn may restrict the variety or amount of food you eat.

4. You may be so busy getting ready for the baby that you neglect your own nutrition needs.

5. You may be trying to cut food expenses to accommodate costly necessities for your baby.

The third-trimester menus in this book are designed with these problems in mind. Look over the list that follows and refer to Chapter Fifteen for details.

Now is a good time to prepare some foods to freeze for those first few days or weeks with your new baby.

Menus

- Using Leftovers with Flair
- Meals in Minutes
- Feel Full Menus
- Best Bite Snacks
- Vegetarian Budget Menus

CHAPTER SIX

Vegetarian Eating

What you will find in this chapter:

- *Vegetarians: The Healthy Minority*
- *The Pregnant Vegetarian*
- *Nutrients of Special Concern*
- *The Eating Expectantly Vegetarian Eating Plan*
- *Vegetarian Shopping List*
- *Vegetarian Food Planning*
- *Eating Out Vegetarian-Style*
- *Vegetarian Convenience-Food Choices*
- *Eating after Delivery*

This chapter answers such questions as:

- *How can I get enough calcium in my diet if I'm vegetarian?*
- *I'm diabetic; how do vegetarian foods fit into my diet?*
- *How can I get vitamin B$_{12}$ in my diet if it is only found in animal foods?*
- *Must I buy special vegetarian foods to have a good diet?*

Vegetarian eating is on the rise as more people realize the benefits of eating plant proteins. (See Chapter Four for more on soya protein.) Even if you just 'lean' toward vegetarian eating, you can receive many of the same health benefits.

Most people eat some vegetarian foods without even thinking about it. The teen who picks up a bean burrito is doing it, the parent who makes pasta with marinara sauce and cheese is doing it, and of course the vegan who eats no animal products is doing it, too. People eat vegetarian for a variety of reasons: because eating vegetarian is healthy, because they're concerned about the environment or animal rights, or simply because vegetarian food is tasty and cheap.

The Food Guide Pyramid depicts a healthy eating pattern for everyone. What many people don't realize is that a vegetarian

Food Guide Pyramid
Suggested Daily Servings

KEY
☐ Fat (naturally occuring and added)
☑ Sugars (added)
These symbols show fats and other sugars in foods.

Fats, oils, and sweets — **Use sparingly**

Milk, yogurt, and cheese — **2–3 servings**

Vegetables — **3–5 servings**

Meat, poultry, fish, dry beans, eggs, and nuts — **2–3 servings**

Fruit — **2–4 servings**

Bread, cereal, rice, and pasta — **6–11 servings**

Source: U.S. Department of Agriculture/U.S. Department of Health and Human Services.

diet (based on grains, fruits, and vegetables, with smaller amounts of protein, dairy, fat, and sugar) exemplifies this eating pattern.

▼

Vegetarians: The Healthy Minority

Many people would like to have the health records that vegetarians have. Vegetarians have lower body mass index (BMI), lower cholesterol, and lower risk of heart disease than meat eaters have. They may also have lower risk of constipation, diverticular disease (an intestinal condition), gallstones, and appendicitis.[1] It appears that vegetarians are also less likely to have adult-onset diabetes, cancer, and high blood pressure.[2] Research shows that a low-fat vegetarian diet along with stress management and exercise can actually reverse coronary heart disease.[3] Vegetarians are generally closer to their ideal body weights than are non-vegetarians. Some studies show that vegetarians have lower rates of osteoporosis, cancer and kidney stones.

Good genes? Not necessarily. Most vegetarian diets are low in saturated fat and thus can prevent high cholesterol levels and heart disease. Vegetarians eat many fruits and vegetables; this increases their intake of healthy phytochemicals and fibre, both of which are thought to be cancer fighters. Lacto-ovo vegetarians have adequate calcium in their diet, which may be protective against colon cancer. Vegetarians may also have beneficial lifestyle habits that contribute to good health, such as regular exercise and abstinence from tobacco and alcohol. Maintaining ideal body weight can reduce the risk of heart disease, high blood pressure, and diabetes.

The position of the American Dietetic Association states, 'Appropriately planned vegetarian diets are healthful, are nutritionally adequate, and provide health benefits in the prevention and treatment of certain diseases.'[4] The key word here is *planned*. Even a vegetarian diet can be unhealthy if it contains too much fat and sugar or if it doesn't include a variety of foods, especially protein sources. If you are currently a vegetarian, your diet is probably on its way to meeting the dietary guidelines. If you are contemplating becoming vegetarian, you can become part of the healthy minority, too!

▼

The Pregnant Vegetarian

Some pregnant women turn to vegetarian foods when they find they can't tolerate meat. Sometimes eggs, cheese, or black beans go down a lot easier than a steak. Of course, many women are practising vegetarians before they become pregnant. Vegetarianism has several levels:

Vegan

This person is the 'true' vegetarian. A vegan eats no animal products whatsoever and should be sure to consume reliable sources of vitamin B_{12}, which is found only in animal products or fortified foods. The vegan's need for calcium is actually less than that of meat eaters who consume larger amounts of protein. However, the vegan may have to make an effort to consume enough vegetable sources of calcium. Like meat-eating pregnant women, vegan women may also have difficulty getting enough iron. Vegan women living in northern latitudes and those who get very little exposure to the sun in winter may have a problem producing enough vitamin D, which is made in the skin after exposure to sunlight and is also found in dairy products.

Lacto-Ovo Vegetarian

This person eats no red meat, poultry, or fish, but does eat dairy products and eggs. Lacto-ovo vegetarians have little trouble meeting nutrient needs for iron, calcium, vitamin B_{12}, or vitamin D.

No-Red-Meat 'Vegetarian'

This person is someone who avoids red meat but does eat dairy products, fish, and/or poultry. Although people who eat no red meat may call themselves vegetarians, vegetarian organizations do not regard them as such. No-red-meat 'vegetarians' generally have no problem meeting nutrient needs, except perhaps iron, which is found in lesser amounts in white meats.

Comparison of Vegan and Non-vegetarian Diets of Women Ages Twenty to Forty

Expressed in percentages of the Dietary Reference Intakes (DRIs)*

Nutrient	Vegans	Non-vegetarians
Calcium	72	119
Folic acid	231	49
Iron	118	102
Magnesium	141	108
Vitamin B_6	117	101
Vitamin C	310	193
Vitamin A	336	205
Vitamin B_{12}	25	189
Zinc	71	92

*Previously known as RDA

Nutrients of Special Concern

How does pregnancy affect vegetarians? Most pregnant vegetarians can expect to meet or exceed their nutritional needs. In fact, an American study that compared the diets of health-conscious vegetarian women and non-vegetarian women showed that vegetarian non-pregnant women ate more of most nutrients than meat eaters ate, except for vitamin B_{12}, calcium, and zinc.[5] (See the chart above.) This is a cause for concern since B_{12}, calcium, and zinc are very important during pregnancy.

Vegetarians should pay particular attention to a handful of nutrients: vitamin B_{12}, iron, calcium, and vitamin D. Since vitamin B_6 and zinc are nutrients lacking in all women's diets, we'll address them, too.

Vitamin B$_{12}$

Since vitamin B$_{12}$ is found only in animal products and fortified foods such as commercial breakfast cereals, you should make sure that you have a source of vitamin B$_{12}$ in your diet while you are pregnant and breast-feeding. Because product formulations often change, be sure to check labels.

According to Suzanne Havala, M.S., R.D., Nutrition Adviser to the American Vegetarian Resource Group, 'Some vegetarian specialty foods thought by many to be good sources of vitamin B$_{12}$, such as tempeh and spirulina, are in fact not reliable sources. Food labels listing the vitamin B$_{12}$ content of these foods include forms of the vitamin that are not active for humans and may compete for absorption with cyanocobalamin, the form we use.'

If your diet contains neither animal products nor foods fortified with vitamin B$_{12}$, you probably need a vitamin supplement. Ask your doctor.

Vitamin-B$_{12}$-Fortified Cereal

These cereals provide 100% of the Daily Value for vitamin B$_{12}$. However, since product formulations often change, read the label to make sure these products still contain added vitamin B$_{12}$.

Kellogg's Special K

Nestlé's Cheerios

Note: Many other cereals contain 25% of the Daily Value for B$_{12}$, such as Kellogg's Cornflakes and Nestlé's Shreddies.

Source: Manufacturers' labels

Iron

Even though intakes for iron are about the same for vegetarians and non-vegetarians, the type of iron that vegetarians eat may not be absorbed as well as the iron in meat. Vitamin C consumed with non-heme iron (the form of iron found in plant foods) helps increase the absorption of the mineral. Vegetarian diets are usually high in vitamin C.

Although anaemia is no more common among vegetarians than meat eaters, anaemia can occur in any pregnant woman due to the high iron requirement during pregnancy.[6] Thus, a supplement of 30 milligrams of ferrous iron is recommended for all pregnant women. (See page 71 for vegetarian sources of iron.)

Calcium

Calcium isn't usually a challenge for vegetarians unless they are vegan, are lactose intolerant, or just aren't milk drinkers. Since vegetarians generally eat less protein, this may affect how much calcium is lost in their urine. However, since calcium needs have not been established for vegans, it is best to follow the Dietary Reference Intake (DRI) for calcium, which is 1,000 milligrams.[7] If you are lactose intolerant, see page 68 for information on non-dairy foods high in calcium. If you don't like milk by itself, but do eat other dairy products, see page 66 for tips on sneaking calcium into your diet.

Some sea vegetables are good sources of calcium and other minerals. If you eat sea vegetables regularly, be aware that if they come from polluted waters, they could contain heavy metal pollutants. You should make sure your seaweed comes from a controlled source, such as a sea vegetable farm.

Oxalates and phytates, substances found in leafy green vegetables and whole grains, can affect absorption of calcium. The high oxalate content of vegetables like spinach, Swiss chard, rhubarb, and beet greens make the calcium in these vegetables largely unabsorbable. High-fibre foods also high in phytates – especially wheat bran – can decrease the absorption of calcium from milk. But overall, the absorption of calcium from vegetables and legumes is equal to or better than absorption of calcium from milk.[8]

If you are concerned about your calcium intake, talk to a registered dietitian about increasing the calcium in your diet or ask your health-care provider about a supplement.

Vitamin D

The need for supplemental vitamin D is rare because the body can usually produce all that it needs from exposure to sunlight. Few foods are naturally high in vitamin D; milk, soya milk, and some cereals are fortified with it. If you are strictly vegan and you either live in a northern latitude or have very limited sun exposure, you may need a supplement of not more than 100 per cent of the DRI.

Exposing the hands, arms, and face for five to fifteen minutes per day is believed to provide enough vitamin D from sunshine. People who use sunscreen, have dark skin, or live at northern latitudes or in cloudy or smoggy areas may need increased exposure

or may need to get their vitamin D from fortified foods or a supplement.[9] It has been recently proposed that for vegans who get no sun exposure, the current DRI may not be adequate. Ask your doctor for more information.[10]

Vitamin B$_6$

All women seem to have a problem getting enough vitamin B$_6$. Your body needs this vitamin in proportion to your protein intake, so if your diet is especially high in protein foods, you may need even more B$_6$. (See page 82 for a list of vegetarian sources of B$_6$.)

Zinc

Zinc is a very important nutrient for a developing foetus. It is widespread in such foods as legumes, shellfish, whole grains, and cheese. Many people don't have enough zinc in their diet.

One study that evaluated the diets of vegans and lacto-ovo vegetarians found that neither group met the DRI for zinc. The mean intake for vegan women was only 13 per cent of the DRI, while lacto-ovo vegetarian women's average intake was 71 per cent of the DRI. The women's food choices in this study were mostly low-zinc foods such as fruits, salads, and vegetables.[11]

Factors that may affect absorption of zinc include fibre, phytates, and some minerals. To obtain an adequate amount of zinc, vegetarians – especially vegans – must make careful food choices. Consult the list on page 83 to see how much zinc your diet supplies.

Essential Fat

Vegetarian diets don't contain docosahexa-nenoic and eicosapenaenoic acid (DHA and EPA), omega-3 essential fats that are necessary for foetal brain and eye development. Vegetarians generally do have a source of alpha-linolenic acid – a fatty acid that is converted to DHA and EPA. However, vegetarians also have a much higher intake of linoleic acid – another essential fat that can decrease the conversion of alpha-linolenic acid into DHA and EPA. Therefore, it is recommended that the ratio of intake of alpha-linolenic to linoleic acid be between five to one and ten to one. Sources of alpha-linolenic acid include linseed oil, flaxseed, walnuts, canola oil, walnut oil, and soya bean oil. It is also helpful to substitute monounsaturated fats such as canola oil and olive oil for oils that are high in linoleic acids, such as safflower, sunflower, corn, and cottonseed oils.[12]

Protein

Protein is important during pregnancy, and although vegetarians have just a little less protein in their diets than non-vegetarians have, their intake still exceeds the DRI. The list of foods below will give you an idea of foods that can supply you with the 10 extra grams of protein needed daily during your pregnancy. Keep in mind that eating a variety of protein foods throughout the day is important so that your body can utilize the protein for building tissue.

Vegetarian Foods That Contain 10 Grams of Protein:

Black beans (or any legume), 150 g (5 oz)
Brown rice, 300 g (10 oz)
Cashews, 190 g (6½ oz)
Peas, 175 g (6 oz)
Peanut butter, 2¼ tablespoons
Soya yogurt, 1 cup
Tofu (firm), 250 ml (8 fl oz)
Veggie burger, ⅔ to 1 patty

▼

The Eating Expectantly Vegetarian Eating Plan

This diet covers both vegan and lacto-ovo vegetarians and is meant as a guideline only. Eating a variety of high-nutrient foods without following a structured diet will provide the nutrition you need.

8 or more servings of grains
1 serving is 1 slice any type bread; ½ small bagel, pitta, or English muffin; 1 150-mm (6-inch) tortilla; 8 tbsp cooked rice or pasta; 8 tbsp cooked cereal, barley, bulgur or quinoa; 25 g (1 ounce) ready-to-eat cereal; 3–4 savoury biscuits; or 2 biscuits.

Note: 3 or more of your daily grain servings should be wholegrain.

4 or more servings of milk or milk substitute
1 serving is 250 ml (8 fl oz) any type milk, soya milk (calcium-fortified), or yogurt; 40 g (1½ ounces) cheese; or 50 g (2 ounces) processed cheese.

4 or more servings of fruit

1 serving is 1 medium fresh fruit; ½ grapefruit, mango, or papaya; 8 tbsp tinned or chopped fruit; 4 tbsp dried fruit; or 200 ml (6½ fl oz) fruit juice.

4 or more servings of vegetables

1 serving is 8 tbsp cooked vegetables, 250 ml (8 fl oz) leafy vegetables, 1 small potato, or 200 ml (6½ fl oz) tomato or vegetable juice.

Note: Be sure to eat at least one fruit or vegetable that is high in vitamin C and one that is dark green or orange every day.

3 or more servings of legumes, nuts, and meat substitutes

1 serving is 8 tbsp legumes, tofu, tempeh, or textured vegetable protein; 2 eggs; 2 tablespoons nuts, seeds, or nut butter; or 1 veggie burger patty.

Note: Eat ½ more serving for each 250 ml (8 fl oz) of milk or milk substitute that you don't drink.

Fats and sweets: Eat sparingly.

While most vegetarians need to limit fats and sweets, some may need to increase them to supplement their calorie intake.

Sample Vegan Menu

This menu contains about 2,400 calories and exceeds the DRIs for all major nutrients except vitamin D. (It contains 0 per cent of the DRI for vitamin D.) Vitamin D can be produced in the skin with adequate exposure to sunshine.

Breakfast

250 ml (8 fl oz) oatmeal with
    1½ tablespoons molasses and
    2 tablespoons raisins
1 piece wholemeal bread with
    1 tablespoon peanut butter
250 ml (8 fl oz) soya milk

Snack

250 ml (8 fl oz) calcium-enriched orange juice

Lunch

250 ml (8 fl oz) haricot bean soup with
    1 piece wholemeal bread
Broccoli and tofu stir-fry with 250 ml
    (8 fl oz) tofu, 8 tbsp broccoli, and 150 g
    (5 oz) brown rice
250 ml (8 fl oz) soya milk

Snack

1 apple

Dinner

Salad with 150 g (5 oz) cos lettuce,
    ½ tomato, ¼ avocado, and vinaigrette
    dressing with 2 teaspoons canola oil
Stuffed pepper with 8 tbsp bulgur, 75 g
    (3 oz) black beans, and ½ tomato
100–125 g (4 oz) corn
250 ml (8 fl oz) soya milk

Snack

Shake with 250 ml (8 fl oz) soya milk
    and 250 g (9 oz) frozen strawberries

Sample Lacto-Ovo Vegetarian Menu

This menu, which contains eggs and dairy products, contains approximately 2,400 calories and exceeds all of the DRIs for pregnancy.

Breakfast

75 g (3 oz) bran-flakes with 2 tablespoons
    raisins and ½ banana
250 ml (8 fl oz) skimmed milk
1 piece toast with 2 teaspoons peanut
    butter

Snack

25 g (1 ounce) Cheddar cheese
1 apple
25 g (1 ounce) baked tortilla chips

Lunch

375 ml (12 fl oz) split-pea soup
250 ml (8 fl oz) spinach salad with
    ½ tomato, mushrooms, ¼ avocado,
    25 g (1 ounce) grated reduced-fat
    Cheddar cheese, croutons, and
    vinaigrette dressing with 2 teaspoons
    canola oil
1 piece wholemeal bread
1 orange
250 ml (8 fl oz) low-fat yogurt

Snack

250 ml (8 fl oz) milk
2 teacups popcorn
Celery sticks

Dinner

250 ml (8 fl oz) Black Bean and
    Corn Salad (page 254)
1 serving Broccoli Quiche (page 334)
Wholemeal roll with 1 teaspoon
    reduced-fat butter or margarine
250 ml (8 fl oz) skimmed milk

Snack

Strawberry Shake (page 271)

Complemen... An O...

A myth about co...
has been passed d...
recently, vegetaria...
to eat the traditio...
grain with dairy, o...
have a 'complete ...
thinking is that as
eats a variety of f...
calories, he or she...
all the amino aci...
position of the A...
Association on v...
sources of protei...
adequate amoun t...
acids if a variety ...
sumed and ener g...
Research sugges t...
proteins do not ...
the same time.'[13]

Vegetarian...

Now that you are...
ably much more ...
the store. This ha...
reproduced and u...
for more informa...
label reading.)

make sure your seaweed comes from a controlled source, such as a sea vegetable farm.

Oxalates and phytates, substances found in leafy green vegetables and whole grains, can affect absorption of calcium. The high oxalate content of vegetables like spinach, Swiss chard, rhubarb, and beet greens make the calcium in these vegetables largely unabsorbable. High-fibre foods also high in phytates – especially wheat bran – can decrease the absorption of calcium from milk. But overall, the absorption of calcium from vegetables and legumes is equal to or better than absorption of calcium from milk.[8]

If you are concerned about your calcium intake, talk to a registered dietitian about increasing the calcium in your diet or ask your health-care provider about a supplement.

Vitamin D

The need for supplemental vitamin D is rare because the body can usually produce all that it needs from exposure to sunlight. Few foods are naturally high in vitamin D; milk, soya milk, and some cereals are fortified with it. If you are strictly vegan and you either live in a northern latitude or have very limited sun exposure, you may need a supplement of not more than 100 per cent of the DRI.

Exposing the hands, arms, and face for five to fifteen minutes per day is believed to provide enough vitamin D from sunshine. People who use sunscreen, have dark skin, or live at northern latitudes or in cloudy or smoggy areas may need increased exposure

or may need to get their vitamin D from fortified foods or a supplement.[9] It has been recently proposed that for vegans who get no sun exposure, the current DRI may not be adequate. Ask your doctor for more information.[10]

Vitamin B_6

All women seem to have a problem getting enough vitamin B_6. Your body needs this vitamin in proportion to your protein intake, so if your diet is especially high in protein foods, you may need even more B_6. (See page 82 for a list of vegetarian sources of B_6.)

Zinc

Zinc is a very important nutrient for a developing foetus. It is widespread in such foods as legumes, shellfish, whole grains, and cheese. Many people don't have enough zinc in their diet.

One study that evaluated the diets of vegans and lacto-ovo vegetarians found that neither group met the DRI for zinc. The mean intake for vegan women was only 13 per cent of the DRI, while lacto-ovo vegetarian women's average intake was 71 per cent of the DRI. The women's food choices in this study were mostly low-zinc foods such as fruits, salads, and vegetables.[11]

Factors that may affect absorption of zinc include fibre, phytates, and some minerals. To obtain an adequate amount of zinc, vegetarians – especially vegans – must make careful food choices. Consult the list on page 83 to see how much zinc your diet supplies.

Essential Fat

Vegetarian diets don't contain docosahexa-nenoic and eicosapenaenoic acid (DHA and EPA), omega-3 essential fats that are necessary for foetal brain and eye development. Vegetarians generally do have a source of alpha-linolenic acid – a fatty acid that is converted to DHA and EPA. However, vegetarians also have a much higher intake of linoleic acid – another essential fat that can decrease the conversion of alpha-linolenic acid into DHA and EPA. Therefore, it is recommended that the ratio of intake of alpha-linolenic to linoleic acid be between five to one and ten to one. Sources of alpha-linolenic acid include linseed oil, flaxseed, walnuts, canola oil, walnut oil, and soya bean oil. It is also helpful to substitute monounsaturated fats such as canola oil and olive oil for oils that are high in linoleic acids, such as safflower, sunflower, corn, and cottonseed oils.[12]

Protein

Protein is important during pregnancy, and although vegetarians have just a little less protein in their diets than non-vegetarians have, their intake still exceeds the DRI. The list of foods below will give you an idea of foods that can supply you with the 10 extra grams of protein needed daily during your pregnancy. Keep in mind that eating a variety of protein foods throughout the day is important so that your body can utilize the protein for building tissue.

Vegetarian Foods That Contain 10 Grams of Protein:

Black beans (or any legume), 150 g (5 oz)
Brown rice, 300 g (10 oz)
Cashews, 190 g (6½ oz)
Peas, 175 g (6 oz)
Peanut butter, 2¼ tablespoons
Soya yogurt, 1 cup
Tofu (firm), 250 ml (8 fl oz)
Veggie burger, ⅔ to 1 patty

▼

The Eating Expectantly Vegetarian Eating Plan

This diet covers both vegan and lacto-ovo vegetarians and is meant as a guideline only. Eating a variety of high-nutrient foods without following a structured diet will provide the nutrition you need.

8 or more servings of grains

1 serving is 1 slice any type bread; ½ small bagel, pitta, or English muffin; 1 150-mm (6-inch) tortilla; 8 tbsp cooked rice or pasta; 8 tbsp cooked cereal, barley, bulgur or quinoa; 25 g (1 ounce) ready-to-eat cereal; 3–4 savoury biscuits; or 2 biscuits.

Note: 3 or more of your daily grain servings should be wholegrain.

4 or more servings of milk or milk substitute

1 serving is 250 ml (8 fl oz) any type milk, soya milk (calcium-fortified), or yogurt; 40 g (1½ ounces) cheese; or 50 g (2 ounces) processed cheese.

4 or more servings of fruit

1 serving is 1 medium fresh fruit; ½ grapefruit, mango, or papaya; 8 tbsp tinned or chopped fruit; 4 tbsp dried fruit; or 200 ml (6½ fl oz) fruit juice.

4 or more servings of vegetables

1 serving is 8 tbsp cooked vegetables, 250 ml (8 fl oz) leafy vegetables, 1 small potato, or 200 ml (6½ fl oz) tomato or vegetable juice.

Note: Be sure to eat at least one fruit or vegetable that is high in vitamin C and one that is dark green or orange every day.

3 or more servings of legumes, nuts, and meat substitutes

1 serving is 8 tbsp legumes, tofu, tempeh, or textured vegetable protein; 2 eggs; 2 tablespoons nuts, seeds, or nut butter; or 1 veggie burger patty.

Note: Eat ½ more serving for each 250 ml (8 fl oz) of milk or milk substitute that you don't drink.

Fats and sweets: Eat sparingly.

While most vegetarians need to limit fats and sweets, some may need to increase them to supplement their calorie intake.

Sample Vegan Menu

This menu contains about 2,400 calories and exceeds the DRIs for all major nutrients except vitamin D. (It contains 0 per cent of the DRI for vitamin D.) Vitamin D can be produced in the skin with adequate exposure to sunshine.

Breakfast

250 ml (8 fl oz) oatmeal with
   1½ tablespoons molasses and
   2 tablespoons raisins
1 piece wholemeal bread with
   1 tablespoon peanut butter
250 ml (8 fl oz) soya milk

Snack

250 ml (8 fl oz) calcium-enriched orange
   juice

Lunch

250 ml (8 fl oz) haricot bean soup with
   1 piece wholemeal bread
Broccoli and tofu stir-fry with 250 ml
   (8 fl oz) tofu, 8 tbsp broccoli, and 150 g
   (5 oz) brown rice
250 ml (8 fl oz) soya milk

Snack

1 apple

Dinner

Salad with 150 g (5 oz) cos lettuce,
   ½ tomato, ¼ avocado, and vinaigrette
   dressing with 2 teaspoons canola oil
Stuffed pepper with 8 tbsp bulgur, 75 g
   (3 oz) black beans, and ½ tomato
100–125 g (4 oz) corn
250 ml (8 fl oz) soya milk

Snack

Shake with 250 ml (8 fl oz) soya milk
   and 250 g (9 oz) frozen strawberries

Sample Lacto-Ovo Vegetarian Menu

This menu, which contains eggs and dairy products, contains approximately 2,400 calories and exceeds all of the DRIs for pregnancy.

Breakfast

75 g (3 oz) bran-flakes with 2 tablespoons raisins and ½ banana

250 ml (8 fl oz) skimmed milk

1 piece toast with 2 teaspoons peanut butter

Snack

25 g (1 ounce) Cheddar cheese

1 apple

25 g (1 ounce) baked tortilla chips

Lunch

375 ml (12 fl oz) split-pea soup

250 ml (8 fl oz) spinach salad with ½ tomato, mushrooms, ¼ avocado, 25 g (1 ounce) grated reduced-fat Cheddar cheese, croutons, and vinaigrette dressing with 2 teaspoons canola oil

1 piece wholemeal bread

1 orange

250 ml (8 fl oz) low-fat yogurt

Snack

250 ml (8 fl oz) milk

2 teacups popcorn

Celery sticks

Dinner

250 ml (8 fl oz) Black Bean and Corn Salad (page 254)

1 serving Broccoli Quiche (page 334)

Wholemeal roll with 1 teaspoon reduced-fat butter or margarine

250 ml (8 fl oz) skimmed milk

Snack

Strawberry Shake (page 271)

Complementary Proteins: An Old Myth

A myth about complementary proteins has been passed down for years. Even recently, vegetarians have been advised to eat the traditional legume with grain, grain with dairy, or nut with grain to have a 'complete protein'. Current thinking is that as long as a vegetarian eats a variety of foods with enough calories, he or she will have enough of all the amino acids. According to the position of the American Dietetic Association on vegetarian diets, 'Plant sources of protein alone can provide adequate amounts of essential amino acids if a variety of plant foods are consumed and energy needs are met. Research suggests that complementary proteins do not need to be consumed at the same time.'[13]

Vegetarian Shopping List

Now that you are pregnant, you are probably much more aware of what you buy at the store. This handy shopping list can be reproduced and used weekly. (See page 195 for more information about shopping and label reading.)

Produce

Vegetables: asparagus, artichokes, aubergine, broccoli, Brussels sprouts, beets, cabbage, carrots, cauliflower, celery, courgettes, corn, garlic, green beans, lettuce (cos, soft leaf, iceberg), mushrooms, onions (white, red), peppers (green, red, yellow), potato (sweet, white, new), rhubarb, spinach, squash, swede, Swiss chard, tomatoes, turnips, winter squash

Fruit: apples, avocados, bananas, blueberries, canteloupe melon, cherries, grapes, grapefruit, honeydew melon, lemons, oranges, pears, peaches, plums, pineapple, raspberries, strawberries, watermelon

Other: _____

_____

Note: Fruits and vegetables that aren't in season should be bought frozen.

Dry/Bulk Foods

Grains/flour/etc.: barley, bulgur, nutritional yeast, oats, wheatgerm, wheat pastry flour, wholemeal flour

Rice: basmati, brown, instant, long- and short-grain, wild

Dried fruit: apricots, dates, prunes, raisins

Nuts and seeds: almonds, cashews, peanuts, sesame seeds, walnuts

Breads: rye, wholemeal, bagels, English muffins, pittas, tortillas (corn, flour)

Pasta: wholemeal, durum wheat

Snack foods: rice cakes, savoury biscuits, corn cakes, pretzels, digestive biscuits, granola bars, biscuits

Mixes: falafel, hummus, burgers

Other: _____

_____

Tinned Goods/Jar Goods/Packaged Items

Beans: adzuki, black, kidney, haricot, pinto, chickpeas

Non-fat evaporated milk

Fruit: peaches, pears, pineapple

Spreads/dips: chutney, jam, peanut butter, tahini spread

Soups

Tomatoes: paste, sauce, spaghetti sauce, whole

Vegetarian specialty foods: veggie burger mix, sea vegetables, miso

Other: _____

_____

Refrigerated Foods

Cheese: processed, low-fat Cheddar, low-fat cottage cheese, mozzarella, soya, Swiss

Tofu

Milk: semi-skimmed, skimmed, soya

Yogurt: dairy, soya

Eggs

Fresh pasta

Biscuits

Spreads: butter, margarine

Other: _____

_____

Oils/Condiments

Flavoured vinegar

Low-fat salad dressings

Low-sodium soy sauce, tamari sauce, mayonnaise, mustard

Oils: olive, canola, walnut

Spices: _____

_____

Sweeteners: honey, molasses, sugar (brown, white)

Frozen Foods

Frozen meals _____

_____

Fruits _____

_____

Meat substitutes _____

_____

Pancakes, waffles _____

_____

Sorbet, frozen yogurt _____

_____

Vegetables _____

_____

Veggie burgers, hot dogs _____

_____

Tempeh

Wraps, burritos

Drinks

Juices: frozen, bottled (vegetable, fruit)

Sparkling water

Decaffeinated coffee, tea

Other: _____

_____

Nonfood Items

Paper goods

Soaps

Toiletries

Other: _____

_____

▼

Vegetarian Food Planning

In Chapter Fifteen, you will find two weeks of budget menus modified to fit pregnancy needs.

▼

Eating Out Vegetarian-Style

As more people eat meatless, restaurants are adding vegetarian and vegan options to their menus. Some restaurants are very accommodating and will put together vegetarian meals that aren't even on the menu. Below are some healthy vegetarian entrées you're likely to find at various kinds of sit-down restaurants. Not all meatless entrées are vegan, so if you are concerned about animal-derived ingredients, you should consult the restaurant manager.

Vegetarian Entrées at Restaurants

Asian/Chinese

Any tofu (also called bean curd) dish
Egg foo yung
Noodle dish with vegetables and/or tofu

Bistro

Veggie burger
Vegetable platter
Spinach-and-artichoke dip
Veggie wrap
Stuffed potato

Continental

Quiche
Ratatouille
Vegetable risotto
Bean soup

Indian

Vegetable curry dish
Lentils
Spinach paneer

Italian

Cheese- or vegetable-stuffed ravioli or manicotti
Stuffed aubergine
Pasta primavera
Pasta e fagioli (pasta-and-bean soup)
Cheese or veggie pizza
Vegetarian lasagna

Mexican

Bean burrito
Huevos rancheros
Cheese or green chilli enchilada
Bean Tostadas

Middle Eastern

Falafel (ground chickpea fritters often served in pitta bread)
Hummus (chickpea dip)
Tabouli (bulgur salad)
Baba ghanouj (aubergine dip)
Ful medames (fava bean and chickpea dish)

Steak House

Vegetable or bean soup
Salad bar
Baked potato bar
Steamed vegetables

Thai

Vegetarian basil rolls
Vegetable boat
Tofu mussaman curry

Vegetarian Fast Food

Only a handful of fast-food restaurants offer vegetarian options besides ordering a sandwich or burger without the meat. Veggie burgers are common in restaurants, but they are still not on menus at the big burger chains – except at Burger King. Progress may be made if many people contact the corporate offices of fast food chains to request more vegetarian choices.

Salad bars are also a good option, as are hearty bean soups and vegetarian chillis.

For more information on vegetarian options in restaurants or about ingredients in restaurant foods, contact the Vegetarian Resource Group (VRG). This non-profit organization publishes a booklet called *Vegetarian Journal's Guide to Fast Food*. It also publishes *Vegetarian Journal* and many other resources, including vegetarian dining guides for major cities. Visit VRG's website at www.vrg.org.

▼

Vegetarian Convenience-Food Choices

Going meatless is getting popular, and vegetarian foods are now widely available at supermarkets and health food shops. The fat in some products is still surprisingly high, though, so be sure to read labels if fat is a concern for you. On the next page is a table that lists the nutrient information for some products currently available. The nutrient contents given are per serving as listed on labels.

Following are just some of the frozen entrées, either vegetarian (containing cheese or milk) or vegan, found in most grocery shops. To make a complete meal, add milk or yogurt, vegetable, fruit, and in some cases beans or another protein source.

Lean Cuisine Angel Hair Pasta
Lean Cuisine Cheese Ravioli
Lean Cuisine Fettuccini Primavera
Lean Cuisine Macaroni and Cheese with Broccoli
Weight Watchers Kung Pao Noodles and Vegetables
Weight Watchers Parisian-Style White Beans with Vegetables
Weight Watchers Pasta and Spinach Romano
Weight Watchers Paella Rice and Vegetables
Weight Watchers Peking-Style Rice and Vegetables
Weight Watchers Pilaf Florentine
Weight Watchers Risotto with Cheese and Mushrooms
Weight Watchers Santa Fe-Style Rice and Beans

In addition, the larger supermarkets have their own brands of vegetarian meals.

Here are some ideas for convenience foods you can buy at the grocery shop or supermarket to form the foundation of a vegetarian meal.

Bird's Eye Meal Starter Oriental Stir Fry
Bird's Eye Meal Starter Primavera
Bird's Eye Meal Starter Teriyaki Stir Fry

Again, as with the vegetarian convenience entrées, the larger supermarkets have their own brand of convenience foods which can be used as the foundation of a vegetarian meal.

▼

Eating after Delivery

If you stay in hospital long enough to require a meal make sure you choose the vegetarian option on the menu. Many hospitals have options for vegetarians, but they usually aren't vegan.

See page 169 for more information about eating after delivery.

Eating after Surgery

If you have a caesarean section, you may not eat solid food for a day or so, depending on the type of anaesthesia you receive. The progression from 'nothing by mouth' to 'regular diet' usually starts with clear liquids, such as clear juices, soup, coffee, tea, and mineral water. As your tolerance increases, your diet will progress to a full liquid diet, which includes such foods as thinned hot cereals, cream soups, and dairy products.

You should be able to omit the non-vegetarian foods and eat double portions of the other foods. Again, make sure that you request vegetarian meals once you can eat solid food.

? Questions You May Have

Q: I just found out I have gestational diabetes. How can I fit vegetarian foods into my meal plan?

A: Actually, a vegetarian diet fits very well into a diabetic diet. Depending on your blood sugar, your dietitian may want you to eat less carbohydrate and more fat. To do this you could increase your intake of nuts, avocado, peanut butter, and cheese. Visiting a registered dietitian can help in planning a vegetarian diet to meet your specific needs. On the next page you will find a table of some typical vegetarian foods with their diabetic exchanges.

Q: Is a vegetarian diet lower in fat than a diet containing meat?

A: Generally, yes, but not always. For example, lacto-ovo vegetarians may eat a lot of cheese, eggs, and low-fat or full-cream dairy products, which raise the fat content of the diet. A diet that is not well planned can have as much fat (including saturated fat) as the typical Western diet.

A vegan diet can also be high in fat, although most of the fat would be unsaturated (unless you regularly use coconut products and palm or palm kernel oil). For example, nuts, tahini, avocado, and nut butters, staples for some vegetarians, are very high in fat. Other hidden fats can find their way into the diet through such goodies as tofu ice cream and carob.

The important feature for any type of diet is that high-fat foods – especially those high in saturated fat – be eaten in moderation.

Q: I'm worried about being able to eat vegetarian while I'm in the hospital. Any advice?

A: When you go to the hospital in labour, you will probably be allowed to eat only ice chips or perhaps clear liquid, such as apple juice. This is because if you need anaesthesia, your stomach should be empty. During this time, you might want to remind your doctor that when you *can* eat, you would like a vegetarian diet. You might even want to write down your request before you go to the hospital.

After you have your baby, you will probably be allowed to eat a 'real meal'. Your

Exchanges for Special Vegetarian Foods

Food	Serving Sizes	Exchanges
Beans, dried, cooked	8 tbsp	1 starch + 1 very lean meat
Brewer's yeast	3 tbsp	1 starch
Bulgur, cooked	8 tbsp	1 starch
Carob flour	2 tbsp	1 starch
Miso (a bean and grain paste)	3 tbsp	1 vegetable
Seaweed, cooked	8 tbsp	1 vegetable
Soya flour	8 tbsp	1 lean meat + ½ bread
Soya grits, raw	2 tbsp	1 lean meat
Soya milk	250 ml (8 fl oz)	1 milk + 1 fat
Tahini	1 teaspoon	1 fat
Tempeh	125 g (4 oz)	1 starch + 2 lean meats
Tofu, soft	8 tbsp	1 medium-fat meat
Tofu, firm	8 tbsp	2 medium-fat meats
Wheatgerm	3 tbsp	1 starch

Source: Modified from *Vegetarian Journal Reports*, Vegetarian Resource Group.

meal may depend on what's left in the kitchen, which in turn depends on what time your baby is born. Babies seem to love arriving at off hours, and that may mean slim pickings for a very hungry new mother! A simple meal would be a cheese sandwich, fruit, and juice. For vegans, the selection may be very limited after hours. You may want to bring some non-perishable snacks from home for after delivery.

CHAPTER SEVEN

Special Care for High-Risk Pregnancies

What you will find in this chapter:

• *Expect the Unexpected*
• *Dealing with Your Emotions*
• *Pre-existing Diabetes*
• *Gestational Diabetes*
• *The Diabetic Eating and Exercise Plan*
• *High Blood Pressure*
• *Multiple Births*
• *Coping with Bedrest*
• *Older Mothers*
• *Teen Pregnancy*

This chapter answers such questions as:

• *What kind of diet should I follow if I have gestational diabetes?*
• *Should I cut my salt intake if I have high blood pressure during pregnancy?*
• *How can I prepare and eat healthy meals if I'm on bedrest?*
• *Are artificial sweeteners safe?*
• *How much weight should I gain if I'm expecting twins?*
• *How many calories should I eat if I'm seventeen?*
• *Should I eat differently if I'm over thirty-five?*
• *What are some healthy snacks for a diabetic diet?*

Expect the Unexpected

The unknown can be awfully scary – especially when you're pregnant. To equip you for the unexpected, this chapter tells you how some special conditions may affect you and your baby and what you can do to deal with them. There are other complications associated with pregnancy, but this chapter will discuss only those that can affect or can be affected by your diet. Being informed is the key to taking charge of your health and having the healthiest pregnancy possible.

Dealing with Your Emotions

When you discover that you have a high-risk pregnancy, you will probably find yourself on an emotional roller coaster. You may experience guilt, fear, anger, denial, depression, or loneliness. Emotions are sometimes helpful in getting you through rough times, but emotions can be unhealthy if they prevent you from taking care of yourself.

For example, guilt and fear may motivate you to change your lifestyle to protect your baby, and denial may give you time to get used to the idea of a high-risk condition. However, depression and loneliness may alienate you from people who can help you. Identifying your feelings can help you adjust and seek support from others. If any of your emotions hinder you from dealing with your situation or significantly affect your sleeping or eating patterns, speak with your doctor.

When I was put on bed rest for eleven weeks with my second

child, I had many of the emotions mentioned earlier. At one point I got so upset that I was ready to walk out the front door and away from my problems. Of course that wasn't possible, but it did give me an emotional release. (And looking back, the idea of walking away from my own belly is pretty funny!) What helped me the most was the support I received from others and reading about the experiences of women on bedrest.

Whatever happens, and whatever you have to do to carry out your pregnancy, it will be worth it when you see your healthy baby!

You Are Not Alone

One of the hardest aspects of a high-risk pregnancy is feeling like you are the only person with your problem. You're not alone; many women have faced or are facing the same challenges.

In the UK, you can visit the website belonging to The Centre for Study of Multiple Births at www.multiplebirth.com.

The American Diabetes Association is a good resource for information on all types of diabetes. On this organization's website you can find a multitude of resources, including several consumer and professional magazines. Visit www.diabetes.org. You can also visit the British Diabetic Association at www.diabetes.org.uk.

▼

Pre-existing Diabetes

If you were diabetic before pregnancy, you probably already know the importance of managing your diabetes. Before conception and during pregnancy are critical times to control your blood sugar. Before you attempt to become pregnant, consult your doctor, who will want you to be in tight control and will want to monitor you closely.

The Importance of Tight Control

High blood sugar in the first six to ten weeks of gestation is related to birth defects. Consequently, babies of women who have diabetes are at a higher risk for birth defects. However, mothers who maintain acceptable blood sugar control are at no more risk for having babies with birth defects than the general population.[1]

The American Diabetes Association suggests that *before* conception, diabetic mothers-to-be keep fasting (overnight fast) and just-before-meals blood sugars between 70 and 100 milligrams, one-hour-after-meals blood sugars less than 140 milligrams, and two-hours-after-meals blood sugars under 120 milligrams. Be sure to work out your individual goals with your doctor.[2]

The Health-Care Team

Before we go further, we should talk about a group of people who are very important to the health of your baby: the health-care team. You will need some specialized professionals to help in your care. If you are not already working with these health professionals, you can find them by asking your family doctor.

Your doctor/general practitioner is someone you should talk to before you become pregnant to make sure you are in good control of your diabetes. Your GP can also refer you to a diabetic nurse.

Some obstetricians specialize in high-risk pregnancies and have experience working with pregnant women with diabetes. Some women consult an obstetrician before they get pregnant if they have had previous problems in pregnancy.

An endocrinologist is a physician who specializes in caring for people with diabetes and who treats other conditions that involve hormones. Your obstetrician or doctor may refer you to one to help manage your diabetes during pregnancy.

A certified diabetic nurse is a registered nurse and is someone who has many hours of experience working with people who have diabetes and who has also passed a certification exam. This will probably be the person with whom you work closely for day-to-day management of your diabetes.

A registered nutritionist is someone who will develop an individual eating plan for you. An individual plan is important because it is designed with your specific activity level, work schedule, lifestyle, and favourite foods in mind. The nutritionist usually works closely with the diabetic nurse. Your nutritionist can also work with you after you have your baby to help with diet for breastfeeding and weight loss.

A neonatal paediatrician or neonatal nurse is someone who provides medical care for your newborn baby. Since babies of diabetics sometimes have health problems, a neonatal nurse (who specializes in newborns up to six weeks old) might be needed.

You are the most important member of your health-care team. You are responsible for the day-to-day management of your diabetes, including contacting other members of the team to let them know how you are doing or when you need help.

What to Expect

If you are taking insulin, you will probably have to adjust your doses with the help of your health-care team. Some pregnant women need to adjust their insulin dosages as often as every five days because of increased need.[3] If your diabetes was controlled with diet or oral medications (type II or noninsulin-dependent) before pregnancy, there is a good chance you will be put on insulin during pregnancy. However, after you have your baby, you will likely return to your prior mode of treatment, especially if you return to your ideal body weight and exercise regularly.

Some women take injections before every meal to keep their sugar under control. Others use a pump. Be prepared to take more shots if needed. Taking more shots will probably mean checking your blood sugar more often.

Possible Effects on Mother

Women with pre-existing diabetes have a higher risk of pre-term birth, C-section, and hypertension. Their risk of pre-eclampsia is also higher, and the risk increases with the severity of diabetes.[4]

What to Watch For:

Some common conditions of pregnancy can be a real challenge for women with diabetes. And some common conditions for women with diabetes are more challenging during pregnancy.

Insulin resistance: As pregnancy progresses, especially around the twenty-fourth to twenty-eighth week, a hormone produced by the placenta resists insulin. Therefore, the body needs much more insulin. Diabetic mothers-to-be may need twice the insulin they usually take.

Sign of Insulin Resistance
  increased blood sugar

Ketoacidosis: Ketones are byproducts of fat breakdown and are a sign that glucose is not available and the body is breaking down fat stores for energy. As ketones increase in the bloodstream (usually as a result of high blood sugar from not having an adequate dose of insulin), the pH level of the blood changes and ketoacidosis occurs. Because of changing insulin needs and energy requirements during pregnancy, ketoacidosis can occur more quickly and if not treated, can lead to coma.

Signs of Ketoacidosis
If you have any of these signs, seek medical attention fast! Some symptoms are similar to signs of hyperglycaemia, but are much more intense.

  excessive urination
  excessive thirst
  fruity, acetone, or alcohol breath
  listlessness, total lack of energy
  nausea
  abdominal pain
  vomiting
  laboured breathing

Hypoglycaemia (low blood sugar):
Low blood sugar can occur because of increased activity, inadequate meals or snacks, excessive exercise, foetal energy demands, too much time between meals, or too much insulin. Always have glucose tablets or glucose gel with you, or keep in your purse a food that is a quick source of energy, such as chewable sweets, fruit juice, or non-diet soda. Be sure to have a more substantial snack, such as a half sandwich or cheese and biscuits, about a half-hour later. Add milk for an even more substantial snack.

If you have low blood sugar more than once a week, report it to your doctor. If you can pinpoint the cause of your low blood sugar, try to remedy it with the guidance of your health-care team. Preventing low blood sugar is often just a matter of eating before exercise, eating a bigger meal, or adding a snack. You may, however, need a different insulin schedule. Many people are surprised to find that they have been giving their injections incorrectly, even though they may have been doing it for years. This could also affect your blood sugar.

Signs of Hypoglycaemia
These signs may develop very quickly.

  nervousness
  shakiness
  dizziness
  perspiration
  cold, clammy skin

hunger

headache

disorientation, difficulty paying attention

irritability, sudden mood changes

pale skin

Hyperglycaemia (high blood sugar):
Hyperglycaemia is elevated blood sugar. It can be caused by changes in how your insulin is being used (see insulin resistance); by being less active, by being under mental or physical stress (such as illness); by eating more food or different types of foods than usual; or by a combination of any of these factors. Elevated blood sugar can cause your baby to grow larger and fatter than normal (macrosomia), which may lead to a difficult delivery.

Signs of Hyperglycaemia
These signs occur gradually.

blurred vision

dry, itchy skin

frequent urination

increased thirst

headache

fatigue

Infections: Even minor infections can increase blood sugar and change insulin requirements. This can cause a breakdown of fat and lead to ketoacidosis (see definition on page 106). If you have the symptoms of ketoacidosis, seek medical attention immediately!

Sick-Day Rules

If you are sick with a virus or infection, your blood sugar will increase, even though you may not be eating much. The following rules are important to remember:

▶ **Contact a member of your health-care team.**

This is the first sick-day rule during pregnancy, especially if you are vomiting or have diarrhoea.

▶ **Continue to take your insulin.**

Talk to your physician to see if you should take the same dose. You may actually need more.

▶ **Check blood sugar more frequently.**

Your doctor will let you know how often. This will prevent any potential problems of high blood sugar and ketoacidosis. Your doctor may also want you to check your urine for ketones more frequently.

▶ **Prevent dehydration.**

Do this by drinking at least half a cup of fluid each hour. If you can't keep much food down and you are taking insulin, you must have carbohydrate in liquid form; this will give your body energy and will prevent dehydration. Examples of liquids (as well as some easy-to-digest solid foods) that contain 10 to 15 grams of carbohydrate are:

Fruit Juice or Sweetened Drinks
90 to 125 ml (3½ to 4 fl oz) apple juice
125 ml (4 fl oz) orange juice
90 to 125 ml (3½ to 4 fl oz) soft drink or fruit punch (not diet)
60 to 90 ml (4 to 6 tbsp) lemonade

Solid Foods Easy to Digest
4 saltine biscuits

½ Popsicle

300 ml (10 oz) chicken-noodle soup

300 ml (10 oz) chicken-and-rice soup

250 ml (8 fl oz) cream-of-mushroom
soup (prepared with water)

▶ **If you can eat solids, drink plenty
of calorie-free drinks to avoid
dehydration.**

Good examples are water, soup, decaffeinated tea, sugar-free and caffeine-free soft
drinks, sugar-free fruit drinks, or Popsicles.

▶ **Replenish lost sodium or potassium.**

If you are losing a lot of fluid through vomiting or diarrhoea, you will need to replenish your body with these important minerals. Here are good sources:

Sodium: Soup, tinned soups, salted biscuits.

Potassium: Orange juice, melon, papaya,
banana, orange-pineapple-banana juice,
pineapple juice, tomato juice, vegetable
juice, and dried fruits.

How Diabetes May Affect Your Baby

Blood sugar crosses the placenta from you
to your baby. High blood sugar causes the
baby to produce more insulin. Large amounts
of sugar and insulin can cause serious risks,
including a greater chance of stillbirth.
However, stillbirth is not common.

Birth defects occur more often in babies of
mothers who are diabetic. Fortunately, pre-
pregnancy planning, early prenatal care, and
keeping blood sugar in a narrow range can
dramatically decrease that risk. If possible,
seek medical counselling before you consider pregnancy.

Women with diabetes are prone to having bigger babies (macrosomia). High levels of blood glucose in the mother, especially during late pregnancy, are thought
to be responsible. After thirteen weeks gestation, your baby can start producing its
own insulin in response to high blood glucose levels. Insulin acts as a growth hormone, causing baby to deposit excess fat,
and the increased size may make a C-section necessary.

Babies of women with diabetes sometimes
have hypoglycaemia (low blood sugar)
immediately after delivery and must take
glucose or sugar water. They are also prone
to having higher bilirubin levels, or jaundice, which is easily treated with special
lights in the hospital. Babies of diabetic
mothers may have a higher chance of respiratory distress syndrome.[5]

Children of diabetic mothers are at
increased risk of obesity and impaired glucose tolerance by the time of puberty.
Breastfeeding is encouraged because it
decreases the risk of obesity and in some
populations decreases the risk of diabetes.[6]

If your diabetes is advanced and you have
some blood vessel damage, you may have
restricted blood flow to the placenta, so your
baby may have problems growing and may
be small for gestational age.

What You Can Do

To Keep Your Diabetes under Good Control during Pregnancy:

▶ **See your doctor before you become pregnant.**

The American Diabetes Association recommends a pre-pregnancy care programme, which involves evaluation by your health-care team to improve your chances of becoming pregnant as well as the outcome of your pregnancy.[7]

▶ **Eat more high-fibre foods and whole grains.**

Soluble fibre helps keep blood sugar under control by slowing digestion. Foods high in soluble fibre include oatmeal, peas and other legumes, barley, fruits, and vegetables. The antioxidants and insoluble fibre-found in whole grains have additional benefits, such as preventing constipation.

▶ **Monitor your blood sugar.**

Your physician will give you the blood sugar range within which you should stay. The blood sugar range during pregnancy is much stricter than when you are not pregnant. Remember that blood glucose values reflect what has happened in the last one to three hours.

▶ **Eat regular meals and snacks.**

You will want to eat balanced meals at regular intervals. Most pregnant women need 2,000 to 2,400 calories per day, divided between carbohydrate (40 to 50 per cent), fat (30 to 40 per cent), and protein (20 to 25 per cent).[8] Your calories should be divided among three meals and three snacks, with a space of two to three hours between meals and snacks. You may be instructed to use carbohydrate counting alone or in addition to exchanges. It is best to avoid combining milk and fruit alone for a snack. Including protein in snacks is recommended. Especially important is the bedtime snack, which should contain carbohydrate, fat, and protein. Eating a snack before bedtime (especially one that contains protein) can prevent hypoglycaemia in the middle of the night. Some women even need a snack in the middle of the night (such as a glass of milk) to keep their blood sugar up.

▶ **Exercise.**

You should ask your doctor about specific guidelines for frequency and duration of exercise and when NOT to exercise (such as when blood sugar is too low or too high). Regular exercise can decrease your need for insulin and can also make you feel more energetic. When you exercise, always take glucose gel or tablets, fruit juice, or hard sweets with you, and eat a snack or a meal before you begin. Never exercise when you know your blood sugar is low or when ketones are present. Also, don't give your insulin injection in an area that you will use immediately in exercise. For example, don't give it in the leg if you will take a brisk walk immediately afterward. (See page 182 for other tips on exercising.)

Labour and Delivery

Many doctors will induce labour for pregnant women who are diabetic. With all the high-tech equipment available, your obstetrician can tell just when the baby is developed enough to enter our world. About one-half of all women with diabetes need caesarean delivery because their babies are too big to fit through the birth canal or because of other complications.[9]

During the first twenty-four to forty-eight postpartum hours, your insulin requirements can drop dramatically. You may need to watch for signs of hypoglycaemia. Within a week after delivery, your insulin needs should return to pre-pregnant levels.

How to Cope

▶ **Keep stress low.**

Remember that stress can also raise blood sugar. Learn techniques to handle your stress, such as relaxation, visualization, and advance planning. Again, seek cooperation from others to help reduce your stress.

▶ **Remember that the extra hassle and discomfort you experience now will only last nine months.**

When you have your healthy baby, it will all be worth it.

▶ **Seek out a diabetes support group, preferably one for pregnant women.**

Research shows that women who have more social support can follow their dietary and self-monitoring regimens better.[10]

▶ **You and your family need to be committed to your pregnancy and to the unborn child.**

Everyone should learn how insulin works, the importance of dietary management, and what to do in case of hypo- or hyperglycaemia. You'll also need your family's emotional support and understanding.

'It was really tough to put myself first,' says Cindy, a woman who has been diabetic for fifteen years. 'When I was pregnant with my second child, I felt guilty when I had to stop whatever I was doing to get myself something to eat because of low blood sugar. But I learned that I had to put myself first for the sake of my baby.'

▶ **Learn to recognize the early warning signs of hypoglycaemia, hyperglycaemia, and ketoacidosis so you can take action.**

▶ **Always be prepared to handle a low blood sugar reaction.**

See page 106 on how to treat hypoglycaemia.

▼

Gestational Diabetes

About 4 per cent of all pregnant women will have diabetes of pregnancy, or gestational diabetes mellitus (GDM).[11] Diabetes mellitus is a disorder that prevents the body from using a simple sugar called glucose. GDM is a type of diabetes that occurs only during pregnancy and usually disappears after delivery.

Glucose is a simple sugar that is the final

product of carbohydrate digestion. Carbohydrate is found in all starchy foods, such as bread, potatoes, and corn, and also in milk, fruits, and vegetables. Forms of simple carbohydrate that enter the bloodstream more quickly are found in sweets, jam, syrup, honey, and table sugar. Your body can also make glucose from protein and stored carbohydrates. Every cell in the body uses glucose for energy.

Insulin is the hormone produced by the pancreas that allows glucose to enter your body's cells. A trace mineral called chromium is necessary for insulin to work. Supplementation studies have shown that chromium improves glucose tolerance in women with gestational diabetes and people with type II diabetes. While chromium supplementation is not recommended, it couldn't hurt to eat more foods high in chromium: brewer's yeast, processed cheese, whole grains, apples with skin, spinach, oysters, carrots, and chicken breast.[12]

During pregnancy, women need two to three times more insulin. This is due to increased body weight and increased levels of hormones that work against insulin. These hormones peak during the twenty-fourth to twenty-eighth weeks. When the body cannot produce the insulin it needs, high blood sugar and diabetes are the result.

Effects on Mother

Many women have no symptoms of GDM. Some of the symptoms are also the typical signs of pregnancy, such as fatigue and frequent urination, so it may be hard to tell them apart. Some women have the symptoms of high blood sugar or low blood sugar listed on pages 106–107.

Women with GDM have increased risk of high blood pressure, pre-eclampsia (a hypertensive disorder of pregnancy), and urinary tract infections. Symptoms of urinary tract infections include burning during urination and frequent urination.[13]

Effects on Baby

The most common problem is macrosomia, delivering a large baby, which may make for a difficult delivery, trauma to the baby during delivery, and/or increased need for a C-section.

Less common problems sometimes seen in babies of mothers with GDM include premature delivery, hypoglycaemia (low blood sugar) at birth, increased bilirubin in the blood (jaundice), and respiratory distress syndrome.[14]

One study showed that intensified management of blood glucose resulted in similar rates of macrosomia, C-section, stillbirth, and respiratory complications in children of diabetic and non-diabetic women.[15]

Children of women with gestational diabetes are at increased risk of obesity and impaired glucose tolerance by the time of puberty. Breastfeeding is encouraged because it decreases the risk of obesity and in some populations decreases the risk of diabetes. You should inform your child's doctor that you had GDM so he or she can recommend preventive measures.[16]

Who Is at Risk?

For Gestational Diabetes

Risk factors for gestational diabetes include overweight, family history of diabetes, and adverse pregnancy outcomes such as stillbirth, miscarriage, and congenital malformations. Risk also increases with age and with each subsequent pregnancy.[17]

For Type II Diabetes

Unlike type I diabetes, which generally begins during childhood and requires insulin treatment from then on, type II diabetes is usually diagnosed during adulthood and does not as a rule require insulin injections.

It is estimated that half of all people with diabetes haven't even been diagnosed. Your chances of becoming diabetic are greater if you:[18]

- have a close blood relative who is diabetic.
- were diagnosed with GDM in a previous pregnancy.
- are more than 20 per cent over your ideal body weight.
- have had a baby that weighed 4 kilograms (9 pounds) or more at birth.
- are of African or Asian descent, or a Pacific Islander.
- are over forty-five years old.
- have been previously diagnosed with impaired glucose tolerance or impaired fasting glucose.
- have high blood pressure.
- have high-density lipoprotein (HDL) cholesterol less than 35.
- have a triglyceride level over 250.

Are You at Risk?

Take a test that shows your level of risk at www.diabetes.org/ada/risktest.asp.

Testing for Diabetes

When you are between the twenty-fourth and twenty-eighth weeks of pregnancy, your doctor will ask you to take a glucose challenge test that looks for sugar in the blood. This test is done without special preparation, such as fasting or eating certain foods. First, you will be asked to drink a very sweet drink called glucose (it tastes like cola syrup before the carbonated water is added). One hour later your blood will be drawn, and the amount of sugar (or glucose) in your blood will be tested. If your blood sugar is over 140 milligrams, this is considered a positive, or abnormal, test. You may be asked to:

- see a registered nutritionist for meal-planning guidance

OR

- take a glucose tolerance test, which is similar to the glucose screening test but lasts three hours. You will need to follow a special high-carbohydrate diet for three days prior to the test. Your doctor will give you specific instructions. After drinking the glucose, a health professional will draw your blood every hour for three hours.[19]

If your doctor diagnoses you with GDM, you may be referred to a specialist, such as an endocrinologist or obstetrician. However, your doctor may decide to treat the diabetes aspect of your pregnancy by working closely with a nutritionist, who will give you a diabetic meal plan, and a diabetic nurse, who will teach you about monitoring your blood sugar.

Keys to Controlling Gestational Diabetes

▶ **Eat balanced meals at regular intervals.**

See a registered nutritionist to make a personal meal plan.

▶ **Keep your activity level up.**

Talk to your doctor about recommending a daily exercise programme; most doctors approve of walking or swimming.
Note: DON'T exercise if your blood sugar is elevated or if ketones are present in your urine; contact your doctor. (See Chapter Eleven: Fitting Fitness In for more information on exercise during pregnancy.)

▶ **Divide the food you eat daily into three meals and two to three snacks.**

The bedtime snack is especially important. It should include some starch, protein, and fat.

▶ **Keep a handle on weight gain by making wise food choices.**

Choose foods that are low in saturated fat.

▶ **Avoid emotional eating, such as eating when you are sad, angry, or stressed-out.**

▶ **Eat more wholegrain foods and legumes.**

Avoid concentrated sweets such as biscuits, sweets, puddings, sugar, honey, and chocolate. Also, limit or avoid fruit juices, even unsweetened ones. They contain concentrated amounts of fruit sugar, which can raise your blood sugar.

▶ **Expect to monitor your blood sugar; your midwife will teach you how to do this.**

Your blood sugar level will show you how your diet is affecting the amount of glucose in your blood and will be used to adjust your diet and exercise regimen.

At first, your doctor will ask you to test your blood sugar as often as four to five times per day for the first week. This could include testing in the middle of the night, when blood sugar sometimes drops. When your blood sugar is under good control, you will probably test less often.

▶ **Keep your diet high in fibre.**

Fibre helps stabilize blood sugar. So stay away from foods made with white flour as much as possible. Try to eat raw (instead of cooked) fruits and vegetables. Eat high-fibre cereal with milk as a snack. (See page 51, 'Focus on Fibre'.)

▶ **Smile!**

You have a unique opportunity to improve your family's diet! Try to make the changes permanent.

The Diabetic Eating and Exercise Plan

Many people think that going on a diabetic diet means they must give up all their favourite foods. This is just not true!

The diabetic eating plan is simply a way of eating that includes balanced amounts of carbohydrate, fat, and protein in each meal. All foods are allowed except simple sugars like table sugar, honey, jam, and syrup and foods that contain a lot of sugar like cakes, puddings, biscuits, and sweets. However, foods with small amounts of sugar are allowed in moderation. For example, digestive biscuits, animal crackers, and angel food cake are allowed in moderation when your blood sugar is under good control.

The goal in managing your diabetes is to keep your blood sugar within a certain range. General guidelines are listed on page 104 under 'Pre-existing Diabetes'. However, your doctor may have individual recommendations for you. You can control your blood sugar by not eating too many carbohydrates at one time and balancing your meals with protein and fat. The protein and fat slow digestion and cause a slow, gradual rise in blood sugar, instead of a fast rise that would occur if you ate a carbohydrate food by itself.

Carbohydrate is found in starchy foods like bread, savoury and sweet biscuits, rice, potatoes, corn, milk, yogurt, dried beans, fruit, and fruit juice. Carbohydrate is also found in smaller amounts in nonstarchy vegetables like green beans, carrots, and squash.

The Sweet Success Program in California recommends staying away from fruit juices and processed and refined starch products such as instant potatoes, instant noodles, instant hot cereals, cold processed cereals, tinned soups, and packaged stuffing. It also recommends avoiding sugar-containing sauces such as teriyaki and barbecue. On the other hand, it encourages eating whole-grain breads, non-instant oatmeal, legumes, and lentils because of their small effect on blood glucose.[20] Of course, any food containing concentrated sugars also provides concentrated sources of carbohydrates and should be avoided.

Your meal plan will be arranged with your current eating pattern, individual lifestyle, and activity level in mind. The calories, carbohydrate, protein, and fat that you need in a day will be calculated and then divided between your meals and snacks. Snacks are important because they allow you to eat smaller meals and prevent your blood sugar from dropping too low. (See page 117 for snack ideas.) Follow-up visits with a dietitian are important because assessing the energy needs and eating patterns of a person is difficult in just one visit. Your meal plan may need adjusting as your activity level increases or decreases.

Your Meal Plan

A common meal pattern is one that contains three meals and three snacks comprising 40 to 45 per cent carbohydrate, 20 to 25 per cent protein, and 30 to 40 per cent fat. Hormones sometimes cause higher blood sugar in the morning. For this reason, a low-carbohydrate breakfast (for example, two eggs and one to two pieces of toast) containing 15 to 30 grams of carbohydrate is recommended. Fruit, fruit juice, and milk should be avoided in the morning because of their high simple sugar content. However, fruit and milk are encouraged the rest of the day.

Bev Spears, R.D., of The Diabetes Center of New Mexico in the US starts her GDM patients with just one serving of a starchy food (such as one piece of toast) at breakfast. If the blood sugar testing shows that the amount is well tolerated, the carbohydrate is increased. The preliminary diet excludes milk and juice, because many diabetic women are sensitive to the simple carbohydrates found in these drinks. Milk may be added back into the diet as tolerated.[21] Generally, fruit juices (even ones with no added sugar) should be avoided, since they can increase blood sugar at any time. Vegetable juice and tomato juice are okay.

Your diet will probably be based on the exchange method for meal planning or the carbohydrate counting method.

Carbohydrate counting is a relatively new method of meal planning in the US, but it has been the primary approach in the UK for years. Its focus is balancing the amount of carbohydrates eaten at meals and snacks.

The exchange method of meal planning uses a combination of foods from six food groups: starch, fat, milk, meat, fruit, and vegetable. Each food serving within a group has approximately the same number of calories and other nutrients, so the foods within a group can be exchanged for each other. For example, one serving of starch has 80

calories and 15 grams of carbohydrate. You won't have to worry about those numbers, but do get to know the serving sizes. See page 116 for an abridged exchange list.

The following meal plan has about 2,200 calories and is an example of a meal plan that your dietitian might develop for you. Your calorie needs will vary depending on your size, ideal body weight, and activity level. An individualized diet developed just for you is very important. The sample below is an example only and is not intended to replace individual counselling.

Breakfast

1 medium-fat meat = 1 egg
2 starches = 1 piece wholemeal toast, 8 tbsp old-fashioned oatmeal
2 fats = 2 teaspoons tub margarine
1 milk = 250 ml (8 fl oz) sugar-free or 200 ml (6½ fl oz) natural yogurt

Snack

1 starch = 19 g (¾ oz) wholegrain biscuits
1 fruit = 1 small apple
1 medium-fat meat = 25 g (1 oz) Cheddar cheese
1 skimmed/very-low-fat milk = 250 ml (8 fl oz) sugar-free low-fat fruit yogurt

Lunch

3 starches = 2 slices wholemeal bread, 25 g (1 oz) pretzels
2 very lean meats = 2 ounces tuna packed in water
1 fat = 1 tablespoon reduced-fat mayonnaise
2 vegetables = 1 sliced tomato, raw veggies, cos lettuce
1 skimmed/very-low-fat milk = 250 ml (8 fl oz) milk

Exchange List	
1 starch =	1 piece bread; 1 tortilla; 6 crackers; 8 tbsp pasta, bulgur, corn, potatoes, or hot cereal; 6 tbsp rice; 8 tbsp beans, peas, or lentils (also counts as 1 very lean meat); or 40 g (½ oz) flaked cereal
1 fat =	1 teaspoon margarine, oil, mayonnaise, or butter; 1 tbsp diet margarine (30 to 50% oil) or low-fat mayonnaise; 1 tbsp salad dressing or 2 tbsp low-fat dressing; ⅛ avocado; 20 small peanuts; 8 large olives; 2 tbsp soured cream; or 1 slice bacon
1 milk =	*Skimmed/very-low-fat:* 250 ml (8 fl oz) skimmed milk; ½ or 1%-fat milk or buttermilk; 250 ml (8 fl oz) non-fat or low-fat sugar-free yogurt; or 200 ml (6½ fl oz) natural non-fat yogurt
	Low-fat: 250 ml (8 fl oz) semi-skimmed milk or 200 ml (6½ fl oz) low-fat yogurt
	Full-fat: 250 ml (8 fl oz)
1 meat/meat substitute =	25 g (1 oz) unless specified
	Very lean: fish; shellfish; chicken or turkey breast; fat-free cheese; sandwich meats with 1 gram or less fat per ounce; 4 tbsp non-fat or low-fat cottage cheese; or 8 tbsp cooked dried beans, peas, or lentils (also counts as 1 starch)
	Lean: round, sirloin, or flank steak; pork tenderloin; ham; veal; leg of lamb; dark meat of chicken (no skin); cheese and lunch meats with 3 grams fat or less per 25 g (ounce)
	Medium fat: most other beef; mozarella cheese; cheese with less than 5 grams fat per 25 g (ounce); 1 egg; dark-meat chicken with skin; salmon; tuna in oil (drained); ground turkey; or 8 tbsp tofu
	High fat: spareribs, sausage, regular cheese, hot dogs, or sandwich meats with 8 grams fat or less per 25 g (ounce)
1 fruit =	1 medium fresh; ½ banana; 12 cherries; 15 grapes; or 8 tbsp tinned, unsweetened
1 vegetable =	8 tbsp cooked vegetables; 125 ml (4 fl oz) vegetable juice; or 250 ml (8 fl oz) raw vegetables

Source: *Exchange Lists for Meal Planning,* The American Diabetes Association and The American Dietetic Association, 1995.

Snack
1 starch = 19 g (¾ oz) baked corn tortilla chips
1 fruit = 1 orange

Dinner
3 lean meats = 75 g (3 oz) grilled tenderloin steak
2 vegetables = 8 tbsp each broccoli and carrots
2 starches = 1 small baked potato, 1 wholemeal roll

2 fats = 1 teaspoon tub margarine or butter, 2 tablespoons soured cream
1 skimmed/very-low-fat milk = 250 ml (8 fl oz) milk
1 fruit = ½ frozen banana

Bedtime Snack
1 starch = ½ wholemeal bagel
1 very lean meat = 2 tablespoons peanut butter
1 fruit = 275 g (10 oz) berries

After You Start a Diabetic Diet

Don't be alarmed if you have a small weight loss after you start a diet to control your blood sugar. This is fairly common, especially if you are now eating fewer carbohydrate foods than you did previously. Just remember that weight loss should be temporary, lasting no more than about five days. If the weight loss continues, talk to your doctor or dietitian.

You may be asked to self-monitor your blood glucose to find out how much sugar is in your blood. Some doctors randomly test blood sugar during office visits.

Blood sugar monitoring involves pricking your finger and letting a drop of blood fall on a test strip. The test strip is placed in a tiny machine that reads the blood glucose level and displays it on a panel. Your blood sugar and ketone testing records are good tools to see if you are eating enough food. Go over these records with your health-care team.

If you find that your blood sugars are consistently low at certain times of the day, try to figure out why. Some possibilities are:

- You didn't eat enough food at the previous meal or snack.
- You need to add a snack two hours or so before your sugar is low.
- You're not eating the right kind of snack. (Read on for good snack ideas.)
- You are more active or are exercising close to this time and need more food.

Healthy Snacks

A diabetic snack should contain some carbohydrate, fat, and protein. You may be able to have a carbohydrate snack alone, as long as it is not juice. Your lifestyle, activity level, and weight gain will dictate the type of snacks you need. Again, your individual snack needs should be discussed with your diabetic nurse or doctor.

Balanced Snacks

Each snack equals one starch or one fruit, one meat, and one fat exchange. To add a milk exchange, add 250 ml (8 fl oz) milk or natural or sugar-free yogurt.

> 25 g (1 oz) Swiss cheese and 6 rye biscuits
> 2 tbsp peanut butter and 2 corn cakes
> 1 piece wholemeal bread and 25 g (1 oz) light cream cheese
> 1 small bran muffin and 4 tbsp cottage cheese
> 1 pear and 25 g (1 oz) Cheddar cheese
> ½ ham sandwich on rye bread with 1 teaspoon mayonnaise
> 1 apple with Caramel Dip (see recipe on page 319)
> 6 tbsp beans with 25 g (1 oz) cheese
> 2 tbsp peanut butter and ½ small banana
> Raw veggies, 25 g (1 oz) cheese dip, and 6 savoury biscuits

Starchy Snacks

Each snack is equal to one serving of starch.

> ½ wholemeal pitta bread
> 6 rye biscuits
> 2 rice cakes
> 5 wholemeal biscuits
> 8 tbsp tabouli (bulgur salad)
> 8 tbsp black beans
> 25 g (1 oz) baked tortilla chips

'Free' Snacks

These foods have very few calories, so they can be eaten as desired when you don't have any exchanges left in your meal plan. Do not eat these snacks alone before exercise, because they will not affect your blood sugar.

> Raw vegetables with 2 tablespoons fat-free dressing
> Sugar-free Popsicles (if your doctor allows artificial sweeteners)
> Vegetable stock
> Lettuce and raw greens
> Cucumbers
> Celery

Exercise: A Shot in the Arm

Imagine something that makes you feel more energetic and relaxed, makes your body muscular instead of flabby, allows you to eat more without gaining too much weight, and reduces your long-term risk of heart disease. This something also helps you avoid taking insulin or reduces your dose. Would you go out and buy it by the bucketful? Exercise is this wonderful something, and it is strongly recommended for women who have diabetes.

Doctors generally recommend that you exercise twenty to thirty minutes daily, and at least three times per week; some suggest a daily walk or water exercise. However, you should talk to your doctor to see what specific guidelines he or she has for you. Regular exercise improves the efficiency of your body's insulin, which can help control blood sugar levels so that you don't have to take insulin.

A study done at the Sansum Medical Research Foundation in Santa Barbara, California, found that regular exercise normalized fasting and postprandial (after-meal) glucose levels, which prevented the need for insulin. The women worked out on arm ergometers (stationary bicycles that use the arms to pedal) three times per week for six weeks.[22] Lois Jovanovic-Peterson, M.D., writes in her book *Managing Your Gestational Diabetes,* 'If your doctor tells you to restrict physical activity due to premature labour, you may still be able to do upper-arm exercises – such as lifting 900-gram (2-pound) weights while sitting in a chair.' You can do this while watching the news or your favourite soap! You can do such exercises on a daily basis, split between two ten-to-twenty-minute sessions.[23]

We would all like to exercise regularly, but may have trouble finding time for exercise in our busy schedules. The solution is to *make* exercise a priority and *make* time for it regularly. (See Chapter Ten: Fitting Fitness In for tips on 'exercising without exercising'. Also found in Chapter Ten are exercise guidelines for pregnancy.)

If you start exercising when your blood sugar level is normal, you could have low blood sugar when you finish. Here are some tips for avoiding low blood sugar during exercise:[24]

- If you know your blood sugar is low, delay exercise until after you have had a meal or snack.
- If your blood sugar is within normal range, eat one serving of fruit before a thirty-minute activity.

• If your blood sugar is within normal range, eat one serving of starch and one serving of fruit before an activity that lasts an hour or more.

• If your activity is more strenuous, you may need to increase the amount of food for your snack.

• If your activity (such as a hike) is longer than two hours, eat before you go and also bring snacks to eat along the way.

• Always carry hard sweets or glucose tablets with you in case you have low blood sugar or an insulin reaction. Packaged peanut-butter or cheese biscuits are also good to keep in your bag.

The Scoop on Sweeteners

There are three types of sweeteners: nutritive sweeteners, which contain calories; sugar alcohols, which contain fewer calories; and non-nutritive sweeteners (also called artificial sweeteners), which contain virtually no calories. The different types of sweeteners and their use during pregnancy (and as they relate to diabetes) are described below.

For more information about sweeteners, visit the American Dietetic Association at www.eatright.org, or the Center for Science in the Public Interest at www.nutritionaction.org.

Sucrose and Other Sugars

If you have diabetes while pregnant, you should avoid foods with concentrated sugars – even if you could use sugars in your diabetic meal plan before you were pregnant. You can find the different types of sugars on food labels by looking for these words: *sugar (brown, icing sugar, invert, raw, cane, crystallized cane, turbinado), honey, corn syrup, dextrin, fruit juice concentrate, maple syrup, corn sweetener, malt,* and *molasses.* Less-processed sugars like honey, molasses, and brown sugar have the same calories as processed sugars and can have the same effect on your blood sugar. Small amounts of sugar are common in many foods. That's okay; simply choose foods with the least amount of sugar. Keep in mind that 4 grams of sugar is equivalent to 1 teaspoon.

Sugar Alcohols (Polyols)

You may have seen the ingredients sorbitol, mannitol, and xylitol on food labels. These are sugar alcohols, types of sugar that are not completely absorbed in the intestines. Sugar alcohols therefore have fewer calories than sugar and do not raise blood sugar the way regular sugars do. Sorbitol and mannitol, often found in diet sweets, can cause diarrhoea if eaten in large amounts. Isomalt, lactitol, maltitol, hydrogenated starch hydrolysates (HSH), and erythritol are other sugar alcohols that you will be seeing more of in the future. Check with your dietitian about fitting foods with sugar alcohols into your eating plan.[25]

Artificial Sweeteners

If you are avoiding sugary foods and drinks, you may still want an occasional something sweet. Should you eat products sweetened with artificial (non-nutritive) sweeteners? Aspartame with acesulfame K is found in Hermesetas Gold, a granulated sweetener, and also in Sweet 'n' Low.

Aspartame (containing a source of phenylaline) is found in Boots Sweetner, and aspartame is also found in Canderel, both the tablets and the granulated product.

Sodium saccharin is found in Hermesetas Original, Sweetex, and the granulated Sucron.

Boots Fructose powder is a granulated product.

Many doctors would prefer that their patients limit or avoid artificial sweeteners. Moderation is usually a good rule to follow when it comes to food. A moderate intake of artificial sweeteners would be one to two servings per day. Consult with your doctor for individualized recommendations.

Saccharin

Saccharin has been shown to cause bladder cancer in rats and remains somewhat controversial. Because saccharin can cross the placenta and remain in foetal tissues for a while, it has been suggested that women consider careful use of saccharin during pregnancy.[26]

Aspartame

Aspartame is a widely used sweetener. Although aspartame is popular, some people have reported reactions such as dizziness and headaches after ingesting it. People with a metabolic disorder called phenylketonuria (PKU) should avoid it.

How much aspartame is too much? The Acceptable Daily Intake (ADI) set by the US Food and Drug Administration (FDA) is 50 milligrams of aspartame per kilogram of body weight (22.7 milligrams per pound). A 375-ml (12-fl oz) diet soda contains approximately 225 milligrams; a 250-ml (8-fl oz) yogurt or 125-g (4-fl oz) gelatin dessert contains about 100 milligrams; 125 g (4 fl oz) of frozen yogurt contains about 47 milligrams; and a packet of aspartame sweetener contains 37 milligrams. To exceed the ADI, a 68-kilogram (150-pound) woman would have to drink more than fifteen diet drinks in a day!

Most people keep within the ADI for aspartame without even trying. If you have a sweet tooth, though, you should keep an eye on how much aspartame you use. You may find yourself eating a lot of foods sweetened with aspartame.[27] Also, be aware that sometimes aspartame and saccharin are found together in a product. Be sure to read food labels carefully.

Acesulfame K

The safety of consuming acesulfame K during pregnancy was determined by rat studies. Several well-respected scientists have said that the carcinogenicity testing was flawed. Given this possibility and the fact that acesulfame K can cross the placenta, it is best to avoid acesulfame K while you are pregnant.[28] Keep in mind that acesulfame K and sucralose are sometimes mixed in a product, so read food labels carefully.

Sucralose

Sucralose was approved in the United States in 1998 and has been used by millions of people around the world since 1991. It's the only non-nutritive sweetener made from sugar. Sucralose has been approved for use in beverages, baked goods, desserts, syrups, jams, chewing gum, and more. It was determined not to pose any carcinogenic, reproductive, or neurological risks to humans on the basis of one hundred studies conducted over twenty years. According to the Center for Science in the Public Interest (CSPI), a US consumer watchdog group, sucralose is safer than saccharin and doesn't raise the concerns that aspartame and acesulfame K do.[29]

The ADI for sucralose is 5 milligrams per kilogram of body weight (11 milligrams per pound of body weight).

Sweeteners Awaiting FDA Approval

Alitame is currently awaiting FDA approval pending more research. Alitame is approved for use in food and beverages in Australia, New Zealand, Mexico, and the People's Republic of China.

Stevia, which is much sweeter than sugar without the calories, is made from the stevia shrub and has been used for years in South America and Japan. Although it is sold in the United States as a dietary supplement, it has not been approved as a food sweetener by the United States, Canada, or the European Union. European animal tests have indicated fertility and reproductive problems and have deemed stevia unacceptable as a sweetener. It is best to avoid using stevia until it is approved as a sweetener.[30]

Diet Foods

It's not just sugar and calories that diet products may be lacking; some are also missing vitamins and minerals, which are so important for you and your baby. One mineral that diet drinks do have is phosphorus, which can be a problem in large amounts. It is thought that a high proportion of phosphorus to calcium in the diet causes leg cramps during pregnancy.

If you choose to use artificially sweetened products, moderation is the key. What's moderation? Most professionals consider one to two servings per day moderate – a serving being one diet drink (caffeine-free) or one serving of diet jelly pudding, or hot cocoa.

? Questions You May Have

Q: Will I have to take insulin?

A: If your blood sugar can't be controlled by diet and exercise, you will probably take insulin in the form of a self-administered shot. You may take one or several insulin shots daily. Even if you don't take insulin, you will probably be asked to monitor your blood sugar.

Blood glucose monitoring is a great way to see how you are doing with your diet. You may be following your meal plan closely, yet seeing high blood sugars. This is because some foods affect your blood glucose quite differently, even though they are similar in carbohydrate value and calories. Also, some women can tolerate carbohydrates better than other women.

Q: What else can affect my blood glucose?

A: Many other factors can affect your blood glucose or blood sugar level:

- The combination of protein, fat, carbohydrate, and fibre you eat at a meal.
- How much fibre is in your diet. Fibre slows down digestion, causing slower release of glucose into the bloodstream.
- Your activity level. Exercise uses up extra glucose and causes insulin to work more efficiently, thus keeping your blood sugar down and reducing the likelihood that you will have to take insulin.
- Your overall health. Infection and illness can increase blood sugar levels. (See page 107 for 'Sick-Day Rules'.)
- Your stress level. Emotional stress can also increase your blood sugar level.

Q: Can hypoglycaemia harm my baby?

A: One animal study indicates hypoglycaemia in mother does cause hypoglycaemia in baby, and that baby will produce glucose from other sources, such as fat, to meet its energy needs. Recurrent bouts of hypoglycaemia could cause poor growth in baby.[31]

If you take insulin, some doctors recommend having a glucagon kit available for severe hypoglycaemic reactions. (Glucagon is a hormone that increases blood sugar.) Make sure that relatives, friends, and co-workers know what to do for you if you start having the symptoms of hypoglycaemia, including knowing how to use the glucagon kit. Also, be sure to wear a necklace or bracelet that identifies you as diabetic.

Q: What about hyperglycaemia?

A: Hyperglycaemia is more likely to adversely affect your baby. High blood sugar can cause the baby to have increased body fat, which could cause delivery problems. High blood sugar can also increase your baby's risk of being overweight and having impaired glucose tolerance when he or she is older. It has been suggested that if a baby has hypoglycaemia at birth caused by the mother's hyperglycaemia, it could cause long-term neurological dysfunction.[32]

Q: I have gestational diabetes. Will I still have diabetes after my baby is born?

A: Most women's blood sugar levels go back to normal shortly after delivery. Only a small number of women continue to have glucose intolerance.

However, over half of the women who have gestational diabetes will be diagnosed with type II (adult-onset) diabetes ten to fifteen years after their children are born. Women who have GDM with one pregnancy are very likely to have it with other pregnancies, too. The American Diabetes Association recommends having your blood glucose tested six weeks after delivery, and if normal at least every three years thereafter.[33] Can you avoid post-pregnancy diabetes? Very possibly, if you maintain your ideal body weight and exercise regularly. Eating a balanced diet is also beneficial.

Q: What about my next pregnancy?

A: Women with GDM have a very high chance of having GDM with subsequent pregnancies. Losing excess weight between pregnancies, exercising regularly, and eating well can cut your risk.

Q: What if I get sick and can't eat?

A: If you get ill and don't feel like eating or can't keep food down, you should first contact your doctor. Women are usually instructed to continue taking insulin (if applicable) because illness can raise blood sugar levels. You must also continue drinking fluids, so that you don't become dehydrated. (See page 107 for 'Sick Day Rules'.)

Q: Will my baby be diabetic?

A: Not at birth. However, having diabetes (either pre-existing or gestational) does increase your child's risk of being overweight and of having impaired glucose tolerance, which are risk factors for diabetes. Breastfeeding is the first line of defence, since it can decrease the risk of obesity. Your family should also practise a healthy lifestyle, including regular activity, a healthy diet with plenty of high-fibre foods, and close-to-ideal weight.

Q: The week before I had my blood sugar checked, I was eating a lot of sweets and soft drinks. Is that what caused my diabetes?

A: No. However, you may have craved sweets because of the diabetes. When your blood sugar is high, but you don't have enough insulin to use the glucose, your body sends out the signal that you need energy.

Sugar does not cause diabetes. However, excess simple sugar and starches in the diet cause the pancreas to secrete more insulin; and if your body cannot produce the amount of insulin needed, the result is high blood sugar.

▼

High Blood Pressure

Sarah was surprised when she went to her doctor's surgery and found that her blood pressure was elevated. She felt fine! No one in her family had high blood pressure (hypertension), and she had never had a problem with it either. Sarah's condition, called pregnancy-induced hypertension (PIH), is diagnosed in 10 to 20 per cent of women pregnant for the first time.

Sarah was asked to take time to rest. Because she was a salesperson at a local department store, resting was virtually impossible while she was at work. However, she did try to put her feet up for a few minutes when she could and rested a lot in the evenings.

After closely monitoring Sarah's blood pressure for several weeks, Sarah's doctor decided she should be on strict bedrest to prevent her blood pressure from getting worse. She took temporary disability leave, which allowed her to keep receiving some income. After two months on bedrest, Sarah delivered a healthy, blue-eyed boy who weighed 3 kilograms (7 pounds).

For Sarah, following the doctor's orders paid off! Keeping her doctor's appointments and staying in bed kept her blood pressure from going up any more and improved her circulation. The improved circulation allowed adequate blood flow and nutrients to her baby so he could grow adequately.

Had Sarah not taken such good care of herself, the PIH might have escalated into more serious conditions called pre-eclampsia and eclampsia. PIH, pre-eclampsia, and eclampsia are all hypertensive disorders of pregnancy. Each is a stage of the same disease. These disorders are also known as the toxaemias of pregnancy, or simply toxaemia. Because the term *toxaemia* has been used to describe the hypertensive disorders of pregnancy in the past, some people may still use the term.

The following list of definitions will help you understand high blood pressure during pregnancy:[34]

Pregnancy-Induced Hypertension (PIH) or Transient Hypertension refers to high blood pressure caused by pregnancy. PIH may also be called gestational hypertension. Women with PIH usually have no symptoms, and their blood pressure generally goes back to normal after delivery. They are at risk of developing PIH again in subsequent pregnancies and may also develop chronic hypertension later in life.

Pre-eclampsia refers to several complications, including high blood pressure, protein in the urine, and oedema (excessive fluid retention). Kidney and liver damage can occur if untreated.

Eclampsia is a potentially fatal condition in which the mother can go into convulsions or a coma.

Chronic Hypertension is high blood pressure that existed before pregnancy, or that is diagnosed before the twentieth week of pregnancy.

If pre-eclampsia were superimposed upon chronic hypertension, the woman would have high blood pressure and the pre-eclampsia symptoms (protein in the urine and oedema).

What Happens to Blood Pressure during Pregnancy

Blood pressure usually drops during the first half of pregnancy and then rises to normal levels. Women with mild hypertension may also experience that drop and may have normal blood pressure until mid-pregnancy. Not until the third trimester does blood pressure increase to the point where some type of treatment (such as bed rest or medication) may be necessary. Once blood pressure increases, it may not drop back to normal levels until after delivery.

Though the causes of PIH are not fully understood, poor nutritional status is one risk factor. PIH appears to occur at a higher rate among women with poor nutritional intake and no prenatal care.

Your overall food intake, including adequate calories, protein, and certain minerals, appears to be important in preventing high blood pressure. If you don't have enough energy or calories from carbohydrate or fat in your diet, your body will use dietary or tissue protein for energy. This can reduce protein available for tissue growth and can also limit the protein used in fluid balance.

Underweight women who fail to gain weight properly have a higher risk of developing PIH.

You are more likely to develop hypertension during pregnancy if you fall into one or more of these categories:[35]

• You are pregnant for the first time.
• You are expecting multiple foetuses.
• You are diabetic.
• You have kidney disease.
• You were overweight before your pregnancy.
• Your mother had pre-eclampsia.

The information below applies both to women with PIH and to those with chronic hypertension.

Risk to Mother

The biggest danger of high blood pressure during pregnancy is pre-eclampsia. Restricted activity and bedrest are two treatments to control your blood pressure and ensure that adequate blood and nutrients circulate to your baby.

Risks to Baby

Even if you have no symptoms, high blood pressure can reduce blood flow – and thus oxygen and nutrient flow – to your baby. Your baby may not grow properly and may have intra-uterine growth retardation (IUGR). Your physician will probably monitor your baby's heart rate and growth with ultrasound tests. Women with hypertension are also more likely to have a miscarriage or stillbirth. If your blood pressure cannot be controlled, your baby may be delivered prematurely.

What You Can Do

If You Have Chronic High Blood Pressure before Pregnancy:

▶ **See your doctor before you become pregnant.**

Establish good blood pressure control and a base-line reading of your blood pressure.

▶ **Lose weight and start a regular exercise programme before pregnancy.**

Both can help reduce your blood pressure.

▶ **When you become pregnant, see your doctor as soon as possible to start your prenatal care.**

Be sure to keep your appointments with your health-care provider so that you and your baby can be monitored.

If You Are Diagnosed with High Blood Pressure during Pregnancy:

▶ **Get plenty of rest – at least eight hours of sleep per night.**

Also, try to lie down for a few hours during the day on your left side to increase blood flow to your baby. When sitting, elevate your legs above your hips to improve circulation.

▶ **Monitor your blood pressure.**

You may go to your doctor's surgery or antenatal clinic for a blood pressure check or you may check it at home. Keeping track of your blood pressure will give you and your doctor a better idea of your average blood pressure over time.

▶ **Be aware of your sodium intake.**

Because your need for sodium increases during pregnancy, restricting sodium in your diet is not necessary. However, women who are salt-sensitive before pregnancy and follow a sodium-restricted diet may want to continue to watch their sodium during pregnancy. Ask your doctor about your specific sodium needs. Foods with excess sodium include pickles; tinned soups; smoked and cured meats such as bacon, sausage, and ham; and many frozen and ready-to-eat foods. Sodium information can be found on nutrition labels.

▶ **Eat plenty of calcium-rich foods.**

Research has shown that calcium plays a role in reducing blood pressure and may also reduce the risk of pre-eclampsia and premature birth.[36] Though the evidence isn't conclusive enough to recommend supplementary calcium over the Dietary Reference Intake (DRI), getting plenty of calcium through your diet can only help! Try to have at least four servings of calcium-rich foods every day. If you are lactose intolerant or allergic to milk, a calcium supplement from your doctor may be warranted. If you simply don't like dairy products, see page 66 for tips on sneaking calcium into your diet.

▶ **Eat balanced, healthy meals.**

Follow the Eating Expectantly Eating Plan! (See page 53.)

▶ **Watch your activity level.**

Because you will need to restrict your activity or may be on bed rest, you'll need super-speedy meals. (See page 309 for 'Meals in Minutes' and page 136 for eating tips for women on bed rest.)

▶ **Avoid caffeine, alcohol, and cigarettes; these substances can increase blood pressure.**

▶ **Keep your stress level low.**

Cut down on commitments and chores. If you're a type A person, learn to slow down! One study has shown that women in high-stress jobs during the first twenty weeks of pregnancy were more likely to have pre-eclampsia than women in low-stress jobs.[37]

▶ **Continue drinking plenty of fluids, even if you are retaining fluid.**

▶ **Avoid prolonged vigorous exercise, including lifting.**

This is especially important for women with children at home. Instead of picking up your children, squat to their level. Don't bend over with straight knees! Your physician will give you more specific exercise guidelines.

What Can You Expect?

If you have high blood pressure during pregnancy, you may be asked to restrict your activity, be on bed rest, or be hospitalized. Rest has been shown to reduce premature labour, lower blood pressure, and help the body get rid of excess water.[38]

Even if you aren't given special instructions for rest, you should set aside time every day to be off your feet. Making rest a priority on your own may prevent imposed restrictions and medications from your doctor. (See page 135 for 'Coping With Bed Rest' if bed rest or hospitalization becomes necessary.)

Elevated blood pressure and pre-eclampsia may warrant an early delivery of your baby, preferably induced vaginal delivery. However, in cases where a speedy delivery is necessary, a C-section may be done.

In some cases, even bed rest or restricted activity may not adequately control blood pressure. If this happens to you, you may need to be hospitalized, put on medication, or deliver prematurely. For women who have chronic high blood pressure before pregnancy, hospitalization is not uncommon.

Rest during Pregnancy

Tell the typical woman to rest, and she'll say, 'Oh, okay,' and take a fifteen-minute catnap then go back to her very busy lifestyle. Most people don't realize how vital rest is for pregnant women with high blood pressure.

Kathy said her doctor told her to rest, and she did lay down for a rest 'every so often'. She didn't realize exactly what the doctor meant. Eventually she was put on strict bedrest. When she went into labour, her blood pressure became very elevated and she had to have an emergency C-section. She wished that someone had explained what 'rest' really meant!

If you're told to rest, this is what you should do:

▶ **Rest one to two hours off your feet in both the morning and the afternoon every day. Ask your doctor for specifics.**

▶ **With your supervisor, arrange a rest period at work or a reduced work schedule.**

▶ **Enlist older children to help with household duties. You may also need some extra help with child care.**

▶ **Avoid stressful situations that could further increase your blood pressure.**

? Questions You May Have

Q: How will I know if I am developing pre-eclampsia?

A: These are specific signs and symptoms of pre-eclampsia:

• Swelling of hands, face, feet, and legs. Some water retention during the last months of pregnancy is normal. However, if the swelling moves to the upper part of your body, it may be a sign of pre-eclampsia.

• Sudden increased weight gain. If weight gain is not explained by increased food or fluid intake and occurs over a short period of time, this may also be a symptom. If you gain several kilograms or pounds over a few days or in less than a week, check with your doctor.

• Persistent, violent headache. If you have a severe headache that just won't go away, contact your physician immediately. This may be a warning sign of a convulsion.

- Visual difficulty. Blurred vision or partial-to-complete blindness are signs of pre-eclampsia. Again, seek medical attention immediately.
- Stomach pain. This can also be a sign of pre-eclampsia.[39]

Q: Will I still have high blood pressure after delivery?

A: Probably not immediately after delivery, unless you have chronic hypertension. Women who have pregnancy-induced hypertension are very likely to have high blood pressure later in life. You might reduce your risk of hypertension by going back to your ideal body weight after pregnancy, exercising regularly, and eating a nutritious diet containing adequate high-calcium foods. (See page 173 for more information on losing weight after delivery.)

Women with pre-eclampsia have about the same risk of developing hypertension later in life as those who never had the disease.[40]

Q: What about my next pregnancy?

A: If you have PIH, you have about an 80-per cent chance of developing it again in later pregnancies. If you have pre-eclampsia along with chronic hypertension, your risk of having the same problem with other pregnancies can be as high as 70 per cent.[41]

On the bright side: If you do have the same problem with your next pregnancy, you will be a pro at handling it! You will know how to truly rest, how to monitor your blood pressure, and what to expect during your pregnancy.

For more information on coping with chronic disease during pregnancy, I recommend an excellent book titled *Intensive Caring* by Diane Hales and Timothy Johnson, M.D., Crown Books.

▼

Multiple Births

One way to have an instant family is to deliver twins, triplets, or more! In the United States and other countries that have increased the use of fertility treatments, carrying multiple foetuses is much more common than it used to be. In 1996, one in thirty-eight U.S. births produced twins, and in 1997 that rate rose to one in thirty-three. In 1996, 1 in 795 U.S. births produced triplets. Between 1995 and 1996, quadruplet births rose 53 per cent, and pregnancies with five or more foetuses rose 42 per cent.[42] The likelihood of having a multiple birth rises with age; a woman who is between thirty-five and forty is three times more likely to have fraternal twins than a woman who is twenty to twenty-five years old.

What Can You Expect?

Before we discuss the potential problems of carrying multiple foetuses, we need to make an important point: You have more control over your pregnancy and the health of your babies than you may think. Some of the small daily choices you make – like eating the right foods, resting when your body tells you to, and following the advice of your

More Statistics on Multiples	
Twins	Average gestation is 37 weeks. Average birth weight is between 2.25 and 2.6 kilograms (5 pounds and 5 pounds, 11 ounces). 50% of twins are preterm, and 50% are low-birth-weight.
Triplets	Average gestation is 33 to 34 weeks. Average birth weight is 1.75 kilograms (3.9 pounds). 75% of triplets are preterm, and 90% are low-birth-weight. Average hospital stay is 29 days.
Quadruplets	Average gestation is 30 weeks. Average birth weight is 1.7 kilograms (3 pounds, 12 ounces).

Sources: Brown, J. "Nutrition and Multifetal Pregnancy." Journal of the American Dietetic Association, 100, 3, March 2000. Luke, B. and T. Eberlein. *Expecting Twins, Triplets or Quads*. New York: HarperCollins, 1999.

doctor – can significantly affect your babies' well-being.

Multifoetal pregnancies are considered high-risk, and here's why: Newborn multiples tend to be preterm, low-birth-weight, and small for their gestational age. Multiple deliveries accounted for 3 per cent of U.S. births in 1997, but 21 per cent of all babies that were low-birth-weight.[43] Birth defects, respiratory distress syndrome, cerebral palsy, and other complications are more common among multiples. During a multifoetal pregnancy, a woman is more likely to have pre-eclampsia, iron-deficiency anaemia, hyperemesis gravidarum (persistent, excessive nausea and vomiting), placenta previa (abnormal placement of placenta), and kidney problems.[44] Many women carrying multiple foetuses are given tocolytic agents (medication to stop labour) and put on bedrest.

Does this mean that you will have the problems above? No. You may have some – or you may be lucky and have minimal problems. Many women at the University of Michigan Multiples Clinic in the US have beaten the odds. Two-thirds of the mothers at this clinic deliver at thirty-six weeks or later – compared with only two-fifths nationwide. Triplets born in this clinic's program weigh 35 per cent more than the national average birth weight for triplets. Two-thirds of the clinic's newborns weigh more than 2½ kilograms (5½ pounds), and one-fourth of the clinic's newborns weigh more than 3 kilograms (6½ pounds). That's double the average birth weight of multiples.

What do all these numbers mean? It bears repeating: Careful attention to your health while you're pregnant can significantly affect your babies' well-being.

What Factors Affect the Birth Weights of Multiples?

• Your pre-pregnancy weight and height (Shorter and lighter mothers are more prone to having smaller babies.)
• How much weight you gain
• The pattern of your weight gain (Weight gain in early pregnancy is important.)
• How long your pregnancy lasts (gestation)

- Your diet (Quality counts!)
- Whether the babies are identical or fraternal (Identical foetuses – produced from one egg that splits – generally weigh less.)
- Number of foetuses (The more there are, the less they will usually weigh.)
- Sex (Girls tend to be lighter.)

The Most Important Factor: Weight Gain

As with single-foetus pregnancies, the amount of weight gained during a multifoetal pregnancy is directly related to the babies' birth weight. And because multiples tend to be delivered early and tend to be smaller, weight gain during multifoetal pregnancy is even more important.

The Subcommittee on Nutritional Status and Weight Gain during Pregnancy in the US has concluded that a weight gain of 16 to 20 kilograms (35 to 44 pounds) produces the healthiest twins.[45] A study done in Washington state found a weight gain of about 20 kilograms (44 pounds) was associated with optimum outcome of pregnancies lasting at least thirty-seven weeks and babies weighing over 2.5 kilograms (5.5 pounds).[46]

The chart below outlines weight gain suggested by Dr. Barbara Luke at the University of Michigan Multiples Clinic.

The pattern of your weight gain also affects your risk of pre-term delivery and low birth weight. That is: Gaining weight consistently throughout pregnancy is related to a healthier outcome. And early weight gain has a great effect on birth weight, as was found in a large study of twins.[47]

Another twin study revealed that underweight women who gain at least 513 grams (1.13) pounds per week during the first twenty weeks of pregnancy and 811 grams (1.92 pounds) after twenty weeks of pregnancy were more likely to have twins that weighed at least 2.5 kilograms (5.5) pounds. Normal-weight women who gained 680 grams (1.5) pounds per week after twenty weeks were more likely to have babies that weighed at least 2.5 kilograms (5.5 pounds).[48]

The suggested pattern of weight gain above will help you make short-term, intermediate, and long-term weight-gain goals. You and your doctor will probably work out an individual plan for you. Remember to keep your eye on the prize: healthy babies!

Recommended Weight Gain Pattern for Multifoetal Pregnancy				
Type of Pregnancy	Weekly Goal before 24 Weeks g (lb)	Goal by 24 Weeks kg (lb)	Weekly Goal after 24 Weeks g (lb)	Total Goal kg (lb)	Average Gestation (weeks)
Twins	450 (1)	10.9 (24)	900 (2)	18–22.5 (40–50)	36
Triplets	680 (1.5)	16.3 (36)	1100 (2.5)	22.5–27 (50–60)	32
Quadruplets	900 (2)	22.7 (50)	1360 (3)	29.5–36 (65–80)	30

Source: Luke, Barbara, and Tamara Eberlein. *When You're Expecting Twins, Triplets, or Quads.* New York: HarperCollins, 1999.

Your Diet

Very little research has been done regarding exact nutrient needs of women pregnant with multiples. Calorie needs increase immensely, and the need for some vitamins and minerals increases, too – though no one is sure how much. One thing we do know is that nourishing foetuses takes a lot of good food. Following are some guidelines modified from the University of Michigan Multiples Clinic. Keep in mind that your doctor or dietitian may want to develop a more individualized plan for you.

The Need for Specific Nutrients

Calcium

Magnesium sulfate is a common tocolytic agent for multiple pregnancies. Although it is very effective in preventing pre-term labour, it alters calcium metabolism, causing large amounts of calcium to be lost in the urine.[49] For one women pregnant with triplets, a postpartum fracture was thought to be due to osteoporosis after bedrest and therapy with magnesium sulfate.[50] Because of magnesium sulfate's effect on calcium metabolism, additional calcium (dietary or supplemental) may be necessary for women on magnesium sulfate therapy.

Iron

Iron is needed in even greater amounts for multifoetal pregnancies because of the increase in blood volume. Iron is best absorbed from animal sources. See page 33 for iron-rich and zinc-rich foods. Liver is the best source of iron and is recommended in the University of Michigan program. However, liver contains large amounts of vitamin A, which can cause birth defects in early pregnancy, which is why you will not find it in any of the food lists in this book.

Eating for Multiples								
Type of Pregnancy	Total Calories	Dairy (servings)*	Meat, Fish, Poultry (servings)†	Eggs (servings)‡	Vegetables (servings)§	Fruits (servings)‖	Grains (servings)*	Fats (servings)**
Twins	3,500	8	10	2	4	7	10	6
Triplets	4,000	10	10	2	5	8	12	7
Quads	4,500	12	12	2	6	8	12	8

*Serving size: 250 ml (8 fl oz) milk or ice cream, 25 g (1 oz) hard cheese.
†Serving size: 25 g (1 oz). Concentrate on beef and pork, since these are highest in iron.
‡Serving size: 1 egg.
§Serving size: 110 g (4 oz) cooked or 225 g (8 oz) raw.
‖Serving size: 1 medium fresh fruit, 75 g (3 oz) raw, 150 g (5 oz) berries, 40 g (1½ oz) dried fruit, 175 ml (6 fl oz) juice.
*Serving size: 1 slice bread, 25 g (1 oz) cereal, pasta, or rice.
**Serving size: 1 teaspoon oil, margarine, or butter; 1 tbsp salad dressing or mayonnaise.

Source: Modified from *When You're Expecting Twins, Triplets, or Quads* by Dr. Barbara Luke and Tamara Eberlein. New York: HarperCollins, 1999.

Vitamin D

Vitamin D appears to be used in larger amounts during multifoetal pregnancies. Vitamin D is made in the skin with exposure to sunlight. Since a woman may not get any exposure to the sun during the last half of a multifoetal pregnancy, she needs to get adequate vitamin D from fortified foods (milk and some breakfast cereals) or a supplement.[51]

Essential Fatty Acids

Essential fats (discussed in detail in Chapter Two), are important for development of the nervous system (including the brain) and retina. This development occurs at the end of pregnancy and throughout the first two years of life. The amount of essential fatty acids in the bloodstreams of multiple foetuses is significantly less than in a single foetus. This indicates that women pregnant with multiples need to consume more essential fats – although the specific amount is not known.[52] See below for some good sources of essential fatty acids.

Good Sources of Omega-3 Fatty Acids

These fatty acids are particularly important for brain and retina development.

Animal Sources:
- Fatty fish, especially cold-water fish like salmon, mackerel, tuna, sardines, and lake trout
- Eggs
- Meat (Although meat is not high in essential fats, it has been shown to be a significant source when consumed in large amounts.)[53]

Plant Sources:
- Flaxseed oil and flaxseed
- Canola oil
- Soybean oil

Good sources of Omega-6 Fatty Acids
- Sunflower oil
- Safflower oil
- Corn oil

The best approach is to eat cold-water fish like salmon several times a week, cook with canola oil, and use margarines and salad dressings and that are made with canola or sunflower oil.

What about Supplements?

The US Institute of Medicine recommends a supplement containing the nutrients listed below. Most prenatal vitamins contain at least these amounts.

Iron:	30 milligrams
Zinc:	15 milligrams
Copper:	2 milligrams
Calcium:	250 milligrams
Vitamin B_6:	2 milligrams
Folate:	300 micrograms
Vitamin C:	50 milligrams
Vitamin D:	5 micrograms

Dr. Luke, however, teaches her clients how to get most of the nutrients above from food. With the exception of calcium, magnesium, and zinc, minerals show promise in reducing preterm birth.[54] Speak with your doctor about what supplement is best for you.

A Twin Success Story

At the Montreal Diet Dispensary, a special programme called the Higgins Nutrition Intervention Program was used to try to decrease some of the risks apparent in disadvantaged mothers of twins. The programme consisted of individualized risk assessment, determination of dietary needs, nutrition education based on clients' eating patterns, and regular follow-up. Women not able to afford the prescribed diet were given a supplement of milk and eggs.

The programme, which had previously proven successful with mothers expecting one baby, also produced positive results with mothers of twins. The twin infants of mothers who participated in the programme weighed almost 75 grams (3 ounces) more than the infants of non-participating mothers. The programme infants had a 25-per cent-lower rate of low birth weight and a 50-per cent-lower rate of very low birth weight. (Babies with very low birth weight are usually the sickest babies, who require intensive care.) Also, the preterm delivery rate was 30 per cent less. This intervention program included eating 1,000 extra calories and 50 extra grams of protein above non-pregnant needs after twenty weeks. Women who were underweight before pregnancy and those with special risk conditions, such as a poor outcome of a prior pregnancy, received additional instructions.[55]

What Can the Higgins Program Do for You?

One researcher has found that women who had multiple gestations ate about the same amount as those pregnant with just one foetus.[56] That means you probably need to take a close look at what you're eating. Better yet, seek the services of a registered dietitian, who can give you individualized dietary advice. Increased calories and protein seem to be a significant factor in preventing low birth weight and prematurity in certain groups of women.

To achieve the 16- to 20.25-kg (35- to 45-pound) weight gain, you will need to gain about 675 g (1½ pounds) per week during the second and third trimesters. This may require an additional 500 to 600 calories per day more than your pre-pregnant diet. Based on the Higgins research, you could need up to 1,000 extra calories per day.

How Can I Possibly Eat More Food?

While some women enjoy pigging out on healthy foods (plus a few splurges), others have trouble getting all that extra food down. What to do?

First, make sure your diet has all the essentials—especially protein, fruits, and vegetables. (See page 53, 'The Eating Expectantly Eating Plan'.) Then add extra foods to boost your calorie intake. The foods most concentrated in calories are fat and sugar — the usual no-nos. However, to get all the calories you need with what seems to be an ever-shrinking stomach, you must give yourself permission to eat no-nos.

The easiest extra to add is fat. Concentrate on adding vegetable fat. You may need to eat as much as 40 per cent of your calories as fat to gain enough weight. Put nuts, olives, and avocado in your salads and sandwiches. Eat guacamole! Add butter to your vegetables, more salad dressing to your salads, extra oil when cooking, and so on. Eat more salmon; it is high in fat, and the fat is important for your babies' brain and eye development. Another way to add more calories to your diet is by eating high-sugar foods. By that I don't mean you should drink a soft drink and eat a chocolate bar every day! Instead, turn to the category of foods I call the 'good extras', which includes milk shakes, puddings, peanut-butter cookies, and other foods that are high-calorie but will also provide nutritional basics. (See page 247 for high-energy snack choices.)

Six Ways to Feed Multiples

1. *Eat your way through the day.* Eat three meals and three to four snacks per day. Balanced meals and mini-meals that contain protein are best.

2. *Say good-bye to guilt!* Gaining weight is critical for the health of your babies – and that means eating much larger quantities of food (and fat) than you may be used to. Milk shake, anyone?

3. *Where's the beef?* Hopefully in your fridge and freezer. Dr. Luke recommends eating red meat twice a day for the iron. Boost iron absorption more by cooking with an iron or aluminum pan and eating a vitamin-C-rich food with each meal. Also, avoid drinking coffee and tea within an hour of a meal.

4. *Drink, drink, drink!* Dehydration can bring on preterm labour, so drink often. Eight 475-ml (16-ounce) glasses of water per day is recommended.

5. *Get in the slow lane.* Since it's important to slow down to allow your body to nurture your babies, you may need to let some things go, such as cooking. Use the quick and easy menus on page 234. Encourage your partner to go crazy in the kitchen. Let your good-hearted friends fill your freezer with ready-to-eat meals. Treat yourself to gourmet takeout or restaurant delivery. (Remember that you may need to fill in some fruits and veggies.)

6. *Drink your snacks from a tin.* Some women find nutritional supplements to be lifesavers. Often given to people in the hospital who need extra nutrition, these drinks contain balanced nutrition with added vitamins and minerals – plus they have lots of calories. They come in different flavours and are often good over ice or blended with ice cream and fruit.

Resources for Parents of Multiples

Book
Cooper, Dr Carol. *Twins and Multiple Births.* Vermilion, 1999.

Organisations
Twins and Multiple Birth Association (TAMBA), PO Box 30, Little Sutton, South Wirral L66 1TH
Tel: 0151 348 0020

On-line Resources

The American Dietetic Association
www.eatright.org

MOST (Mothers of Super Twins)
www.mostonline.org

National Organization of Mothers of Twins
Clubs
www.nomotc.org

The Center for Study of Multiple Birth
www.multiplebirth.com

The Triplet Connection
www.tripletconnection.org

Twins Magazine On-line
www.twinsmagazine.com

About.com
www.multiples.about.com/parenting/
multiples/

▼

Coping with Bed Rest

We all dream of having just one day in bed to sleep, watch TV, or catch up on our reading. But spending several weeks in bed may seem more like a nightmare.

Bed rest is prescribed for multiple reasons, including hypertension or pre-eclampsia, multiple gestation (twins or more), premature labour, or poor growth of baby (also called intra-uterine growth retardation, or IUGR). Some women are put on bed rest for several months, which can really give a person cabin fever.

Following is a guide to help you make the most of your rest period. This information was developed by talking to others and also from personal experience. I was on bed rest for eleven weeks for preterm labour. It was all worth it in the end. My son Robert was born healthy and weighed 3.37 kilograms (7 pounds, 7 ounces). My labour even had to be helped along a little!

At first, the days seemed to go on forever. But once I got into a routine and my doctor gave me the okay to get up a little more, time became much more bearable. I wrote most of the following information before I was on bed rest, so I was able to follow my own advice. And it worked! I hope it helps you, too.

Welcome to Club Bed

Setting Up the Room

You will probably want to set up a makeshift bedroom near the place where your family gathers. A family room off the kitchen works nicely. Here are the basic living supplies with which you'll want to furnish your new room:

- Bed with plenty of pillows (Or rent a hospital bed.)
- Phone that will reach to the bed or a portable phone (Think of it as your link to the outside world, and don't forget the phone book.)
- Fridge or mini-fridge for your bedside
- Microwave (depending how strict your bed rest is)
- Large bedside table or a hospital-type table that can be raised or lowered to your level (This can be rented from a

medical supply company. Several TV trays work well, too.)
- Any medicines you are taking, including those taken occasionally for heartburn, constipation, and so on
- Large jug, filled with fresh water daily, and an ice bucket
- Soup tins for doing arm exercises (if your doctor approves)
- An intercom system (Invest early in one for the baby; it will save your voice and save your family lots of trips back and forth fetching for you.)

Eating and Dietary Considerations

Yes, eating is a whole new challenge when you spend all your time on a mattress or couch! Keep in mind that you will need fewer calories than usual since you'll be using very little energy for activity. (If you are taking medication to stop your contractions, it may increase your metabolism, and you may need to eat about the same as you did before.) A potential problem is that the lack of activity may increase blood sugar and lead to gestational diabetes. To help control your risk, avoid concentrated sweets and fruit juices. (See page 110 for more about gestational diabetes, and if your appetite isn't good see page 133, 'How Can I Possibly Eat More Food?' for tips on adding calories. Following is a guide to bedroom cuisine:

▶ **Make shopping lists and menus so your family or friends can shop for you.**

▶ **Keep snacks next to you:**
- A fruit bowl filled with fresh and dried fruit such as apples, figs, and prunes
- A jar of peanut butter
- Individually wrapped cheeses
- Wheat and rye bicuits, digestive biscuits, rice cakes, baked tortilla chips
- Raw veggie sticks in a plastic container with ice
- Cheese food that doesn't need refrigeration
- Nuts

Note: Beware – convenience foods that need no refrigeration are often high in fat and salt. Eat sparingly!

▶ **If possible, keep a microwave next to you.**

If you have a microwave nearby, you'll also want:
- Low-fat popcorn
- Decaffeinated tea, decaffeinated instant coffee, hot-chocolate mix, and mugs
- Tins of hearty single-serving soups such as split pea, chunky chicken-vegetable, and beans with ham

▶ **If you are allowed to get up briefly to make a meal, the following can be prepared in six to seven minutes from scratch or with leftovers:**
- Scrambled eggs on toast
- Frozen microwave dinners (See page 230 for healthy choices.)
- Vegetarian beans, corn tortilla toasted in oven, cheese, lettuce, and tomato
- Salad with prepared lettuce in the bag – you just add the tomato, cheese, ham, turkey, and veggies
- Bean soups in a cup
- Chicken salad with pineapple

- Chicken fajitas or burritos
- Chicken curry over bulgur
- Chicken taco
- Chicken-English-muffin melt
- Chicken sandwich
- Pasta with tomato sauce (bottled)
- Pasta salad with tuna
- Pasta primavera
- Turkey tetrazzini
- Quick tuna casserole
- Chinese takeaway or delivery
- Pizza delivery (also delivered sandwiches, pastas, and so on)

Bed rest joke: The best and worst thing about bed rest: You aren't the cook and you aren't the cook! (From *Sidelines* newsletter, Winter 1992.)

Entertainment to Keep Handy

You may have to be creative with this!

- Radio or stereo
- TV and VCR with remote control (Be sure you have a *TV Guide*.)
- Mini-library set up with magazines, books, stationery, and photo albums
- Diary to keep track of your days
- Calendar
- Computer with which to play games, keep track of finances, and write letters (You can also borrow your kid's Nintendo or Game Boy!)
- Large notebook for making all kinds of lists – things to do, things for others to do, things to buy, things to make, bills to pay, what's on sale where, and so on
- Word games
- Crafts such as cross-stitch, embroidery, knitting, and so on

- Books on tape for when you get tired of reading

Eleven Activities to Keep Your Mind Alive

1. *Volunteer by phone.* Have you always wanted to volunteer, but never had the time? Here's your chance. You could do fundraising or check on elderly people unable to go out. Or you could create your own network of bed-bound mothers. Check the local paper or the Red Cross for volunteer opportunities.

2. *Enhance your skills.* Take a correspondence course. Learn a new computer programme.

3. *Increase your vocabulary.* Several good books are available, such as *30 Days to a More Powerful Vocabulary.* Crossword puzzles and other word games can also help. Keep a dictionary nearby.

4. *Learn a language. Parlez vous Français?* Many language courses are available by mail. Your new language could be the start of a dream trip to Monte Carlo or Madrid.

5. *Interact on-line.* If you have a computer with Internet access next to you, you'll have the world at your fingertips. You can:

- Read the news.
- Invest on-line and track investments.
- Bank and pay bills on-line.
- Chat on-line.
- Play interactive games on-line with people from around the world at:
  www.altavista.com
  www.yahoo.com
  www.aol.com
  www.thehouseofcards.com

- Shop! Most Internet service providers have many links to on-line shopping. This may be particularly useful for buying groceries or baby clothes, furniture, and other supplies

6. *Learn to cook, craft, or decorate.* Check out shows on television.

7. *Have a makeover.* You may not feel like putting on makeup, but just for a change, you might have someone come over and give you a new look.

8. *Become a financial wizard.* Plan your retirement. Send for information on all those great-sounding mutual funds. Keep up with the stock market. Plan how you'll pay for your baby's university tuition.

9. *Make a quilt, afghan, or rug.* You can order kits by mail.

10. *Start your Christmas shopping, even if it's March.* Use your TV, computer, or catalogues or start making the presents by hand.

11. *Create new recipes.* No kidding! I met a soldier who was in a national cooking contest. It turns out he developed his recipe while he was stationed in Saudi Arabia during Operation Desert Storm. I was wondering how he ever found access to a kitchen or found time to cook. He thought about cooking and wrote down all his ideas for ingredients. When he got back home, he experimented with a few and sent them to the contest.

Exercise and Activity

Your activity level is a very individual matter that should be discussed with your doctor. However, you should ask about doing isometric exercises and/or arm exercises using light weights or 350-gram (12-ounce) tins. Such exercises will help you keep some muscle tone and help you avoid feeling sore from lack of movement. Remember that you can always practise your pelvic floor exercises!

Also ask about turning from side to side often during the day. This will help prevent soreness in muscles and skin.

Other Survival Tips

▶ **Make a schedule of what you'll do during the day.**

This will make the day seem shorter and less monotonous.

▶ **Enlist others' help. If you have children, make a poster of chores for them to do.**

This may be a good time for your children to learn to do the laundry, dishes, and even cooking – depending on their ages. If you don't have children, you'll need to depend on your partner, family (if they live close by), or friends. Although asking others to do things for you will be tough, make a list of all the little things that need doing and delegate them to different people. Hire a helper if necessary.

▶ **Remember it's okay to let the housework go. (In your case, it's a must!)**

You have only one priority: for your little one to grow as much as possible for as long as possible. Whether the floor is mopped or the carpet is vacuumed really isn't important. Investigate getting household help from an agency. A home-care assistant can take care of your children, cook, clean, run errands, and so forth.

▶ **Think positive.**

You might want to invest in a 'positive thought for the day' type of book. Though the time in bed might be rough, having a premature or sick baby would be much worse. Make the most of your time.

▶ **Find other women in the same boat.**

Ask your doctor for names of other women in his or her practice who are on bed rest. When I was on bed rest, Norma, a friend of mine who had been on bed rest, called regularly for support. Get the word out among friends and co-workers or at your place of worship, and folks who have been where you are will likely step forward with a comforting word or a helping hand. You can also call your local antenatal clinic and see if anyone else is on bedrest.

▶ **You would be surprised at the number of services that will come to your home!**

I had a massage therapist visit my home weekly because I had a lot of soreness from lying around. I think it improved my circulation and I know it pampered me. You can also find someone who will cut your hair in your home, a pedicurist or chiropodist who will come and attend to your feet and nails, a beautician who can give you a facial and

so forth. Though these are really splurges, it's little things like these that can help you make it through the tough times.

▼

Older Mothers

In the past, most women started their families in their early twenties. Now many women are waiting until they are over thirty-five or into their forties. Waiting to start a family can have both advantages and disadvantages. Some women find that thirty-something is the perfect time for them. They are financially stable, have spent time developing a career, and are ready to start on the 'mother track'. On the other hand, they may be more set in their ways and may be less physically ready for pregnancy and motherhood.

Barbara never really thought about having children until she was thirty-five years old. Then her biological clock started ticking loudly and suddenly Barbara wanted to join the ranks of mothers. She had heard that older mothers-to-be had a few more risks compared to their younger counterparts, so she visited her doctor, who assured her she was in great physical shape. She worked out five times a week, didn't smoke, had no chronic diseases, and had already cut out caffeine. She did, however, skip meals and often ate on the run.

Her doctor explained that she was on the right track in improving her lifestyle, but that she should work on her diet. He told her that slight nutrient deficits could affect fertility. She then consulted a registered dietitian who, after looking at a three-day food diary, made some suggestions about how Barbara could improve her diet.

The dietitian suggested Barbara continue taking her mulitvitamins (which contained folic acid) and advised her to add supplements of nutrients that were missing in her diet.

Barbara worked a few months to improve her diet and became pregnant eight months later. She delivered a healthy baby boy weighing 3.4 kilograms (7½ pounds)! She was so thrilled with motherhood that she became pregnant again when her son Brian was eighteen months old.

Stories like Barbara's are becoming common as more women are putting off having a family until their late 30s or even 40s. But this approach does have its risks, so if you are over thirty-five, it's important to be in the best physical condition possible before you become pregnant.

What Can You Expect?

A large study from Sweden showed that women thirty-five or older are more likely to deliver prematurely, have a baby with low or very low birth weight, and have a baby small for gestational age. Women forty or older were also at increased risk for these complications.[57] However, negative outcomes were more likely with first births than with second births.[58] So you can improve your chances of having a healthy baby if you have your first child before age thirty-five, even if you have more children when you are older. Most of the complications associated with older mothers are due to increased rates of fibroid tumours (leiomy-

omas), hypertension, and diabetes in women as they get older.[59]

The likelihood of a caesarean section increases with age and with increasing pre-pregnancy body mass index (BMI).[60] One reason is that older first-time mothers — especially those over forty — may have a long history of infertility; both patients and physicians may be anxious to avoid a poor outcome and thus may be more likely to resort to caesarean delivery.[61] Older pregnant women also have a higher risk of delivering a baby with Down's syndrome and other types of autosomal trisomy (defects caused by an extra chromosome).[62]

Although there is greater risk for pregnancy complications in women over thirty-five, overall outcome can be good.[63]

What You Can Do

The most important thing you can do to reduce your risk of diabetes, C-section, and other complications is to achieve a body weight as close to your ideal weight as possible before you get pregnant. You should be practising a healthy lifestyle by exercising regularly and eating a well-balanced diet. Start your prenatal care as soon as possible and follow your health-care provider's advice about exercising while you are pregnant.

▼

Teen Pregnancy

Teen pregnancy rates have been dropping since 1992. However, the birth rate for fifteen-to-seventeen-year-olds is similar to the birth rate for women ages thirty-five to thirty-nine.[64] Teen pregnancy is not only psychologically stressful for the teen and her parents, but it is also physically stressful to the teen because she is often still growing. There is some evidence that in pregnant girls who are still growing, the mother and baby may compete for nutrients.[65] Also, teens who are still growing are more likely to have excessive weight gain and deposit more body fat, which may put them at greater risk of being overweight and of developing type II diabetes, cardiovascular disease, and hypertension later in life.[66]

One thing is certain: Teens are not known for having healthy eating habits. A nationwide survey showed that among teens aged twelve to nineteen, only 22 per cent ate the recommended two daily servings of dairy, only 19 per cent ate the recommended two daily servings of fruit, and only 32 per cent ate the recommended 150 to 200 grams (5 to 7 ounces) of protein foods each day.[67] Nearly one-fourth of the vegetables eaten by adolescents are French fries.[68] Adolescent girls consume the largest amount of added sweeteners as a percentage of total calories of any age group; one-third comes from soft drinks.[69]

Adolescent girls also tend to practise unsafe weight-loss methods. One study indicated that many white female secondary school students who smoke report using smoking to control their appetite and weight. A national survey of fifth and sixth form students found that 32 per cent skipped meals, 22 per cent fasted, 7 per cent used diet pills, 5 per cent induced vomiting after meals, and 3 per cent used laxatives to lose weight.[70]

Clearly, many teens may start their pregnancies malnourished.

What Can You Expect?

Infants of teens are twice as likely to have low birth weight and are five times more likely to die in the first twenty-eight days after birth than infants of adults. Among infants born to teens sixteen or younger, 14 per cent are born prematurely (before thirty-seven weeks gestation).[71] However, you can give birth to a healthy, normal baby; it all depends on you. By eating the right foods, gaining enough weight, taking a prenatal vitamin, practising good health habits, and visiting your doctor regularly, you can have the healthiest baby possible.

What You Can Do

Get help. You may be facing problems that you can't solve by yourself. There are many people you and your parents can turn to for help. Your school counsellor or nurse or doctor will give you some guidance. Your minister or a close family friend may be able to give you advice. The local antenatal clinic provides free medical care. Remember that having social support can mean a healthier baby. A study in Mexico City showed that pregnant teens who received psychological support from the twentieth week (supposedly reducing anxiety levels) gained significantly more weight than pregnant teens who received no support.[72]

Gain enough weight. Weight gain is one of the best predictors of a healthy baby. The suggested weight gain is 11.5 to 18 kilograms

(25 to 40 pounds); most teens should gain toward the upper end of the recommendation. If you were underweight before pregnancy or are still growing, adequate weight gain is even more important to ensure that you have a healthy baby. It is also critical to gain weight from the very beginning of pregnancy and gain weight consistently throughout pregnancy.[73] Talk about your weight gain goal with your doctor.

See your doctor regularly. Getting adequate prenatal care is associated with having a healthier baby. The Toronto Healthiest Babies Possible Program showed that nine to eleven visits with a doctor throughout pregnancy helped prevent low-birth-weight babies.[74]

Cut back on sweets. High-sugar foods are often zero-nutrient foods and often take the place of healthier foods. One study in New Jersey has shown that pregnant teens with high-sugar diets have a greater risk of having a baby that is small for its gestational age.[75]

Take a prenatal vitamin supplement (or at least a multivitamin supplement containing 400 micrograms of folic acid) as soon as you think you are pregnant. If you eat one serving or less of dairy products (milk, yogurt, cheese) per day, take a calcium supplement containing 600 milligrams of calcium. Tums is an inexpensive choice.

Get ready to eat right. Take the food quiz on page 62. Add up the totals and compare to the Eating Expectantly for Teens Plan opposite.

Follow the Eating Expectantly for Teens Plan. Make sure not to skip meals and try to eat three snacks every day. Try to make every bite count – for your baby's sake!

Eating Expectantly for Teens Plan

10 or more servings of grains
1 serving is 1 slice any type bread; ½ small bagel, pitta bread or English muffin; 1 150-g (6-inch) tortilla; 8 tbsp cooked rice or pasta; 8 tbsp cooked cereal, barley, bulgur; 25 g (1 oz) ready-to-eat cereal; 3 to 4 savoury biscuits; or 2 biscuits.

Note: 3 or more servings per day should be wholegrain.

5 or more servings of calcium-rich foods
1 serving is 250 ml (8 fl oz) any type milk or yogurt, 40 g (1½ oz) cheese, 50 g (2 oz) processed cheese, or 250 ml (8 fl oz) calcium-fortified orange juice or soya milk.

4 or more servings of fruit
1 serving is 1 medium fresh fruit; ½ grapefruit, mango, or papaya; 8 tbsp tinned or chopped fruit; 4 tbsp dried fruit; or 200 ml (6½ fl oz) juice.

4 or more servings of vegetables
1 serving is 8 tbsp cooked vegetables, 250 ml (8 fl oz) leafy vegetables, 1 small potato, or 200 ml (6½ fl oz) tomato or vegetable juice.

Note: Be sure to include at least one fruit or vegetable that is high in vitamin C and one that is dark green or orange every day.

3 servings of protein foods
1 serving is 50 to 75 g (2 to 3 oz) cooked lean meat (the size of a deck of cards);

2 eggs; 8 tbsp tuna; 8 tbsp legumes, tofu, or textured vegetable protein; or 2 tablespoons nuts or nut butter.

Note: Eat a variety of protein foods, including fish at least once a week. Eat an additional ½ protein serving for each 250 ml (8 fl oz) of milk that you don't drink.

Fats and sweets: Eat sparingly.

If you are having trouble gaining weight, you may need to increase your fat intake. If you are gaining too much weight, you may need to decrease your fat intake. See page 25 for more advice.

Six Ways to Eat Right

1. *Eat three meals and three snacks each day.* This can help you gain just the right amount of weight, while avoiding nausea and heartburn.

2. *If you eat fast food, have a salad and milk (or a milk shake) with it.* Drink water or fruit juice instead of soft drinks. (See page 239 for choosing nutritional fast-foods.) If your diet contains a lot of fast food, make sure to snack on fruits and vegetables between meals.

3. *If you have trouble gaining weight, eat filling snacks.* These include nuts, peanut butter, boiled eggs, cheese, milk shakes, nachos, and guacamole.

4. *If you can't drink milk, try to eat more yogurt and cheese.* Since your bones may still be growing, calcium is very important. (See page 66 for 'Twelve Ways to Sneak Calcium into Your Diet.')

5. *Snack on fruits and veggies.* Eat fresh or dried fruit, carrots and broccoli with ranch dip, or a sandwich instead of crisps, sweets, or soft drinks.

6. *Start the day with a good breakfast.* If you don't have time for breakfast, try these on-the-go meals:

Tortilla with cheese rolled inside
Bean burrito
Peanut butter, honey, and banana
  sandwich
Granola bar and yogurt
Leftover pizza

How Much Weight Should You Gain?

The US Subcommittee on Nutritional Status and Weight Gain During Pregnancy recommends that you gain 16 kg (35 pounds) if you are considered normal weight for your height. If you were underweight before pregnancy, you should gain about 18 kg (40 pounds). If you were overweight, you should aim for closer to 11.5 kg (25 pounds).[76] Though this may seem like a lot, remember that you have only one chance to make a healthy baby!

Almost as important as *how much* you gain is *when* the weight is gained. Teens who gained little weight in the first six months (less than 4.5 kg [10 pounds] by the twenty-fourth week) had a higher risk of having small babies, even if their weight gain caught up at the end of the pregnancy. Inadequate weight gain also seems to be a factor in preterm birth (birth of a baby before thirty-seven weeks gestation). Girls who gained less than 450 grams (a pound) a week at the end of the pregnancy had more premature deliveries.[77] In a study of pregnant teenagers across the United States, it was found that weight gain of 585 grams (1.3 pounds) per week from week fifteen until delivery resulted in babies that did not have low birth weights and were much less likely to need special care.[78]

The problem with 'premies' is that the babies usually aren't quite ready for our world yet. Their lungs may not be developed, and they can have many other problems. Premies are often kept in the special care unit or intensive care unit for infants and aren't able to go home for a while. This is no fun for a baby, who may have to be fed intravenously and have blood taken frequently. Intensive care could also be necessary.

Other Nutrient Needs

Calcium

All women need calcium in their diets. A low intake of calcium, especially before the age of thirty, increases your risk of osteoporosis (brittle bones). You've perhaps seen older women slumped over; their curved backs are probably due to osteoporosis. Or maybe you know a relative who fell and broke a hip. This is probably also due to the brittle-bone disease. How does that concern you now?

Your diet now actually affects how thick your bones will be when you become forty years old. The thicker and stronger your bones are, the lower your risk for osteoporosis.

Zinc

Zinc is an important nutrient needed for cell growth, cell division, and brain development. In a study of low-income pregnant teens, low dietary intake of zinc was related to a double risk of having a low-birth-weight baby and a threefold risk of very preterm delivery.[79] In women who had inadequate amounts of zinc in their blood, zinc supplementation increased birth weight and infant head circumference significantly. This underscores the importance of a prenatal supplement containing a balance of nutrients, as well as a diet with zinc-rich foods.[80] See page 33 for food sources of zinc.

Iron

Many pregnant teens start pregnancy with low iron stores. Iron deficiency in early gestation has been associated with a 200 to 300 percent increase in risk of prematurity and stillbirth. It is impossible to get all the iron you need from food; you must take an iron supplement or a multivitamin that contains adequate iron, like a prenatal vitamin. You can also boost your intake of iron-rich foods. See page 33 for more information.[81]

What you will find in this chapter:

- *My Experiences with Breastfeeding*
- *The Feeding Decision: It's Up to You*
- *Why You Should Consider Breastfeeding*
- *Possible Obstacles*
- *A Note to Dad*
- *Preparing for Breastfeeding*
- *Nutrition during Breastfeeding*
- *Nutrients of Special Concern*
- *Drugs and Breastfeeding*
- *Breastfeeding for Special Groups*
- *Tips for Formula Feeding*
- *About Bonding*

This chapter answers such questions as:

- *Who can answer my questions about breastfeeding?*
- *How will I know if I have enough milk for my baby?*
- *What if my husband isn't supportive of my decision to nurse?*
- *Can I drink coffee while breastfeeding? What about alcohol?*
- *Should I try to lose weight while nursing?*
- *What if my baby is premature – can I still nurse her?*
- *What about PCBs in breast milk?*

CHAPTER EIGHT

Considering Breastfeeding

My Experiences with Breastfeeding

When my first son, Nicolas, was born, I never wondered which feeding method I would use. In fact, this decision had been made long before I even met my husband! As a health professional who knew all the physical benefits of breastfeeding and had recommended breastfeeding to thousands of women, I had to breast-feed.

The pressure was on! The most difficult week of my life was that first week after Nicolas was born. I had a long labour and a difficult delivery. Nicolas and I didn't catch on to the fine art of breastfeeding right away. When Nicolas did not breast-feed for twenty-four hours, I felt guilty and gave permission for him to have a bottle. It was a big mistake!

Nicolas continued to receive bottles in the hospital. At home, our breast-feeding attempts failed again; during a feeding, he would latch on and pull away more times than I could count (or bear). As a last resort I called our paediatrician, who referred me to a lactation consultant. She was our saviour.

We had two problems, Nicolas and I. He had nipple confusion. (Sounds like the making of a good joke!) That explained his frequent latching on and pulling away. He had gotten used to a plastic nipple in the hospital, so he couldn't get the hang of mine. And I wasn't positioning him correctly. A week or two after seeing the lactation consultant, we started to learn how the special process of breastfeeding works.

If I hadn't known about the benefits of breastfeeding, recommended it to so many women, and been under financial pressure from quitting my job, I would surely have quit breastfeeding that first week. That's why I feel compassion for all the women who want to breast-feed and are having difficulties.

Looking back, I'm so glad I hung in there and nursed Nicolas. The time we spent together was wonderful. And Nicolas was never sick while I was nursing him. One of my most memorable nursing sessions took place at an outdoor jazz concert that my husband Frank, Nicolas, and I attended when Nicolas was three months old. I felt perfectly comfortable feeding him under the privacy of a blanket. Actually I felt proud, because we were enjoying our own little routine. I didn't feel embarrassed about breastfeeding in public, as I had at first, and I liked feeling self-sufficient: no packing up bottles, trying to keep them cold, or looking for a place to warm them.

When my second son, Robert, was born, we had a totally different experience. I nursed Robert very soon after delivery, and he caught on immediately! I made it clear that Robert was not to have any plastic nipples while in the nursery, so he never had nipple confusion. At home, Robert continued to eat very well. Because I felt like a pro, I was comfortable breast-feeding him anywhere – with or without a blanket. Breast-feeding was especially convenient when we travelled overseas to visit our relatives; we didn't have to worry about packing formula.

I would never trade the experiences of nursing my children – both were special. More and more studies are citing the benefits of breastfeeding, so I urge you to give it a try!

▼

The Feeding Decision: It's Up to You

You may have been pondering how you'll feed your baby since the day your pregnancy was confirmed. Or through personal observations, you may have made your decision long ago. In any case, try to ensure that your decision is based on what is best for your baby, you, and your family.

Breastfeeding undoubtedly offers the most benefits for baby and mother. However, whatever method you decide to use, make a decision *you* feel good about.

Keep in mind that you can both breast-feed and formula-feed. Many women find this combination convenient, especially if they are going back to work. Even if you breast-feed for a short time, your baby will still benefit. If you do decide to combine breast- and bottlefeeding, introduce the bottle only after breastfeeding is well established to avoid nipple confusion.

Since this is a nutrition book for mothers, this chapter will be primarily devoted to breastfeeding. However, if you decide to combine breastfeeding and formula feeding, I have listed some hints for formula feeding on page 167.

▼

Why You Should Consider Breastfeeding

Breastfeeding has been shown to greatly improve a newborn's short-term and long-term health. Following are just some of the benefits of breastfeeding.

Benefits to Baby

- Breast milk provides superior nutrition matched to your baby's needs. Colostrum, or first milk, is sometimes called 'first immunization' because it contains important antibodies. As a result, breast-fed babies have fewer allergies, less diarrhoea, a lower risk of serious bowel disorders, and fewer ear infections and respiratory illnesses.
- Research shows that essential fats found in breast milk (but not found in formula) are important to brain development. Studies show that breast-fed children have higher IQs than non-breast-fed children because of critical brain development during the time of breastfeeding. Breast-fed babies accumulate twice as much docosahexanenoic acid (DHA) in their brains as formula-fed babies.[1]
- Breast-fed babies have a lower risk of sudden infant death syndrome (SIDS).[2]
- Breast milk may exert lifelong protection against insulin-dependent diabetes, cancer (including breast cancer), Crohn's disease (a chronic inflammatory disease of the colon), allergic diseases, and other chronic digestive diseases.[3]
- Breastfeeding promotes good jaw and facial development.

Benefits to Mother

- Breastfeeding helps you and your baby get acquainted and develop a close relationship.
- Women who have breast-fed have a lower risk of premenopausal breast cancer and ovarian cancer and a reduced risk of hip fracture later in life due to improved bone-building in the postpartum period.[4] Breastfeeding may also be related to a small but long-lasting reduction in postmenopausal breast cancer risk.
- Breastfeeding uses many calories and helps mothers of newborns lose their 'baby fat'. Mother Nature designed women to gain a certain amount of fat during pregnancy to be used during breastfeeding.
- Breastfeeding helps your uterus return more quickly to its normal size and can also prevent haemorrhage if you breast-feed right after delivery.[5]
- The time you spend breast-feeding gives you a chance to recuperate, relax, and catch up on your reading. Life is fast-paced; perhaps breastfeeding was intended to slow us down to spend more time with our new little ones.
- Breastfeeding is convenient. You always have food for your baby with you, and it's always at the right temperature – no running to the store to buy formula, no

messy mixing, and no worrying about proper refrigeration.

Benefits to the Family

- Breastfeeding saves money. Formula costs for one year can add up! Who couldn't use a little extra cash?
- Breastfeeding may give your family a chance to have quiet time together. If you have other children, you can use some of your nursing sessions as a time to read stories to older children.
- Research indicates that breastfeeding might change genetic predisposition to chronic disease, so breastfeeding may improve the health of your family in generations to come!

Breastfeeding for the Nation

Breastfeeding also offers social and economic benefits for the nation, including reduced health-care costs and reduced absenteeism among employees. Because of these benefits, the US government has worked to increase breastfeeding through its 'Healthy People' objectives. This effort has helped; the number of mothers who breast-feed their infants in the early postpartum period increased from 52 per cent in 1990 to 62 per cent in 1997. The number of women breastfeeding their infants at six months increased from 18 per cent in 1990 to 26 per cent in 1997.[6]

Possible Obstacles

Women who want to breast-feed may encounter obstacles in the people around them. If you plan accordingly, you can remove such obstacles and enjoy a successful nursing experience.

Betty Crase, formerly with La Leche League International, has nursed three out of four of her children. She feels the biggest barrier to breastfeeding is society's attitude. 'Society is still prejudiced against breastfeeding,' she says. 'The breast is still viewed as a sex object instead of for nourishing babies. This attitude can deter a woman from breast-feeding. Women must feel comfortable breast-feeding wherever they are.'[7]

Following are some other barriers and some suggestions on how to overcome them:

Unsupportive Family and Friends

▶ **Point out the benefits of breastfeeding that would most interest the unsupportive person.**

For example, your partner might be interested in saving money or in learning about the scientifically proven benefits of breast-feeding. Be assertive in your beliefs.

▶ **Find friends or relatives who have breast-fed and are willing to help you bring your family around to your way of thinking.**

Knowing someone who can share your experience and offer support may also make learning to breast-feed easier.

▶ **Invite your partner, family member, or friend to go to a breast-feeding class or La Leche League meeting.**

Unsupportive Hospital Staff

Unsupportive hospital staff can be quite problematic for women who are still undecided about breastfeeding. If you have some doubt, and your nurse prefers that you bottle-feed, the battle may already be lost!

Supportive hospitals will have:

- Policies that are conducive to breastfeeding, such as rooming-in for the baby. Having your baby room-in with you helps you establish breastfeeding.
- A lactation specialist or consultant on staff who can visit you right after delivery to get you started. Lactation specialists are usually nurses who have extensive knowledge about breastfeeding; they have all the answers! Midwives or health visitors can make home visits to see how things are going. Check on this while you are pregnant.
- Classes about breastfeeding for expectant mums and families. These highly informative classes may sell your partner, friends, or family on breastfeeding as well as give you lots of answers.
- Breast pumps for rent. These 'industrial' pumps are very efficient and can usually empty both breasts in fifteen minutes.

This comes in very handy for women who work.

- A list of community breast-feeding support groups, such as La Leche League, that you can call on 0207 242 1278 when you have questions. La Leche League meetings are open to pregnant women, and you may learn quite a lot about nursing just by spending time with nursing women. The National Childbirth Trust is a similar organization that can be contacted on 0208 992 8637.

Having Enough Milk

Once a mother is breast-feeding her child, her biggest concern may be whether she is producing enough milk. You can make enough milk; it's a simple process of supply and demand. The more often you nurse your baby, the more milk your body makes. Here are some tips to help you make sure your baby is getting enough breast milk:[8]

▶ **Make sure you have positioned your baby properly: tummy to tummy.**

Your baby should be comfortable and should have a good grasp of your nipple to empty your milk glands. When your breasts are emptied, they'll make more milk to fill the demand.

▶ **Let your baby determine the length and frequency of feedings.**

You should nurse eight to twelve times in a twenty-four-hour period during the first week to help establish your milk supply.

▶ **Weigh your baby to ensure adequate weight gain after the first week.**

A breast-fed infant should gain 100 to 200 grams (4 to 7 ounces) per week or 450 grams (1 pound) per month.

▶ **Monitor wet nappies and bowel movements.**

These are physical signs that your baby is drinking enough milk. There should be six to eight wet nappies and three to five bowel movements per day in the early months.

▶ **Make a habit of drinking a glass of water or other beverage every time you breast-feed.**

Working While Breast-Feeding

Breastfeeding after going back to work is a great way to provide for your baby while you are away. And it's good for your company, too. Since breast milk protects against infection, women who breast-feed miss fewer days of work due to their babies' illnesses. Breastfeeding while working does take a bit of planning, though. Below are some tips. (See Chapter Nine for more advice on going back to work.)

▶ **Check out breast-feeding support at work while you are pregnant.**

Your supervisor or the personnel department are good places to start.

▶ **If your company has no lactation program, look into starting one.**

Corporate lactation programmes are becoming more popular as the business world realizes the benefits of breastfeeding. A lactation

programme usually includes a mother's room for pumping, an electric breast pump available for use, and attitudes supportive of breastfeeding. Medela, a pump manufacturer, offers tips on starting a lactation programme. For more information, visit Medela's website at www.medela.com.

▶ **Investigate flexi-hours or working part-time temporarily.**

▶ **Find a day-care provider close to your workplace.**

This will enable you to feed your baby during your lunch hour.

▶ **Rent an electric pump if your workplace doesn't provide one.**

Breast pumps can be rented or sometimes borrowed from hospitals. Consult with your midwife for advice.

▶ **Be sure to build up a good milk supply before you begin giving your baby breast milk from a bottle.**

You may want to get your baby used to taking a bottle a week or two before you return to work.

▶ **If your workplace doesn't have a refrigerator, bring a coolbag to work so you can store your milk safely.**

Seeking Help

An early visit by the health visitor is a real benefit to nursing mothers. Betty Crase says, 'An early visit builds the mother's confidence and can answer some of her questions.'[9] In the US, the Colorado Breast-

Feeding Task Force is encouraging the American Academy of Pediatrics to make a five-to-seven-day postpartum visit standard procedure for breast-fed babies.[10]

Most authorities on breastfeeding agree that the first two weeks are crucial for long-term breast-feeding success. If you have trouble in the first few weeks, seek help from your health visitor, a specialist, or a local La Leche League leader…fast!

You can reach La Leche League International at www.lalecheleague.org, or the National Childbirth Trust (see page 149).

▼

A Note to Dad

– from Dr. Steven Nafziger, University Family Medical Center, Pueblo, Colorado

I once fancied myself as much of an expert on breastfeeding as anybody, and I thought that the advice on breastfeeding I gave women was always adequate and well taken. When my wife made the decision to breast-feed our first child, I quickly learned that simplistic advice like 'Just keep trying; it will all come together' fell quite short. Every day, I faced some practical but perplexing questions about breastfeeding that made me realize how much I still needed to know about breastfeeding – not only professionally, but also as a father.

I'm sure that most fathers recognize at least some of the merits of breastfeeding. Breast milk is by far the best food for your baby. Breast-fed babies have fewer allergies

Words of Encouragement from an Experienced Mother

Helene, the mother of five children, says, 'The bond between mother and child while the child is being nourished in the womb is not over when the umbilical cord is cut. The bond continues and grows as the mother breast-feeds and holds that new miracle of life in her arms. It is not just a nutritional need that is being met for the baby. It is a psychological, emotional, and physical need for both as well. No sensation compares with nursing your child. Nothing is as satisfying and fulfilling as nursing. I would tell every new mother who is considering breastfeeding to do it.'

and fewer illnesses during the breast-feeding period. Breastfeeding is also economical and convenient.

When mums breast-feed instead of bottle-feed, dads do get out of having to feed and mix formula, but they can do other helpful and thoughtful things. Breastfeeding requires a lot of a woman's time, which prevents her from doing other things, especially in the first few weeks. Doing housework and laundry, cooking, caring for other children, answering doorbells and telephone calls, and bringing baby to mom for feeding are only a few examples of what a father can do. Bathing or walking the baby or spending time playing with him or her will not only free up time for mother but will also create a bond with the child, which is the best gift any parent can give a child.

Of all the things a father can do to help mum while she's breast-feeding, support is probably the key. Many women will make the decision to breast-feed on the basis of how much they're feeling supported. A woman will be more likely to breast-feed if her partner has an enthusiastic, supportive, and positive attitude rather than an indifferent or negative attitude. A partner's support and willingness to help can ease any reservations or fears a mother might have about breastfeeding. Breastfeeding for the first time is a new experience not only for the father, but also for the mother, and it requires a commitment from both of them. A father who realizes this has taken the first and most crucial step toward the mother's successful breast-feeding experience.[11]

▼

Preparing for Breastfeeding

Before You Deliver

Well before your due date, get ready for breastfeeding by following this checklist.[12]

▶ **Attend a breast-feeding information class or a La Leche League meeting.**

Look in the phone book to find a local NCT group or visit www.lalecheleague.org.

▶ **Find someone who has breast-fed whom you can call when you have questions or concerns.**

This person could be a La Leche League leader or member or simply a knowledgeable friend or relative.

▶ **Find a hospital and paediatrician who support breastfeeding.**

The Baby Friendly Hospital Initiative of the United Nations Children's Fund (UNICEF) and the World Health Organization (WHO) recommend, among other things, that infants be nursed within thirty minutes of delivery; that no water, formula, or supplements be given to newborns unless medically necessary; and that babies room-in with their mothers twenty-four hours a day.

Surprisingly, not all paediatricians are supportive of breastfeeding. A recent survey of paediatricians showed that only 65 per cent recommended breastfeeding to their patients as the exclusive feeding method for the first month. It also showed that 72 per cent were not familiar with the Baby Friendly Hospital Initiative.[13]

▶ **Check out on-line resources.**

▶ **If returning to work, find out if your company and boss will support your decision to breast-feed.**

Do whatever you can now to prepare them.

▶ **Prepare yourself for breastfeeding.**

Breast preparation while pregnant is not recommended because it can cause premature labour. (Ask your doctor for more details.) Though nipple soreness during nursing is usually a result of incorrect positioning, some soreness may be due to sensitive skin around the nipple. Alleviating the soreness can be as simple as going braless or topless around the house or not washing your nipples with soap.

▶ **Have these things on hand:**

Nursing pads (washable cloth pads or disposable cotton pads) and a breast pump or access to one (useful if you have trouble with engorgement). I found that a battery-operated pump worked much better than a hand pump. Some women prefer to rent an electric pump.

At the Hospital

When you arrive at the hospital, use the following checklist to get off to a good start with breastfeeding.[14]

▶ **In addition to telling the doctors and nurses you plan to breast-feed, write a note ahead of time that states you plan to breast-feed and give the note to the nurse upon your arrival.**

▶ **Ask to room-in with your baby twenty-four hours a day.**

This enables you to feed your baby on demand more easily. However, some mothers would rather rest, knowing that their babies are well cared for, and have them brought in frequently to nurse. Ask that your baby not receive any bottles when he or she is away from you.

▶ **Tell the staff to keep anaesthesia and other labour medications to a minimum so you and your baby will be alert during breastfeeding.**

▶ **Tell staff you want to breast-feed as soon as possible after delivery – on the delivery table or in the recovery room.**

▶ **Tell staff not to give your baby supplemental water, sugar water, or formula unless medically necessary. Also ask them not to give your baby a dummy, as this can cause nipple confusion.**

According to Dr. Nancy Krebs, a Denver paediatrician, 'Full-term babies don't have to drink very much in the first twenty-four hours or so because most are born relatively well hydrated. Watch for colourless, diluted urine and adequate number of stools, because these are indicators of adequate nutrition. A baby who is very small at birth or who may have had a stressful delivery is more vulnerable to dehydration or low blood sugar.'[15]

If your baby doesn't breast-feed much at first, consult your paediatrician or lactation specialist.

▶ **Ask a lactation specialist or nurse to help you get started.**

Contrary to popular belief, breastfeeding doesn't necessarily come naturally. Most of us need to learn, and some of us need help.

▶ **Nurse your baby as often as the baby wants for as long as the baby wants – the sooner the better.**

Nurse as often as every one to three hours. You may need to wake your baby for feedings.

What Might Happen and What You Can Do

While you're in the hospital, things may happen that make you question your decisions about breastfeeding. Here's some information to help you stay the course.[16]

▶ **The nurses or doctors may tell you that you need your rest.**

Tell them you will not sleep well without your baby and that you need all the nursing practice you can get before you go home and are on your own.

▶ **Your baby may only nuzzle at the first feeding.**

This is okay! It is important for you to get to know each other.

▶ **You may wonder why your milk is thick and yellowish.**

It's supposed to be! This 'first milk', or colostrum, is low in fat and packed with carbohydrates, protein, and antibodies. Feeding your baby as much colostrum as possible will help your baby be as healthy as possible, help you and your baby establish a breastfeeding bond, and help your mature milk come in.

▶ **Breastfeeding may be uncomfortable at first.**

We all have different tolerances for discomfort. However, breastfeeding should not *hurt*. If it does, ask a nurse to help you get your baby properly positioned and latched on.

▶ **The hospital may give you formula or coupons for formula in the discharge packet.**

Hospitals do this because formula companies provide the samples free of charge. This does not mean that your baby will *need* the formula. Your body can make all the milk your baby needs.

▶ **Before you leave the hospital, be sure to ask for a list of names and phone numbers of people in your area whom you can call if you have breast-feeding questions or problems.**

▼

Nutrition during Breastfeeding

The Best-for-Baby Breast-feeding Eating Plan

While breast-feeding, you actually need to eat more than you ate during your pregnancy. And you should continue to make every bite count. Below is a meal plan that will allow you to meet your nutrition needs during nursing. Your daily diet should contain at least some of the following foods, which add up to about 2,400 calories. Remember that you may need more or less than these.

10 or more servings of grains

1 serving is 1 slice any type bread; ½ small bagel, pitta bread or English muffin; 1 150-mm (6-inch) tortilla; 8 tbsp cooked rice or pasta; 8 tbsp cooked cereal, barley,

bulgur; 25 g (1 oz) ready-to-eat cereal; 3 to 4 savoury biscuits; or 2 biscuits.

Note: 3 or more servings should be whole-grain.

4 to 5 servings of calcium-rich foods

1 serving is 250 ml (8 fl oz) any type milk or yogurt, 40 g (1½ oz) cheese, 50 g (2 oz) processed cheese, or 250 ml (8 fl oz) calcium-fortified orange juice or soymilk.

4 or more servings of fruit

1 serving is 1 medium fresh fruit; ½ grapefruit, mango, or papaya; 8 tbsp tinned or chopped fruit; 4 tbsp dried fruit; or 200 ml (6½ fl oz) juice.

4 or more servings of vegetables

1 serving is 8 tbsp cooked vegetables, 250 ml (8 fl oz) leafy vegetables, 1 small potato, or 200 ml (6½ fl oz) tomato or vegetable juice.

Note: Be sure to eat at least one fruit or vegetable that is high in vitamin C and one that is dark green or orange, every day.

3 to 4 servings of protein foods

1 serving is 50–75 g (2 to 3 oz) cooked lean meat (the size of a deck of cards); 2 eggs; 8 tbsp tuna; 8 tbsp legumes, tofu, or textured vegetable protein; or 2 tablespoons nuts or nut butter.

Note: Try to eat fish at least once a week to get your share of essential fat for your baby's growing brain. Eat an additional ½ protein serving for each 250 ml (8 fl oz) of milk that you don't drink. (See pages 25 and 26 for more info on essential fatty acids.)

Fats and sweets: Eat sparingly.

Women who breast-feed for more than six months and have reached their pre-pregnant weight may need to increase their intake of vegetable fats and other healthy extras to maintain their energy and milk supply.

Sample Meal Plan for Breastfeeding

Breakfast

Corn Bran with blueberries
Wholemeal bagel with light cream
  cheese
Milk

Snack

Vegetable juice
Savoury biscuits
Carrot sticks
Turkey

Lunch

Grilled cheese sandwich
Sliced tomato
Peach
Sugar biscuits
Milk

Snack

Fresh fruit salad

Dinner

Grilled chicken
Grilled vegetables
Spinach salad with red pepper and mushrooms
Wholemeal roll
Fresh orange
Milk

Snack

Peanut butter and digestive biscuits
Yogurt with dried fruit

Calorie Needs

Your breast-feeding diet should be similar to your pregnancy diet, except now you need about 200 calories more (or 500 calories more than the amount you ate before you were pregnant). A good way to get the extra calories is to eat an additional snack or higher-calorie snacks. (See Chapter Thirteen for snack ideas.)

The suggested calorie intake for lactation takes into consideration the 100 to 150 calories a day that come from fat stored during pregnancy. For this reason, breastfeeding can help you lose weight; what a wonderful way to do it! The average weight loss for breast-feeding women is 450–900 grams (1 to 2 pounds) per month, after the first month postpartum. If you breast-feed longer than that, you will probably continue to lose weight, but at a slower rate.[17]

While research has shown that the extra 500 calories are needed for successful breast-feeding, you may be less active during your first month or so postpartum.[18]

Therefore, after breastfeeding has been well established, you should evaluate your energy needs based on weight gain during pregnancy, weight loss per week during breastfeeding, and your activity level. You may need more or less than 200 calories above pregnancy needs, but it's a good place to start.[19] To ensure you have a nutritious and adequate milk supply, make sure that your calorie intake does not go below 1,800 calories.

If you breast-feed longer than six months, if you didn't gain much during pregnancy, or if you drop below your usual weight, you may need up to 650 calories per day (or even more) over your non-pregnant calorie needs. Also, if you are very active, you will need more calories than the average woman. If you find that you are losing weight too quickly or are having trouble eating the recommended amount of food, you could see a registered dietitian for some individualized advice.

Protein Needs

Your protein needs also to increase during breastfeeding. You'll need 65 grams of protein per day (or 5 grams more than during pregnancy) during the first six months of breastfeeding. If you nurse longer than six months, you will need about 62 grams of protein per day because your baby will start eating solids and so will drink less milk.[20]

If you can drink or eat the recommended four daily servings of dairy products, you can meet your protein needs by eating just 65 grams (2½ ounces) of protein per day (including the amount of protein in six servings of grain products). This is because each serving of milk contains the same amount of protein as 25 grams (1 ounce) of meat. The Best-for-Baby Breast-Feeding Eating Plan contains a protein boost to ensure that you get enough of the important nutrients like zinc, iron, and vitamin B_6 that are found in some protein foods.

If you prefer not to eat much meat, you will need to choose the rest of your diet wisely. (See pages 70, 71, and 83 for good food sources of iron and zinc.)

Nutrient Needs

Most of your nutrient needs stay the same during lactation; some decrease and some increase. You will need slightly more thiamin, riboflavin, vitamin B_{12}, and magnesium. You will need significantly more vitamin C, vitamin E, niacin, zinc, and selenium. You will need less folic acid and iron than during pregnancy. However, many physicians will recommend that you continue to take an iron supplement to help replace iron deficits from pregnancy or blood loss during delivery.

Be sure to continue getting plenty of fibre in your diet. (See page 51 for 'Focus on Fibre'.) When I experienced some constipation during the first few weeks of breastfeeding, my doctor explained that the hormones associated with breastfeeding can slow down the digestive process.

Don't forget fluids! Although in the past it was thought that women needed to drink a lot of extra fluid to produce breast milk, it now appears that drinking to your thirst will provide you with adequate fluid. However, if you live in a dry climate or exercise in hot weather, your thirst may lag behind your actual fluid needs.

If you were to eat very poorly while breast-feeding, your body would draw from stored pools of nutrients. If you breast-fed for six months and depended entirely on stored nutrients to feed your baby, you would deplete 19 per cent of protein stores, 4 per cent of calcium stores, 14 per cent of iron stores, 46 per cent of vitamin A stores, and close to 100 per cent of folic acid stores. Most of us get more than enough protein.

But if your diet does not include adequate amounts of calcium, iron, vitamin A, and especially folic acid, your own nutritional status could be in danger. Since pregnancy and breastfeeding are such physically demanding jobs, make sure that your own diet is as good as it can be so you'll have all the energy you possibly can.[21]

Calcium Needs

During pregnancy, women are often reminded about their need for calcium. After delivery, calcium in the diet may not seem that important. It is. First, the calcium in bone is often used as a calcium source during breastfeeding, especially if you do not have enough calcium in your diet. Heavy metals (like lead) accumulated in your bones over your lifetime can be released into your bloodstream – and to your baby – if you lose too much calcium from your bones during breastfeeding. Calcium loss during breastfeeding also puts women at risk for developing osteoporosis later in life.[22] The Dietary Reference Intake (DRI) for calcium during breastfeeding is 1,000 milligrams – the same as during pregnancy.[23] However, the US National Institutes of Health recommends 1,200 to 1,500 milligrams per day for pregnancy and lactation. (See pages 68 and 69 for calcium contents of your favourite foods.) If you cannot obtain the recommended amount of calcium through your diet, ask your health-care provider about a calcium supplement.

Nutrients of Special Concern

When we compare average vitamin and mineral intakes of women to the needs of breast-feeding women, we find that intakes of several nutrients are below the DRIs. When a woman eats 2,700 calories per day, only zinc and calcium may fall below the DRI. However, if the diet contains less than 2,700 calories (and the average nursing woman's probably does), intakes of calcium, magnesium, zinc, vitamin B_6, and folic acid will likely fall well below the DRI.

Improved food choices are better than taking a nutrient supplement for several reasons. Most nutrients are absorbed better from foods than from supplements, and foods may contain unidentified nutrients not found in supplements. Also, taking a supplement can give you a false sense of security; you may be tempted to make poorer food choices, thinking that your vitamin will make up the difference.

If you do choose to take a supplement, take one that contains a broad spectrum of vitamins and minerals and contains no more than 100 per cent of the DRI for any of them. Some doctors recommend that you continue taking prenatal vitamins. This is fine, but be aware that their high iron content may worsen constipation. Remember that after pregnancy, a woman's need for iron generally decreases – unless she has lost a lot of blood during delivery or is anaemic. Ask your doctor.

Best Food Sources

Calcium

Milk, cheese, yogurt, tinned or small fish with edible bones (salmon, mackerel, sardines), tofu processed with calcium, Chinese leaves, broccoli, kale, molasses, collard, mustard, and turnip greens.

Zinc

Oysters, seafood, lean red meats, poultry, eggs, wheatgerm, nuts, dried beans and peas, yogurt, and whole grains.

Magnesium

Bran cereal, wheatgerm, Swiss chard, spinach, nuts, seeds, beans and peas, whole grains, dried fruit, prawns, and scallops.

Vitamin B_6

Mustard greens, bananas, poultry, meat, fish, potatoes, sweet potatoes, spinach, prunes, watermelon, some legumes, soya beans, lentils, chickpeas, pinto beans, fortified cereals, and nuts.

Folic acid

Spinach, leafy green vegetables, asparagus, black-eyed peas, lentils, kidney beans, fortified cereals, legumes, broccoli, Brussels sprouts, and orange and grapefruit juices.

Drugs and Breastfeeding

If you must take a medication during breast-feeding, you don't necessarily have to stop nursing. The safety of the medication depends on the drug and its dosage. For example, if you are taking an antibiotic for a breast infection, you are actually encouraged to breast-feed. However, some drugs pose a risk for your baby, including anti-protozoal compounds, antineoplastic drugs, some antithyroid drugs, and synthetic anti-coagulants. Make sure your doctor knows you are breast-feeding before he or she pre-scribes a medication.

If you must take one of the above drugs, pump your milk temporarily to keep your milk supply up. Discard the pumped milk and resume breast-feeding several days after you stop the medication. Ask your health-care provider or pharmacist when the med-ication will leave your system so you can start breast-feeding again. If you take a lactation-suppression drug to stop breast-feeding, don't give your baby any of your milk while your milk supply is dwindling.

Some over-the-counter drugs should not be taken while you are breast-feeding. For example, acetaminophen (such as Tylenol) is usually recommended for pain instead of aspirin. Consult your health-care provider about which over-the-counter medications he or she recommends before the need arises.

Breastfeeding for Special Groups

Mothers of Multiples

If you have given birth to multiple babies, can you still breast-feed? The answer is an enthusiastic 'Yes!' As you may have guessed, breast-feeding multiples is a bit more com-plicated than nursing a single baby. But since multiples are often born smaller than single babies, your breast milk is even more impor-tant to give your babies a healthy boost.

Mothers of single babies need more energy while they are nursing, but according to Dr. Barbara Luke at the University of Michigan Multiples Clinic, mothers of multiples need about 300 calories less.

Some on-line resources for nursing multiples are parentingweb.com/lounge/multiples.htm and www.lalecheleague.org. Books are listed in the Recommended Resources at the back of the book.

Vegetarians

Vegans (vegetarians who eat no animal products) need to plan their diets a little more carefully to make sure their breast milk contains everything their babies need. Vitamin B_{12} must be consumed from a reli-able source; the DRI for breastfeeding is 2.9 micrograms. Vitamin D, calcium, and zinc may also be harder to find in a vegan diet. Please see pages 31, 68, and 83 for food sources of these nutrients.

Another factor that could affect your baby's development is the type of fat in your diet. Amounts of DHA (an essential fat) are lower in the blood of breast-fed infants whose mothers are vegetarian. DHA is not found in vegetarian diets, although alpha-linolenic acid, a fatty acid found in vegetable oils, can be converted to DHA in small amounts. It has been suggested that excess linoleic acid be avoided to support the production of DHA.[24] For more information, visit the Vegetarian Resource Group's website at www.vrg.org. (See also Chapters Six and Seven for more information on vegetarian eating and multifoetal pregnancy.)

Teens

You can give your baby the best possible start by breast-feeding him or her. Breastfeeding has many benefits that may be especially important to you: It is less expensive, it is all-natural, it can help you get your body back in shape, and it can help you bond with your baby. There are also many health benefits, as described earlier in this chapter. One important one is a reduced risk of breast cancer – this applies to teens, too![25] Just remember to continue eating as well as you can, and take a multi-vitamin/mineral supplement.

Mums of Premies

If your baby was born prematurely, breast-feeding can give him or her a vital boost. And breast-feeding a premature infant can be even more rewarding for you than nursing a full-term infant, because you'll know that you are doing all you can to help your baby grow.

New research indicates that breast-feeding the premature infant may provide even more health benefits than feeding a full-term infant; it has been shown to improve short-term and long-term health (by decreasing risk of infections), gastrointestinal function, and neurological development. However, preterm infants often have higher nutrient needs than breast milk can satisfy. A premie's special nutritional needs may be met by the use of multinutrient supplements during the time the infant is being tube-fed. A human milk fortifier like the one made by Enfamil can also add nutrients to your milk so that your baby gets the nutrition he or she needs while still getting the benefits of breast milk.[26]

Your baby may have to stay in the neonatal intensive care unit so he or she can be monitored closely. If so, you will probably be pumping milk to be fed to your baby through a tube. However, skin-to-skin contact (also called kangaroo care) is encouraged to help increase milk production. While you are pumping, it may be helpful to keep a picture of your baby (or babies) next to you. While it may be disappointing not to be able to nurse your baby 'in person', just remember what a special gift you are giving.

Because your baby is extraspecial, your milk should be extraspecial, too. Besides following all the dietary advice in this chapter, you should look at your intake of essential fatty acids and make sure you eat a good source of them on a daily basis. While exact requirements for these fats have not been determined, eating foods rich in them may help your baby's brain and eye development. Please see page 26 for sources of essential fatty acids.

For more information on parenting premies, see *Your Premature Baby and Child: Helpful Answers and Advice for Parents* by Amy E. Tracy. On-line resources include www.lalecheleague.org and the websites for parents of multiples listed on page 135.

On-Line Breast-Feeding Resources

La Leche League
www.lalecheleague.org

Breastfeeding.com
www.breastfeeding.com

? Questions You May Have

Q: I've heard that if I eat gassy foods such as broccoli, onions, and even milk and chocolate, my baby can get wind. Do I have to stop eating all my favourite foods?

A: No. Although strongly flavoured vegetables and spices may give your milk a different flavour or may give your baby wind, to stop eating such foods is not necessary for everyone. After talking to many women, I have learned that baby's reaction to mum's diet seems to be an individual matter. One friend of mine continued eating plenty of garlic while nursing, and her baby had no problem with it. Another friend loved to eat hot peppers, and her baby apparently liked them, too.

Keep in mind that a lot of wind can simply be a result of the baby's immature digestive system. Both my children had problems with wind. I altered my diet in every way possible, but nothing seemed to help. I chalked it up to their own digestive systems and used a lot of over-the-counter infant wind medicine. They finally outgrew it.

If your baby has wind, you might try changing your diet for several days to see if the change makes a difference. Sensitivity to flavours and wind-causing foods seems to vary from baby to baby. If your baby has no problem with wind, you should be able to eat any food in moderation.

Q: We have a lot of food allergies in my family. Can breastfeeding help prevent them in my baby?

A: It's possible, but it hasn't been proven conclusively. Some studies suggest that components of food eaten by the mother can pass into the breast milk and cause allergic reactions in the baby. While avoiding certain foods during breastfeeding is sometimes recommended, one study has shown that there is no difference in the number of allergies among people whose mothers followed restricted diets.[27]

Evidence does show that breastfeeding lowers the risk of both asthma and eczema. A whey-hydrolysate formula (made for infants with allergies) showed similar results.[28]

Probably the best advice for women who have allergies or a family history of allergies is to breast-feed as long as possible and to eat a large variety of foods so that no one food will be passed in large amounts to the baby through the milk.[29]

Q: Can I start drinking coffee again?

A: Your baby will receive about 1 per cent of the caffeine kick that you get in your coffee or other caffeinated beverage. The equivalent of one or two cups of coffee per day is not likely to have a negative effect on baby.[30] However, caffeine can accumulate and cause your baby to be irritable and to have trouble falling asleep. So go easy.

Q: I have gone into premature labour. Though I am now on bedrest and medication to stop the labour, I am concerned that I won't be able to breast-feed if my baby arrives prematurely. Any advice?

A: Breast-feeding a premature infant can be even more rewarding than nursing a full-term infant. One study shows that feeding an infection-prone premature infant with colostrum (first milk) may have even more significant anti-infective effects than feeding it to full-term infants.[31] Another study reports that preterm infants who were tube-fed breast milk in their early weeks of life had significantly higher IQs at seven-and-a-half to eight years of age than those who did not. This difference was still significant after allowing for the mother's education and social class.[32]

If your baby comes very early, he or she may have to stay in a special area of the nursery to be monitored closely and to have the environment kept at a precise temperature. You may have to express milk so that it can then be fed to your baby through a special bottle or tube. In this case, you will need to pump your breasts.

The fact that you are thinking ahead is wonderful; you can arrange to rent a good-quality breast pump or find out whether you can use one while you're at the hospital. Taking pictures of your baby and keeping them near you while pumping may help you express milk. Not being able to breast-feed in person may be disappointing, but think of the benefits you are still able to provide for your baby.

Q: My mother says I should drink a beer before I breast-feed to increase my milk supply. Will it? And is it safe for my baby?

A: This old wives' tale has not been scientifically proven. On the other hand, we do know that alcohol is released in the milk and that excessive drinking can cause problems with letdown, high alcohol level in breast milk, and lethargic babies. There has been one report of lowered psychomotor development scores in babies with increased alcohol exposure.[33] Since foetal brain development continues to occur during the first year of life, avoiding alcohol or drinking only limited amounts makes sense.

A recent study showed that the smell of alcohol could be detected immediately in the breast milk of mothers who had drunk the equivalent of the amount of alcohol in one can of beer. The smell was strongest at thirty to sixty minutes after the mother imbibed. The babies drank less milk during the feeding, possibly due to the change in taste and smell of the milk. Another theory is that alcohol could decrease the mother's milk supply.[34]

Alcohol in breast milk can also significantly change an infant's sleep pattern, causing him or her to sleep less.[35]

If you'd really like to go out on the town and have more than one or two drinks, just pump your breast milk afterward and discard it. You can give your baby some previously pumped milk. Or if you'd just like an occasional drink, use common sense. Don't drink on an empty stomach, as this will speed the flow of alcohol into your bloodstream and your breast milk. Ask your health-care provider for more information.

Q: I still smoke. Can this somehow affect my milk?

A: Nicotine and cotinine (another component of cigarette smoke) have been found in breast milk. No symptoms of exposure to the chemicals have been seen in infants, but nicotine can affect how much milk you are able to produce. Some researchers advise that if you do smoke, you should not smoke for two-and-a-half hours before nursing and avoid smoking while near your baby.[36]

For information on kicking the habit of smoking, call the National Helpline for Smoking Cessation on 0800 169 0169.

Q: If I breast-feed, will my baby have a smaller risk of being overweight when he gets older?

A: Yes. Breastfeeding does seem to decrease your baby's chances of becoming overweight or obese as he or she gets older. The longer you breast-feed, the less your child's risk of becoming overweight.[37]

Q: Should I try to lose weight while breast-feeding?

A: You will probably lose weight without even trying. Instead, you need to focus on eating a well-balanced diet so that your breast milk continues to contain a good supply of the nutrients your baby needs. Losing 450 to 900 grams (1 to 2 pounds) per week is generally safe. However, you should not eat less than 1,800 calories per day. Monitoring the growth and general health of your baby is also a good way to check the quality of your milk.

Most women lose the first 9 kg (20 pounds) quite easily; it's the last 2.25 or 4.5 kg (5 or 10 pounds) that may hang on. This is when you should bring in the reinforcements: aerobic exercise and weight resistance. These exercises help you lose more body fat while keeping muscle. More muscle means burning more calories all the time![38]

Q: I want to have another baby right away. Should I still breast-feed if I get pregnant?

A: In developing countries, mothers commonly continue to breast-feed well into the second trimester of another pregnancy. However, breastfeeding during pregnancy can take its toll on you. Pregnancy and lactation are nutritionally and physically demanding. One study showed that mothers who breast-fed while pregnant had babies that weighed slightly less than the babies of mothers who did not.

Much depends on your nutritional status. If you breast-feed while pregnant, you must meet the nutritional demands of your growing foetus, your growing baby, and yourself. These demands can add up to as much as 900 extra calories a day, depending on the age of your baby. If you aren't able to consume all those extra calories, protein, vitamins, and minerals, you could wind up nutritionally depleted.

Although breast-feeding while pregnant is possible, you may want to wait at least a few months after weaning your baby before conceiving again.[39]

Q: I've heard that women who breast-feed could have a lower risk of osteoporosis later in life. Is that true?

A: Research shows breastfeeding can affect osteoporosis. While it appears that some calcium stored in bone is used during breast-feeding, when you stop nursing, the bone is rebuilt, sometimes with even more calcium. For this reason, your calcium intake during nursing is important, but it may be just as important to have a calcium-rich diet afterwards, when bone rebuilding is taking place.[40]

Q: Does my diet really affect my breast milk?

A: Yes. Breast milk is a constantly changing fluid. It changes from the beginning to the end of a feeding and it changes as an infant gets older. It also can vary according to your diet.

The most variable component in breast milk is fat. The amount of body fat you have can affect the fat in milk. Dietary fat also affects the amount and types of fat in breast milk. Essential fats (necessary for brain and retina development) in your breast milk are related to the amounts of those fats in your diet. So are trans fats. (See page 26 for more info about trans fats.) The amount of vitamins in your breast milk is also related to the vitamins in your diet; vitamins D and K may not always be adequate. On the other hand, minerals in breast milk (except selenium and iodine) do not vary according to diet.[41]

All these facts should motivate you to eat well while you are breast-feeding!

Q: I've heard that PCBs can be in breast milk. Can this affect the safety of my breast milk?

A: Over a lifetime, a person is exposed to environmental pollutants that accumulate in small amounts in the body – mostly in fat. The chemicals of greatest concern are organochlorines, a group of synthetic compounds persistent in the environment. Examples of these are polychlorinated biphenyls (PCBs), a family of industrial chemicals, and dichlorodiphenyl trichloroethane (DDT), an insecticide. Chemical treatment for termites is often associated with these residues. Although some of these chemicals have been banned for years, they persist in the environment and are still used in other parts of the world.

Infants are exposed to these environmental pollutants during pregnancy and through breast milk. In one ongoing study, infants whose mothers' breast milk contained PBB, a chemical related to PCBs, were followed. At ages two to four, children who had higher exposure to the chemical had lower scores on development tests; however, by ages four to six, these differences had disappeared.[42] A study of Dutch children found lower test scores among children exposed prenatally to dioxin (another environmental chemical) and PCBs. However, exposure to these compounds during breastfeeding was not related to forty-two-month cognitive performance.[43]

During pregnancy, a foetus's exposure to chemicals is much higher than during breastfeeding, but since body fat stored during pregnancy is used during breastfeeding, your diet during pregnancy can affect the amount of pollutants in your breast milk.

Should this information affect your decision to breast-feed? No. Betty Crase, former Director of Scientific Information at La Leche League International, says, 'Unfortunately, we live in a contaminated world. However, the known and documented benefits of breastfeeding still outweigh the risks of contaminants that may be found in breast milk. What many people don't realize is that artificial infant formula can also contain environmental contaminants, especially if the water used to prepare it contains lead or other chemicals.'[44] And the foremost researcher of PCBs in breast milk says,

"Breastfeeding is recommended despite the presence of chemical residues.'[45]

Chemicals in our environment are an unfortunate reality. The commonsense solution is to try to limit your present and future exposure to chemicals by following the tips below.

▶ **Avoid recreationally caught fish not caught by you (fish that is caught by friends or sold at a roadside stand). Also, avoid fish from areas you know are polluted.**

These fish are more likely to come from contaminated water. Friends who give you leftovers from their fishing trip may not know you are breast-feeding. You should definitely still eat fish; the omega-3 fatty acids found in fish are important to your baby's brain, which continues to develop during the first year of life.

▶ **Avoid quick weight loss while breast-feeding.**

Toxins from the environment are stored in body fat. If you go on an extreme weight-loss diet, some of these accumulated chemicals can enter your milk in larger amounts as your body fat is released from storage.[46]

▶ **Avoid using pesticides, herbicides, and insecticides (especially chemicals for termite extermination) in your home – even those that claim to be non-toxic.**

▶ **Avoid eating the skin and fat of poultry, meats, and fish. Drink skimmed or semi-skimmed milk. Eat more plant sources of protein.**

Q: I have just had a case of food poisoning. Can the bacteria that caused my illness be passed to my baby in breast milk?

A: According to Dr. Steven Nafziger of the University Family Medical Center in Pueblo, Colorado, 'The bacteria that cause most common types of food poisoning do not pass through the breast milk. However, some rarer forms of food poisoning involve bacteria that make toxins. These toxins can directly affect the baby through the mother's breast milk. I encourage a breast-feeding mother who is experiencing flu-like symptoms to come into the office so I can evaluate her condition and make a specific recommendation.'[47]

Q: I'd like to start a vigorous exercise programme. Can I still successfully breast-feed?

A: Yes. One study showed that among women who did aerobic exercise forty-five minutes per day, five times per week, for twelve weeks, their exercise had no effect on the amount of milk they produced or how much weight their babies gained.[48]

Q: I am a total vegetarian. Is there anything that my milk will be missing?

A: People who eat no animal protein or dairy products sometimes need another source of vitamin B_{12}, since it is found naturally only in animal products. You need to consume foods fortified with vitamin B_{12} or take a B_{12} daily supplement of 2.6 micrograms.[49] (See page 30 for more information about vitamin B_{12}.)

The calcium requirement for vegetarians is thought to be less than for meat eaters because vegetarian diets are lower in protein than the diets of meat eaters.

If you consume no dairy products, you may need to plan your diet carefully to include high-calcium foods or take a calcium supplement. Zinc and iron are other nutrients that may require you to work at getting sufficient amounts. (See page 83 for vegetarian sources of zinc, pages 68 and 69 for calcium, and pages 70 and 71 for iron.) If you have concerns about your diet, discuss them further with your baby's health-care provider or ask a registered dietitian to help you analyze your diet.

Q: Can breastfeeding lower my risk of breast cancer?

A: Yes. Several studies indicate that breastfeeding has a protective effect against breast cancer.[50] Breastfeeding can also cut your child's breast cancer risk when the child grows older.[51] What a special gift!

Q: Does my baby need any special vitamins while I am nursing?

A: Your breast milk contains nearly everything your baby needs. However, a few nutrients are not contained in adequate amounts in breast milk, and some mothers have special dietary considerations that are discussed under 'Breastfeeding for Special Groups'.

Vitamin D and vitamin K have recently been reported not to appear in sufficient amounts in breast milk. If your water does not contain fluoride, or if your family drinks bottled water, your baby may need a fluoride supplement at six months. Ask your paediatrician if he or she recommends a supplement for breast-fed babies.

By six months, your baby will have depleted his or her iron stores. This is the right time for introducing iron-rich foods like fortified cereals and teething biscuits.

▼

Tips for Formula Feeding

If you decide to feed your baby formula or to combine breastfeeding and formula feeding, the following information may be useful:

- If formula is your baby's sole source of nutrition for the first four to six months, the American Academy of Pediatrics recommends you choose one that is iron-fortified to prevent iron-deficiency anaemia.[52]
- If you use powdered or concentrated formula that needs to be mixed with water, make sure your water contains adequate fluoride. You can call your local water department to find out. If your water does not contain enough fluoride, your baby's health-care provider will need to prescribe a supplement.
- Whether you feed your baby breast milk, infant formula, or a combination of the two, you should not give your baby cow's milk or products containing cow's milk until your baby is one year old. The American Academy of

Pediatrics recommends this because, among other effects, the protein in cow's milk may trigger the development of insulin-dependent diabetes.[53]

- If you use formula that has to be mixed with water, make sure that your water doesn't contain too much lead. Three common preparation practices that can increase lead in formula are:
  - Using water that is drawn from the tap first thing in the morning. If your pipes contain lead, water that has been sitting in the pipes for several hours will have a high concentration of lead.
  - Excessive boiling. In just five minutes of boiling, the amount of lead is concentrated threefold.
  - Using a lead-based kettle for boiling.[54]

(See page 38 for more information on lead.)

▼

About Bonding

Bonding is a term often used when discussing breastfeeding. Bonding refers to touching, cuddling, and holding and can be acheived regardless of the feeding method. The long-term effects of bonding are very positive and are thought to affect a child's self-esteem as well as the mother's attitude toward the child.

A breast-feeding mum must remain with the baby while feeding, unless she expresses milk into a bottle. Bottle-fed babies can also bond with whoever is feeding them. However, some parents learn that the bottle can be propped by a blanket, which allows them to go about doing other things. This hands-off feeding is not recommended because of choking danger and also because it does not promote bonding, or developing a close relationship with the baby. Furthermore, if a baby falls asleep with a bottle in his or her mouth, the milk remaining in the baby's mouth can cause tooth decay.

Whatever method of feeding you choose, feeding your baby will be enjoyable – but it can also be stressful. Since babies can't talk to you, figuring out what they need is sometimes difficult. Some great advice about

More Information on Infant Feeding

For more information on infant feeding, see *Healthy Food for Healthy Kids*, the follow-up book to *Eating Expectantly*. *Healthy Food for Healthy Kids* is written in the same easy-to-read style, contains information about feeding kids from birth to school age, and also contains delicious kid-tested recipes. To review an excerpt from *Healthy Food for Healthy Kids*, visit www.healthyfoodzone.com.

infant feeding can be found in *Child of Mine: Feeding with Love and Good Sense* by Ellyn Satter, R.D., M.S. (Bull Publishing). Ms. Satter is a dietitian and a social worker who gives advice about eating and tips on how to encourage a positive feeding relationship with your child.

CHAPTER NINE

Now That You Can See Your Feet Again, or...

The First Weeks with Baby

What you will find in this chapter:

• *What to Expect after Delivery*
• *Menus for the First Week with Baby*
• *Going Back to Work*
• *Your Body Is Changing*
• *Losing That Baby Fat Sensibly*
• *Weight-Loss Plans*
• *Preparing for Your Next Pregnancy*

This chapter answers such questions as:

• *When will I be able to eat if I have anaesthesia during delivery?*
• *How can I possibly eat balanced meals if I'm too tired to cook?*
• *What is the difference between breast- and bottlefeeding?*
• *What's a good weight-loss diet?*
• *How can I tell a good weight-loss programme from a bad one?*
• *How long should I wait before I get pregnant again?*

What to Expect after Delivery

The first few days of postpartum life will likely be spent oohing and aahing over your new arrival and recovering from a very tiring event. You'll need to eat especially well those first few days at the hospital to muster as much strength as possible before you go home.

You may be too tired after delivery to eat a meal; that's normal for some women. You may just feel like drinking some juice or a decaffeinated soft drink for quick energy. Mary never drank sugared soft drinks, but after eighteen hours in labour, she drank 525 ml (18 fl oz) of 7-Up in just five minutes! Some women are so hungry after delivery that they call out for pizza.

High-carbohydrate snacks that might be available at the hospital include English muffins, bagels, toast, bran muffins, raisin toast, canned or fresh fruit, digestive biscuits, milk, yogurt, milk shakes, fruit juices, and soft drinks.

When you do feel like eating, these tips will help you get back on your feet:

▶ **If you select from a menu in the hospital, pick as many high-fibre foods as possible to get your digestive tract back to normal.**

Labour and anaesthesia slow down your digestion immensely. You may also have haemorrhoids from pregnancy or from the pushing stage of labour. Eating high-fibre foods will make your bowel movements softer and easier.

Some high-fibre foods you are likely to see on a hospital menu are Raisin Bran cereal, All Bran, 100% Bran Flakes, wholemeal bread and rolls, apples, oranges, bananas, strawberries, prunes, raw vegetables, salad, baked potatoes, legumes, peas, corn, and sliced tomatoes. Be sure to drink plenty of liquids when eating high-fibre foods.

▶ **Those first few days, eat as much as you want and drink plenty of fluids.**

If you had a long labour, you probably didn't drink much and you'll need to rehydrate. If you are planning to breast-feed, you will need to continue drinking 8 to 10 cups of fluid per day.

▶ **Concentrate on getting your strength back and taking care of your baby those first few weeks.**

Hopefully you cooked some meals ahead of time and froze them. If not, let your partner or other family members cook. Or send them out for fast food or convenience foods. (See Chapter Twelve for healthy, fast, and convenient menus.)

▼

Menus for the First Week with Baby

Those first few days will probably be too hectic to plan menus. Here is a week's worth of quick meals; some include takeout, and some can be made quickly at home.

Day 1
Takeout chicken and Snow Peas, Moo Shoo Prawns
Steamed rice
Fresh fruit
Milk

Day 2
Bacon pizza on wholemeal crust
Tossed salad
Raspberry sorbet

Day 3
Burger on wholemeal bun
Grated carrots with mayonnaise and raisins
Frozen yogurt with strawberries

Day 4
Minute steaks
Mixed vegetables
Easy Microwave Potatoes (page 326)
Cantaloupe melon or tinned peaches

Day 5
Broccoli Quiche (page 334)
Sourdough rolls
Sliced tomatoes with basil
Tropical Pudding (page 272)

Day 6
Bean tostadas
Mexican rice
Avocado-and-tomato salad
Frozen bananas

Day 7
Pasta with Quick Alfredo Sauce (page 260)
Garlic bread
Mixed green salad
Fig bars

Going Back to Work

Because of economic necessity or for personal fulfilment, most women go back to work when their babies are six weeks old. Going back to work can affect your feeding decisions. Unfortunately, many women view going back to work as an insurmountable obstacle to breastfeeding.

During my counselling sessions with pregnant women, I often found that if a woman knew she was going back to work, she threw the idea of breastfeeding right out the window. However, more and more companies are supporting breastfeeding. There's a compelling reason: One study showed that illnesses in breast-fed infants were reduced by 36 per cent and women who breast-fed missed 27 per cent fewer days due to their sick children.[1] You can continue to nurse *and* return to work. Here are three examples of how working women handled their feeding decisions:

- Barb was determined to breast-feed Joshua. Her company supported breastfeeding. She rented a breast pump from the hospital and used it at work. (She used a double pump, which allowed her to empty both breasts at the same time and still have time to run errands or eat lunch. During her lunch break, she came home and fed Josh. Barb found that breast-feeding Josh was just the contact she needed after being away most of the day. I admired Barb for her determination. She carried on

this routine for nine months, until she started daycare in her home. She continued to nurse Joshua thereafter.

- Sarah had a high-stress job. Her boss and company were not very supportive of motherhood. Yet Sarah wanted to breast-feed. She learned that breastfeeding didn't have to be done full-time. She established a good milk supply while she was home with Erin, then she gradually figured out the routine that worked best for her family. She nursed Erin in the morning, Erin's daycare fed Erin two bottles of formula in the early afternoon, then Sarah nursed Erin in the late afternoon while her husband prepared dinner and again before she went to bed. Sarah's milk supply adjusted to Erin's feeding schedule. On the weekend, Erin's dad helped out with the midday bottles to give Sarah a break from feeding.

- Nicole didn't want to have to pump at work, but she wanted to breast-feed. By planning ahead, she and her husband saved some money so that she could work part-time after Sean was born. While at home for ten weeks after her delivery, she built up her milk supply and arranged her schedule to be away four hours each morning. By working part-time, Nicole had the best of both worlds.

If you will be returning to work, your environment at work will influence your feeding decision. Consider the following:

Parental leave time. If your company allows an extended maternity leave, this will give you more time to be with your baby. And if you decide to breast-feed, additional time off will allow you time to increase your milk supply. Even if you decide to breast-feed for just a month, your baby will still receive colostrum, which contains important disease-fighting agents.

Required travel. If your job requires you to travel frequently, you might want to cut your travel time to a minimum whether you breast-feed or not. If you can't cut your travel time, nursing still won't be impossible – but it will require diligent planning. Kristen arranged daycare with a national franchise when she travelled so she could take Katie with her. Not everyone can make such a commitment, but Kristen is a good example of creative problem solving!

Flexible hours. Many companies offer flexible hours, which are useful in many ways. For example, some couples work four ten-hour days instead of five eight-hour days. If both partners can arrange this type of schedule, they would need daycare only three days a week and would both gain time with their baby. Flexible hours can also help a breast-feeding mum. For example, if you can take a long lunch and work later, you might be able to breast-feed your baby at lunch. (On-site daycare makes this even easier.)

Supportive boss and co-workers. Going back to work while your child is an infant may be emotionally difficult. Seek out supportive co-workers – perhaps those who also have children. A supportive boss will understand if you need to take breaks to

pump your breasts or take a little extra time off to feed your baby.

Your Body Is Changing

Welcome to the 'fourth trimester', the twelve weeks after you have your baby. This often-neglected period is important to understand. You are now adjusting from having been pregnant to being a mother. Life is different in many ways, and you are facing many new experiences and emotions. It is important that you take care of yourself physically and mentally. Proper diet and a gradual return to exercise can help you adjust. Listed below are the different changes that will be occurring in different parts of your body.

Uterus

Immediately after delivery, your uterus weighs about 900 grams (2 pounds) and is the size of a grapefruit. In the next six weeks, it will shrink down to normal – around 75 mm (3 inches) long and 50 grams (2 ounces) in weight. Nursing your baby will help your uterus contract and reduce in size. You may feel these contractions for two or three days, especially if this is your second or third baby.

Lochia

Lochia is the vaginal discharge that occurs the first few weeks after delivery. It is your body's way of getting rid of leftover debris from pregnancy. Lochia is a combination of red blood cells, skin cells, mucus, white blood cells, bacteria, and occasionally some of your baby's stool or hair.

Your blood flow will be red and plentiful for the first few days following delivery. Remember that your body generated a greater volume of blood during your pregnancy, and now the excess is being reduced. The amount of blood flow is an individual matter, but within two to three weeks many women return to having a whitish discharge.

If you revert to bright red bleeding, you are being too active. Slow down and enjoy the simple first days of your newborn's life. If your flow remains bright red or has a foul odour, please contact your doctor. Remember that ovulation can occur within weeks after delivery, even if you are breast-feeding. However, ovulation may not occur in the breast-feeding mother until after weaning. The first periods may be heavy and irregular for several months.

Discuss contraception with your doctor if you want to resume having sex within three to four weeks after delivery.

Perineum and Vagina

The area between your vagina and rectum is called the perineum. This area will feel sore due to the tremendous stretching it has undergone, even if you did not have an episiotomy. Ice will be applied in the first twelve hours after your delivery to reduce swelling. After this time, heat will promote healing. Many women take sitz baths (sitting for a short time in warm water).

Pelvic floor exercises will help tone muscles in the perineum. You should have learned how to do them in your antenatal class or prenatal exercise class. If not, consult your midwife.

If you had an episiotomy, your stitches will dissolve by themselves. Your vagina will have decreased mucus until ovulation returns to normal, and intercourse might need additional lubrication. Please note that if you are nursing, ovulation may be delayed for a while, so you may continue to have reduced mucus.

Abdomen

After the birth of your baby, your abdomen will still look very much pregnant, but flabby. This may be one of your biggest disappointments after delivery, unless you are prepared for it. You can start doing exercises to help tighten your abdominal muscles. Remember that good muscle tone will take time and discipline; diet, good posture, and exercise are important. If you have no energy or time to think about exercise in the first few months, tighten your perineum (do a pelvic floor exercise) and abdomen every time you turn on a water tap.

▼

Losing That Baby Fat Sensibly

Are you ready to get rid of the extra weight you gained during pregnancy? Not so fast! Remember that it took nine months to gain the weight; it's not going to come off in a week or two. The key to long-term weight control is a healthy diet combined with exercise.

However, you'd better not exercise vigorously the first six weeks. (Personally, I didn't have to worry about that; I was too tired!) Remember those hormones discussed in Chapter Five: The Third Trimester (the ones that caused your joints and pelvis to become more elastic)? Well, they haven't quite returned to normal yet, so take it easy for a while or you could damage some joints or ligaments. A simple walking regimen is a good start. It's a great way to show off your new baby to the neighbours or meet other new mums at the mall.

Chances are, if you were at your ideal weight before your pregnancy, you won't need any 'diet' at all. And if you are nursing, you shouldn't reduce your calorie intake below 1,800 calories. You may just need to consciously cut back on extras and fat intake (no more middle-of-the-night snacks!) and start moving more. The weight will come off gradually.

Many women want a programme to follow even if they have just 4.5 kg (10 pounds) to lose. Some women were overweight when they became pregnant; they may need something more structured. Later, we will review steps to help you evaluate a weight-loss programme.

Regardless of your situation, my advice is to lose as much of your excess weight as possible before you become pregnant again (that is, if you are planning to have another child). Many of the women I see for weight loss are in their fifties and explain that they never lost all their weight between pregnancies or after their last baby. By the time they see me, they are often forced to lose

weight for a medical reason: diabetes, high blood pressure, or heart disease. Avoid these problems now by controlling your weight sensibly.

I believe many people suffer from yo-yoing weight because they are in a hurry. I've seen this situation over and over in my weight-loss classes. Mary has been overweight for fifteen years, but now she has a class reunion to attend, and all of a sudden she wants to lose her weight *now*. It's human nature.

When we're motivated, we'll do anything to reach our goal quickly. The problem in applying this mindset to weight loss is that most people are easily discouraged and lose the battle before it really begins.

According to some experts, people need almost six months to truly change their habits. Yet Mary expects to do a major overhaul of her diet and lifestyle in two weeks!

When people change their diets drastically, they may at first lose weight quickly because much of it is water. Then, when weight loss tapers to 450 grams (1 pound) or less per week, people feel they're failing and give up. What they forget is that 450 grams (1 pound) per week adds up to 234 kg (52 pounds) per year! That's a lot of weight!

The key to losing weight permanently is determining which diet or lifestyle habits need changing, and then gradually altering eating habits, setting realistic goals, and adopting an exercise programme that you can stick with for life. Remember: Temporary changes may result in temporary weight loss.

Following are some of the characteristics I've observed in people who are most successful in losing weight. People who lose weight successfully . . .

- exercise regularly.[2]
- set realistic goals. When they don't meet their goals, they learn from their experiences instead of giving up.
- have social support from family, friends, co-workers, or support groups.[3] People who complete a weight-loss programme with friends or family lose more weight and are more likely to keep it off.
- work on liking themselves (or already do).
- are motivated to lose weight for internal reasons rather than external reasons.[4] For example, Judy used to lose weight to fit into her old size-six jeans. Now she is losing weight to improve her health.
- concentrate not on the bathroom scales, but on some positive outcome, such as lowered cholesterol or being able to walk further without becoming tired.
- have conquered emotional eating (eating when bored, angry, depressed, or stressed) or are working on it.[5]
- have learned to eat sensibly at restaurants, at parties, while travelling, and so on.
- work at self-monitoring. This may mean keeping a food diary, tracking the amount of fat eaten in a day, or logging those exercise hours each week.
- control their diet; they don't let their diet control them! They make educated, conscious choices about the food they eat. If they want to splurge for a special occasion, they do. They are honest with themselves about the reasons they eat.

▼

Weight-Loss Plans

Diet plans and diet books are abundant, but beware! Many of them promote quick weight loss, which is unhealthy. Others may recommend unbalanced diets, which leave out one or more foods or food groups. Some can be downright dangerous. Virtually all diets work – for the short term. However, many diets fail over the long term. Repeated weight loss and weight gain, often called weight cycling or yo-yo dieting, can be harmful to the body and devastating to the self-esteem.

Evaluating Weight-Loss Plans

The steps below can help you evaluate a weight-loss plan.

1. *Does the plan promote a balanced diet, allowing all foods in moderation? Does it omit certain foods or food groups?*
A balanced plan should allow all foods, even the so-called 'bad' ones, at some point in the programme.

2. *Does the plan include exercise?*
Exercise is so important to weight loss. Most people who lose weight lose some muscle along with fat. However, if you exercise, you will lose little or no muscle mass. Maintaining muscle mass helps you lose more weight, since muscle uses more calories than fat – even when you are sitting in front of the TV! A combination of aerobic and weight resistance exercise is very effective for losing weight and shaping up.

3. *Does the plan include behaviour modification (changing current behaviours)?*
For long-term weight loss, you must identify your problem behaviours so you can work to change them. Some tools used for behaviour modification might include self-monitoring (keeping a diet record) or exercises that promote an awareness of eating patterns.

4. *Does the plan use trained professionals as counsellors or people whose only qualifications are that they have lost weight?*
Many plans use people who have lost weight or are good salespeople as counsellors. Though these people may be good motivators, they may give out inaccurate information unintentionally.

There are lots of quacks out there trying to make a quick dollar. Beware of anything that sounds too good to be true; it probably is. Look for counsellors who are licensed, registered, or have a degree from an accredited college or university.

5. *Does the plan involve buying special foods or supplements?*
Personally, I feel that learning how to eat 'real' food is better for long-term weight loss. However, some people like the convenience of packaged foods.

6. *Does the plan provide a foundation for good future eating habits?*
Hopefully, the plan teaches you how to cook healthfully, plan menus, and eat sensibly in social situations.

The Moderate Approach

The recommended post-pregnant weight loss is about 450 grams (1 pound) or less per week. You're probably thinking, 'So little a week! I'll never lose this weight!' Consider the importance of long-term success, which means keeping the weight off. People who lose weight slowly seem to keep it off the longest.

To lose 450 grams (1 pound) per week, you can cut your food intake by 500 calories per day, use more calories by exercising, or combine eating less and exercising more. For example, Colleen walks about 2 miles every evening, which uses approximately 200 calories. She has also cut 300 calories of extras out of her diet. Colleen's diet-and-exercise approach works best for long-term weight maintenance. Besides being good for muscle tone, cardiovascular health, and endurance, exercise is also good for your mental health! Following is an example of a good fitness programme. Most of these activities can be done with a baby nearby or in a front pack. Postnatal exercise programmes often encourage baby participation. As you can see, fitness doesn't have to be boring!

Suggested Activity Programme for Colleen
Height: 5'4"
Weight: 72.5 kg (160 pounds)
Goal Weight: 54.5 kg (120 pounds)
Activity Goals: Aerobic activity 5 hours per week, strength training ½ hour twice per week

Monday: 1 hour of postnatal exercise class

Tuesday: 30-minute walk at lunch, 30 minutes of strength training after dinner

Wednesday: 1 hour of postnatal exercise class

Thursday: 30-minute walk with baby in front pack, 30 minutes of strength training

Friday: Colleen's day off

Saturday: 1-hour hike with baby in front pack

Sunday: 1 hour of gardening

By following this activity programme, Colleen burns over 1,700 calories! To lose 450 grams (1 pound) per week, she also needs to reduce her diet by 1,800 calories per week or about 250 calories per day. (Please note that the numbers of calories burned are calculated specifically for Colleen.)

The chart below lists a few of the extras Colleen eats that she can easily cut from her diet. These changes add up to a reduction of over 700 calories per day. Colleen will only need to follow half the proposed changes to lose 450 grams (1 pound) per week.

Depending on your weight, height, and activity level, you will probably want to eat between 1,200 and 1,800 calories per day to lose 1 pound per week. Eating under 1,200 calories is usually not advised unless you have a petite build.

Lose Weight by Leaning toward Vegetarianism

Cutting down on animal protein is one good way to cut calories and fat, which can lead to weight loss. Leaning toward vegetarianism, or even becoming vegetarian, might be a good idea. While testing meatless recipes for the book *Make the Change for a Healthy Heart,* I was losing weight without even trying. I had to consciously eat extra snacks to avoid losing weight! (See Chapter Six for more on vegetarian eating.)

Here are two good sources to help vegetarians with weight loss: *Simple, Low-Fat, and Vegetarian* by Suzanne Havala, M.S., R.D.

Low-Fat Food Substitutions			
Food	**Calories**	**Action**	**Calories Saved**
1 tablespoon margarine	100	Substitute low-fat spread	100
1 cola drink	150	Substitute diet cola	148
2 chocolate-chip cookies	140	Substitute 1 peach	100
1 cinnamon roll	230	Substitute 1 Quaker Caramel Corn Cake	180
3 cups full-cream milk	450	Substitute semi-skimmed milk	90
3 tablespoons blue cheese dressing	180	Substitute low-fat dressing	120

(Vegetarian Resource Group, 1994) and *Vegetarian Weight Loss Guide* by Suzanne Havala, M.S., R.D., published in *Vegetarian Journal Reports* (Vegetarian Resource Group, 1990).

Lose That Baby Fat Eating Plan

This meal plan has about 1,500 calories and is meant to be a rough guideline for healthy weight loss. While some women prefer a structured plan, many women do well just concentrating on eating more fruits and vegetables and cutting back on extra fats. This meal plan does not contain enough calories or nutrients for breast-feeding mothers.

7 servings of starches/grains
1 serving is 1 slice any type bread, 1 flour tortilla, 8 tbsp pasta, 8 tbsp rice or legumes, 6 savoury biscuits, or 8 tbsp potato.

3 servings of fruits
1 serving is 1 medium piece fresh fruit, ½ banana, 8 tbsp tinned fruit in its own juice, 250 g (8 oz) melon or berries, 2 plums, or 2 nectarines.

3 or more servings of vegetables
1 serving is 8 tbsp any nonstarchy vegetable or 65 g (2½ oz) lettuce.

5 protein equivalents
1 protein equivalent is 25 g (1 oz) lean meat, 25 g (1 oz) reduced-fat cheese, 4 tbsp cottage cheese, 8 tbsp tofu, 2 tbsp peanut butter, 8 tbsp cooked dried beans, or 1 egg.

2 to 3 servings of dairy products
1 serving is 250 ml (8 fl oz) skimmed or semi-skimmed milk or low-fat yogurt.

If you have just stopped breast-feeding, aim for 4 servings per day to help boost bone mineralization.

3 servings of fat
1 serving is 1 teaspoon margarine or butter or 2 teaspoons reduced-fat margarine, 1 teaspoon mayonnaise or 2 teaspoons reduced-fat mayonnaise, 1 slice bacon, 15 g (½ oz) cream cheese, 1 tablespoon soured cream, ⅛ avocado, 10 peanuts, or 5 olives.

For more information about weight loss or healthy eating, see the Recommended Resources in the back of this book.

? Questions You May Have

Q: I've never been much of a breakfast eater, but I've heard that it's good for you. Is it?

A: You may have heard that breakfast is the most important meal of the day. In many respects, that's true. A recent study showed that people who skipped breakfast had trouble working on tasks that required concentration. Diane Odland, nutritionist at the U.S. Department of Agriculture Human Nutrition Information Service, says, 'When you consider it's been eight or nine hours since you've had a meal, it's obvious that refuelling at breakfast will make you feel and perform better during the day.'[6]

Eating breakfast can also help you lose weight. People who skip the first meal of the day often make up for it later by eating larger meals or snacking on high-fat, high-sugar foods. Whether you stay home with a child or work outside the home, eating breakfast will definitely improve your energy level.

Q: Will I lose all my pregnancy weight without really trying?

A: It depends on how much you gained. In one study, women who gained more than 9 kg (20 pounds) retained from 2.25 to 4.5 kg (5 to 10 pounds) between pregnancies. Those who gained over 18 kg (40 pounds) were an average of 7.75 kg (17 pounds) heavier at the start of their next pregnancy. Since the current recommendation for weight gain is over 11.5 kg (25 pounds), you will probably have to make an active effort to lose the weight.[7]

Q: How long will it take me to lose my baby fat?

A: Again, it depends on how much you gained, how much you eat, and how active you are. A lucky few fit into their pre-pregnancy clothes right after delivery, though that wasn't the case for me or any of my friends.

The amount of time needed to lose the weight and get your old body back is probably a big surprise to every mother. Much to my disappointment, I needed almost nine months to return to my normal weight. I thought I'd be back to my old self within a few months. Doing aerobics three times a week made the biggest change in the way my body looked and helped me lose those stubborn last 2.25 kg (5 pounds).

When I surveyed other dietitians about this book, several suggested that I outline some realistic expectations for weight loss and body size after pregnancy. Here are some things you should expect:

- Very few people go back to wearing their 'skinny' clothes right after delivery. Expect to wear your maternity clothes for a few more months – even though you probably feel like burning them!
- You may need to buy a few outfits one size bigger than you wore before pregnancy to wear until you get your shape back.
- Your body may have reproportioned itself. For example, Kate weighs the same as she did before pregnancy, but her hips are a few inches wider. Most of us continue to have a little tummy unless we diligently practise abdominal exercises. Some women find their rib cages permanently expanded and need to wear a larger bra size. Believe it or not, some women even wear a larger shoe size after pregnancy.
- If you are breast-feeding, you may feel as though you are bursting out of your blouses. Judy was exasperated because, for the first few months of breastfeeding, the only shirts she could wear were her husband's T-shirts and her old maternity shirts. Sandy, however, was glad to have an excuse to buy new clothes!
- Many women lose the last bit of weight after they stop breast-feeding.
- Exercise can't be emphasized enough. It will help you lose baby fat and tone up some of the muscles you haven't used in quite a while.

• Overall, be patient. I clearly remember asking my aerobics teacher how fast I could get into shape after the baby came, if I worked out regularly. I wanted *real* numbers. She said it could be done in six to eight weeks, but I might need time for recovery. 'Not me,' I thought. I was going to be Supermum! Well, after a tough labour and delivery and a long adjustment to motherhood, months passed before I had the time and energy to restart my exercise programme. After my second son was born, I didn't have a problem losing the weight. I breast-fed him longer and I was much more active chasing two kids around.

▼

Preparing for Your Next Pregnancy

Sometime after your labour anaesthesia wears off and before you send out birth announcements, someone will ask, 'So when are you going to have another baby?' You may not be ready to answer that question for a long time. On the other hand, you may want another baby right away. I recommend waiting at least eighteen months before you become pregnant again. A study of nearly 300,000 infants showed that women with less than eighteen months between pregnancies were 14 to 47 per cent more likely to have very premature and moderately premature infants than women with intervals of one-and-a-half to five years.[8] In the meantime, consider getting back to your ideal body weight and following the advice on page 208 for reducing environmental pollutants in your diet. Most importantly, enjoy that baby of yours! The time passes quickly! When you are ready to think about getting pregnant again, turn to Chapter One: Contemplating Pregnancy to learn what you can do for a healthy pregnancy *before* you conceive.

No matter when you decide to have another baby, or even if you decide not to, don't lose the good habits you established during pregnancy. A healthy diet is one of the most important things you can do to ensure good health for you and your children, and teaching your children good eating habits is one of the most precious gifts you can give them.

CHAPTER TEN

Fitting Fitness In

What you will find in this chapter:

- *Benefits of Exercise*
- *What Every Pregnant Woman Should Know about Exercise*
- *Fitting Fitness into Your Busy Lifestyle*
- *Exercise after Pregnancy*
- *Tips for Getting with the Programme after Your Baby Is Born*

This chapter answers such questions as:

- *What if I don't have time for exercise?*
- *Should I exercise differently while I'm pregnant?*
- *How can I relieve back pain?*
- *How does exercise fit in for those on bed rest?*
- *How can I get back in shape after I have my baby?*

Benefits of Exercise

Throughout this book I've mentioned exercise over and over again. I'm hoping repetition will bring home the message that exercise is one of the most important things you can do for your present and future health. Regular exercise can bring you numerous benefits from a small time investment.

While you are pregnant, exercise offers even more benefits:

- Exercise helps battle the fatigue many women feel during pregnancy.
- Exercise makes you physically fit and helps your body get ready for labour.
- Exercise helps you feel better about your expanding body.
- Once you've established a fitness routine, resuming exercising after you have your baby (when you're trying to lose weight) will be easier.
- If you have diabetes, exercise can help you control your blood glucose. But always check with your doctor for exercise advice.
- Exercise classes for pregnant women can help you find interaction and support from a group that understands what you're experiencing.
- Regular exercise will help you sleep better. You may need all the sleep you can get during those last few weeks of pregnancy!
- Exercise will probably help you feel better all over. You'll have a better emotional outlook and you may have improved immunity.

A former couch potato says, 'I was never interested in exercising, but when I became pregnant, my doctor suggested I get involved in an exercise programme for pregnant women at the YWCA. I went to an aerobics class mostly for my baby, and much to my surprise, I began to really enjoy it. I shared labour and delivery stories with other mums-to-be and began a mummy network. Toward the end of my pregnancy, exercise really helped me sleep better. Also, I felt much less tired than I did with my first pregnancy. I had more energy and felt vivacious.'

If you didn't exercise before you were pregnant, you should ask your health-care provider about exercising. He or she may have some special guidelines for you, depending on your current situation. If you exercised routinely before pregnancy, you can probably continue your exercise program with some modifications.

▼

What Every Pregnant Woman Should Know about Exercise

Note: For the most part, these guidelines also apply to the postpartum period.[1]

▶ Don't do too much at first.

Have you ever watched the Olympics and gotten so inspired that you wanted to jump up, drive to the gym, and work out for an hour – even though you hadn't done any exercise in months? Don't! Start out slowly and exercise as little as five minutes per day, and don't forget to warm up and cool down.

▶ Be kind to your joints.

The hormones of pregnancy make joints very elastic, which prepares them for childbirth. Exercise that involves lots of bouncing, jerky movement, jumping, or quick changes in direction could cause joint pain or injury. You should also avoid deep flexing or extending your muscles. Use gentle stretches to cool down instead of stretching to the limit.

▶ Avoid ironman marathons and other rigorous events unless you are already an athlete and you have your doctor's permission.

Stay away from competitive sports. Stick to walking, swimming, or low-impact aerobics (preferably aerobic classes developed just for pregnant women).

▶ Do kinder, gentler exercise.

The extra weight gain in pregnancy changes your body's centre of gravity, so you should avoid sports like downhill skiing, skating, and skateboarding that involve a high risk of falling. Exercise on a wooden floor or a securely carpeted surface to reduce shock and to provide sure footing.

▶ Be consistent.

Regular exercise is best, even if it's only a few minutes per day. Thousands of people are would-be exercisers with good intentions. Their homes are full of treadmills, stationary bikes, rowing machines, and weight sets. Unfortunately, many collections of exercise paraphernalia serve as dust collectors and clothes racks. Their owners would be much better off if they simply set aside fifteen minutes a day to go for a walk.

▶ Warm up and cool down.

Always begin with a five-minute warm-up period of low-intensity exercise, such as slow walking, cycling, or water walking for swimmers, to warm up your muscles, followed by ten minutes of stretching. Strenuous exercise should last fifteen minutes, unless you were exercising before you were pregnant; in that case, check with your doctor. Follow a period of intense exercise with ten to fifteen minutes of cool-down and stretching.

▶ Exercise at least three times per week.

Exercising just twenty minutes a day, three times per week, is much better for you than being a weekend athlete.

▶ Measure your heart rate during exercise.

Exercising too intensely can increase your body's internal temperature and harm your foetus. Measure your pulse at the peak of your activity and also before cool-down. To measure your pulse, place your index finger at your carotid artery on your neck. Keep moving. Count your heart rate for either six or ten seconds. A pregnant woman's heart rate should not exceed 140 beats per minute (fourteen beats in six seconds or twenty-three beats in ten seconds). Check with your health-care provider for alternate guidelines.

▶ Take your time.

Get up from the floor slowly to avoid dizziness or fainting caused by a sudden drop in blood pressure.

▶ Drink, drink, drink!

Drink water before, during, and after exercise to prevent dehydration. Drinking will also help cool you off. Take a plastic bottle filled with water on your walk or to aerobics.

▶ Stay out of the heat.

Don't do any vigorous exercise in hot, humid weather or when you have a fever.

▶ Watch out for danger signs.

Stop your activity immediately and call your doctor if any of these symptoms occur: pain, bleeding, dizziness, shortness of breath, rapid heartbeat, back pain, pubic pain, and/or difficulty walking.

▶ Be kind to yourself.

Think of exercise as a special time for you. You may not always agree, but exercise is a way to pamper yourself!

▶ Eat enough food.

During pregnancy, blood sugar levels are usually lower than non-pregnant levels, and your body uses carbohydrates at a greater rate. So you might have low blood sugar during strenuous exercise. Make sure you don't exercise on an empty stomach. You may want to have some savoury biscuits, fresh or dried fruit, or juice before your workout for more energy.

If you worked out regularly before pregnancy and continue to have a vigorous workout schedule, keep in mind that you will need to increase your calories accordingly.

Your weight gain will let you know if you're eating enough.

Following are some reasons why exercise should be toned down during pregnancy.

- Your resting heart rate is higher than a non-pregnant woman's, and it also rises more quickly during exercise. So watch the intensity of your exercise.
- Your body temperature may rise more rapidly than a non-pregnant woman's. And since your baby's body temperature is always 1°F warmer than yours, elevating your body temperature could mean trouble for your baby. Be careful of how hard and how long you exercise.
- After your fourth month, your uterus may compress your inferior vena cava – the main blood vessel returning blood to your heart. This could interfere with blood flow to your baby. (After your fourth month, don't do any exercise while lying flat on your back.)
- Some hormones relax joints and connective tissue in preparation for delivery and can make joints susceptible to injury. Treat your joints gently by doing slow stretches daily and don't forget to warm up and cool down!
- Some studies have shown that vigorous activity can cause contractions, which may lead to premature labour. One study done with women who had gestational diabetes showed that the safest exercises were those that used mostly the upper body or those that applied little stress below the waist. Researchers found that walking on a treadmill was fine, but jogging was likely to cause contractions. Exercising on a conventional stationary bike caused contractions in half of the women, and exercising on a recumbent bicycle (one in which you sit back with your legs in front of you, not under you) caused no contractions. The upper-arm ergometer proved to be the safest exercise machine. It is similar to a stationary bicycle but is pedalled with the arms.[2]

For more specific information about exercise, ask your doctor or antenatal clinic. Always check with your doctor before starting an exercise programme, especially if you haven't recently exercised.

When You Shouldn't Exercise

According to the American College of Obstetricians and Gynecologists, several conditions totally restrict you from exercising vigorously.[3] If any of these conditions apply to you, consult your doctor before exercising.

- History of three or more miscarriages
- Ruptured membranes
- Premature labour
- Diagnosed multiple gestation (twins, triplets, or more)
- Incompetent cervix
- Bleeding or a diagnosis of placenta previa
- Diagnosed cardiac disease

Some conditions may require you to limit strenuous exercise.[4] If any of these conditions apply to you, be sure to talk with your doctor before starting an exercise programme.

- High blood pressure
- Anaemia or other blood disorder
- Thyroid disease
- Diabetes
- Cardiac arrhythmia or palpitations
- History of premature labour
- History of intra-uterine growth retardation (slowed growth of foetus)
- History of bleeding during current pregnancy
- Breech position of baby in last trimester
- Excessive obesity
- Extreme underweight
- History of extremely sedentary lifestyle

▼

Fitting Fitness into Your Busy Lifestyle

Some people don't exercise regularly because they don't think they have time. It's true: We live in a very fast-paced society. Yet most of us probably have fifteen minutes a day that we waste. Here are a few ideas for fitting fitness into your lifestyle:

▶ **Take a walk every morning before work.**

If you happen to have a treadmill, you can walk while watching the morning news.

▶ **Make more trips up and down the stairs.**

For example, you could unplug the downstairs phone so that every time the phone rings, you need to go up and down the stairs once. Tricks like this will give you more activity, but remember that such activity uses only short bursts of energy and won't improve your overall fitness much.

▶ **Use half your lunch hour to take a walk.**

I did this on the days I didn't go to aerobics. The funny part of it was that I had to turn down many rides. Everyone must have felt sorry for the big pregnant woman walking down the street!

▶ **Write your exercise dates on your calendar and keep them!**

▶ **Exercise with your partner or a friend.**

▶ **Walk the dog; your pooch will love you for it!**

▶ **Sign up for an exercise class just for pregnant women.**

Sometimes, if you pay for a class, you are more motivated to go.

▶ **On the weekend, take a drive to the country where you can walk while admiring scenic views.**

▶ **Get the whole family into exercising!**

Take walks or hikes together.

▶ **Rent or purchase an exercise video just for pregnant women.**

Your Personal Exercise Schedule

Take a moment to write your exercise plan overleaf.

My goal is to exercise _____
times per week, for _____
minutes each time.

My Exercise Schedule:

Monday _____
(time)

Tuesday _____

Wednesday_____

Thursday _____

Friday _____

Saturday_____

Sunday _____

Ten Sneaky Ways to Exercise

Not everyone truly enjoys exercising. If you cringe at the idea of a daily workout, you can increase your physical activity without a planned exercise routine.

▶ **Walk the dog.**

▶ **Shop 'til you drop.**

Or you can walk around the entire mall and window-shop.

▶ **Go dancing!**

Ballroom, country-western, or even square dancing will do. Or put on your favourite music at home and cut a rug!

▶ **Take a stroll around a scenic place like a lake, a tree-lined avenue, or a forest trail.**

▶ **Go canoeing or paddleboating.**

▶ **Do arm exercises using 450-gram (1-pound) weights or tins of soup while watching your favourite show.**

▶ **Go to the pool and just walk from side to side.**

Bring a friend. You won't notice the time passing as you chat away.

▶ **Try aerobic lawn mowing.**

Cut your grass with a push mower and start a fad in your neighbourhood.

▶ **Plant a garden.**

A bonus of gardening is enjoying the fruits of your labour. If you don't care for gardening, clean your house often; vacuuming *can* be aerobic.

▶ **Set a walking date with a neighbour or co-worker.**

Once you get to talking, you'll hardly notice the time or the exercise.

▼

Exercise after Pregnancy

Women often face weight problems after having children. Those last 2.25 kg (5 pounds) just don't seem to come off. If you add another 2.25 kg (5 pounds) with another pregnancy, before you know it, you're 7 to 9 kg (15 to 20 pounds) overweight.

Research has shown that people who exercise regularly lose more weight and have the best odds of keeping it off. Other benefits of exercising include improved cardiovascular fitness, lowered heart rate, lowered blood pressure, decreased blood lipids, decreased blood sugar, toned muscles, less body fat, improved immunity, and more!

After you have your baby, it may be a while before you feel motivated to exercise. That's okay. You have just gone through one of life's biggest events. You may need some time to get used to having a baby in the house and to set up a new routine. (I needed four months to adjust!) Remember those hormones that made your joints more elastic so that your pelvis could stretch for childbirth? Weeks will pass before those hormones drop to their normal levels. Most doctors will approve an exercise programme after the six-week check-up. Until then, walking is generally fine.

A new mother says, 'I was one of those people who thought I would be out of the house and back to exercising within days after delivery. Surprise, surprise! After a week, I still had trouble walking! My neighbour had a C-section, and she was taking her baby on a walk in the stroller when he was just four days old! I was jealous!'

Women have unique labour experiences. Some breeze through labour in a few hours. Other labours last a day and a half. If you had a long labour, it may have taken a lot out of you. If you had stitches, haemorrhoids, or both, it may be even longer before you'll feel okay walking and sitting. Be prepared for the best or worst situation, and remember that this, too, shall pass.

You Don't Have to Be a Race Walker to Lose Weight!

One study compared the effects of low-intensity and high-intensity exercise. Women who walked four days a week for twelve weeks lost 2.25 kg (5 pounds) of body fat, whether they exercised slowly or vigorously. Women in both groups burned 300 calories during each workout. Low-intensity walkers lost more body fat in the abdomen and buttocks, so if those areas are a problem for you, you may want to exercise at a slower rate.[5]

▼

Tips for Getting with the Programme after Your Baby Is Born

▶ **Start at your own pace, no matter how slow it seems.**

▶ **Stretching is important, even if you don't feel like exercising.**

▶ **Find activities you enjoy and include other family members if possible.**

▶ **Join a fitness class for mothers and babies.**

You won't feel as though you are the only one out of shape in such a class. You can meet other mums there, and you won't have to find daycare.

▶ **Schedule your time.**

While you are at home the first six weeks, the days seem to drift by. A schedule that includes some activity will give you a sense of purpose.

► **When you have time during baby's naps, pop in an exercise video.**

Thousands of exercise videos are now available. The most important aspect of exercising is simply doing it. Do whatever it takes to get started, but just do it! (See the Recommended Resources section at the back of this book for more fitness resources.)

► **Check out these on-line fitness resources:**

Fit Pregnancy Magazine
www.fitpregnancy.com

American College of Sports Medicine
www.acsm.org

American Academy of Family Practice
www.aafp.org

? Questions You May Have

Q: Won't exercise make me more tired?

A: At first you may feel a little more tired after exercising while pregnant. This tiredness is a result of the extra weight you are carrying and the extra blood that must be pumped through your heart. (During the first trimester, hormonal changes can also cause fatigue.) However, since exercise increases endurance, you will gradually feel less tired as your body gets accustomed to exercise. Of course, if you are already exercising, you shouldn't feel as tired. If you do, you may not be eating enough foods or the right foods.

Q: How will I know if I'm eating enough while exercising during pregnancy?

A: The rule of thumb here is to eat when you're hungry and to watch your weight gain. If you're not gaining enough, you need to eat more. If you have a busy schedule and just can't seem to eat enough, you may need to slow down. (See page 247 for high-energy snack ideas.)

Q: I'm on bedrest. How can I prevent my body from turning into flab?

A: Pregnancy often causes us to make changes in our lifestyle and habits. Bedrest takes this to the extreme. You *will* lose your level of fitness while on bedrest. However, by stretching and doing isometric exercises (if approved by your doctor), you can retain some of your muscle tone. Ask your doctor for a list of suggested exercises to keep yourself limber and for permission to do arm exercises. And remember that after you have your baby, your endurance for exercise will be very low. You'll need to start out slowly. I thought I would need practically *forever* to get back into shape after I was off bedrest. In just a few weeks, my endurance returned to normal. Your body *will* bounce back, and you *can* become fit again, so think of your situation as a temporary one.

Q: My back hurts all the time lately. What can I do?

A: I can sympathize with you. During the last two months of my pregnancy, I couldn't sweep and mop the kitchen floor in the same afternoon because my back hurt so much. I finally wised up and gave that job to my husband.

Your back undergoes a great deal of stress during pregnancy. Most traditional back-strengthening exercises are not recommended during pregnancy because you perform them lying on your back. One that is recommended is the pelvic tilt. If you are attending an exercise class for pregnant women, you probably already know this exercise. If not, here's a quick tutorial:[6]

How to Do a Pelvic Tilt

1. Stand with feet shoulder-width apart and knees slightly bent.

2. Contract the muscles of the buttocks and abdomen and gently thrust your pelvis forward, rotating your pubic bone upward. Hold this position for ten seconds and release.

3. The pelvic tilt can be done while lying or squatting on your hands and knees.

You should try to do the pelvic tilt as often as possible during the day. Keep in mind that after your delivery, lifting and carrying can still be painful. Continue doing pelvic tilts and other back-strengthening exercises to improve your back health. Keeping your stomach muscles strong will support the back muscles and will prevent back strain. Stomach crunches (or half sit-ups) are a great tummy exercise for the postpartum period.

For more information on exercise, I recommend *Essential Exercises for the Child-bearing Year*, an excellent book by Elizabeth Noble.

Section II

Shopping, Cooking, and Eating Out

CHAPTER ELEVEN

Stocking the Pregnant Kitchen

What you will find in this chapter:

• *Check Out Your Kitchen*

• *A Peek in My Kitchen*

• *Reading Food Labels*

• *Eating on a Budget*

• *Stocking the Kitchen Toolbox*

• *Keeping the Vitamins in Your Vegetables*

• *The Essential Guide to Food Safety*

• *How to Lower Your Risk*

• *Food Safety Reports: Whom to Believe?*

• *Food Safety in a Nutshell*

This chapter answers such questions as:

• *How can I start shopping more healthfully?*

• *What do 'lite', 'light', and 'low-fat' mean on a food label?*

• *Is homemade eggnog safe to drink?*

• *Should I avoid fish?*

• *Why is a variety of foods so important?*

• *How can I eat well if I have a limited food budget?*

• *How can I avoid food poisoning?*

So, now you're motivated to eat well! If your diet is already good, you may not need much help. But if you're turning over a new leaf nutritionally, you may be thinking, 'Where do I begin?'

The best place to start improving your diet is, of course, your own kitchen. First, you need to identify your shopping and eating patterns so you can change them if necessary.

Check Out Your Kitchen

1. What takes up the bulk of room in your freezer? Frozen vegetables? Ice cream? Frozen juice? Fish, chicken, or meat? Fish fingers? Frozen dinners? Frozen pies or cheesecakes? Pizza?

2. Does the top shelf of your fridge hold milk or soft drinks?

3. Are your produce drawers bulging with fresh fruits and veggies, or do they contain only a few lonely, shrivelled carrots?

4. Does your pantry hold many convenience foods? Tinned vegetables and fruits? Potato crisps? Sweets?

5. Do you keep on hand a mix of grains, such as brown rice, pasta, bulgur, wholemeal flour, wheatgerm, oats, and barley, or just white flour, rice, and pasta?

6. Do you keep a variety of vegetables in the house or do you regularly eat your two favourite vegetables and fruits?

▼

A Peek in My Kitchen

People are always curious about how I, a registered dietitian, eat at home. I think they envision my family eating perfectly all the time. They don't realize that we are just like any other family; we have our habits, our likes, and our dislikes. To show you how my family eats and shops, I'll let you take a peek in my kitchen.

In My Cupboards

Tinned tomatoes, tomato sauce, tomato paste

Spaghetti sauce without meat

Tinned sweetcorn, peas, sweet potatoes, pumpkin

Tinned black beans, vegetarian refried beans, kidney beans

Cup o Soup (bean or lentil)

Dried lentils, split peas

Tinned tuna, salmon

White and wholemeal flour

Skimmed evaporated milk

Yeast, sugar, brown sugar, molasses, honey

White rice, brown rice, bulgur, barley, and lots of pasta

Sun-dried tomatoes

Raisin Bran, All Bran, economy-size old-fashioned oatmeal, low-fat granola or muesli

Raisins, mixed dried fruit

Canola oil, olive oil, soy sauce

Many miscellaneous spices

Apple cider vinegar, red wine vinegar, tarragon wine vinegar

Digestive biscuits, corn cakes, pretzels

Toblerone or Cadbury chocolate (My motto: Buy the best, but eat one piece at a time!)

Baked potato crisps, baked tortilla chips, Guiltless Gourmet Oil-Free Tortilla Chips

In My Freezer

Miscellaneous frozen juices

Nutri-Grain waffles

Fish fingers

Trout, salmon, sole, prawns

Chicken, turkey breast

Mashed bananas (to use in banana bread or pancakes)

Chopped spinach or broccoli, mixed vegetables, peas

Frozen healthy entrées

In My Refrigerator

Skimmed milk, eggs, processed cheese, part-skimmed mozzarella cheese, reduced-fat or fat-free Cheddar, fresh Parmesan cheese, Diet Coke, decaffeinated iced tea

Miscellaneous meat, fish, or chicken, thawing

Flavoured low-fat yogurt, fat-free soured cream

Ham or turkey breast deli meat

Yogurt Spread, I Can't Believe It's Not Butter! (light)

Peanut butter

Mayonnaise, fat-free mayonnaise, homemade vinaigrette dressing, homemade dip or dressing (almost fat-free), fat-free herb dressing, barbecue

sauce, teriyaki marinade, ketchup, hoisin sauce, grated ginger, chopped garlic in a jar, Dijon mustard, capers, horseradish, lemon juice, wheatgerm and wheat bran (to prevent rancidity)
Various leftovers

In My Produce Drawers

Summer: all kinds of berries, cantaloupe melon, watermelon, apricots, nectarines, peaches, mangos, pineapple, lemons, tomatoes, carrots, cucumber, courgettes, aubergine, red and green peppers, sprouts, ready-to-eat salad mix, cos or soft leaf lettuce

Winter: apples, bananas, pears, grapes, oranges, grapefruit, dates, figs, aubergine, acorn squash, butternut squash, carrots, leeks, cabbage, broccoli, cauliflower, tomato, lettuce, cucumber

▼

Reading Food Labels

Chances are, you are more concerned about what you eat now than you were just a few months ago. Your favourite new pastime may be studying food labels. Why should you read labels? It's the perfect way to put your nutrition knowledge into practice and make informed purchases.

What Can You Learn from a Label?

In 1990 the US Congress passed the Nutrition Labeling and Education Act, and in 1991 the Food and Drug Administration (FDA) proposed label revisions in accordance with the new law. According to Dr. David Kessler, then Commissioner of the FDA, the old food labels placed consumers at a disadvantage. The new labels 'take the guesswork – and the element of chance – out of food labelling'.

Food labels now contain a gold mine of information. For example, by looking on my box of Raisin Bran, I can see how many calories, how many grams of fibre, and how much sugar or sodium a serving contains. I can find how much protein and fat it has. I can also check out how vitamin A, vitamin C, calcium, and iron in a serving of Raisin Bran stack up. Suppose I'm allergic to milk protein. I can look for it on the list of ingredients.

Following is a list of everything required on a food label:[1]

- Total calories
- Calories from fat
- Total fat
- Saturated fat
- Cholesterol
- Sodium
- Total carbohydrate
- Dietary fibre
- Sugars
- Protein
- Vitamins A and C, calcium, and iron
- Nutrient information (listed in customary serving sizes using household measures)

It has been proposed that the amount of trans fat be included on food labels and in defining nutrient content and health claims. Trans fats are formed when liquid oils are hydrogenated to form solids like margarine and shortening. Trans fats can raise serum cholesterol the same way saturated fat does and can increase the risk of coronary heart disease.

You'll also find that certain terms have standard meanings:[2]

Fat-free: Less than ½ gram of fat per serving and no added fat.

Low-fat: Contains 3 grams of fat or less per 100-gram (3½-ounce) serving.

Light: Has at least ⅓ fewer calories than or ½ the fat of a comparable product. Can also mean that a low-calorie, low-fat food has had its sodium reduced by 50 per cent. May mean light texture or colour.

Reduced: Has at least 25 per cent less of a nutrient or calories than the regular product.

Low in saturated fat: Contains 1 gram or less of saturated fat per serving.

Lean: Has less than 10 grams of fat, 4½ grams of saturated fat, and 95 milligrams of cholesterol per serving.

Extra lean: Contains less than 5 grams of fat, 2 grams of saturated fat, and 95 milligrams of cholesterol per serving.

Cholesterol-free: Has less than 2 milligrams of cholesterol and 2 grams or less of saturated fat per serving.

Low in cholesterol: Contains 20 milligrams or less of cholesterol and 2 grams or less of saturated fat per 100-gram (3½-ounce) serving.

Per cent fat-free: Can only be used on low-fat or fat-free products.

Low sodium: Has less than 140 milligrams of sodium per 100-gram (3½-ounce) serving.

Very low sodium: Contains less than 35 milligrams of sodium per 100-gram (3½-ounce) serving.

Calorie-free: Has fewer than 5 calories per serving.

Sugar-free: Contains less than ½ gram of sugar per serving.

High in: Has 20 per cent or more of the daily requirement for a particular nutrient.

Good source of: Contains 10 to 19 per cent of the daily requirement for a particular nutrient.

Nutrition and Health Claims

Health claims describing the relationship between a food or nutrient and the risk of a disease or health-related condition are allowed on food labels. The health claim must meet certain requirements and must be phrased so that consumers can understand the food-disease relationship. Some such relationships are:

- Folic acid – neural tube defects
- Calcium – osteoporosis
- Sodium – hypertension
- Dietary saturated fat and cholesterol – risk of coronary heart disease
- Fruits, vegetables, and grain products

that contain fibre (particularly soluble fibre) – risk of coronary heart disease
• Dietary fat – cancer
• Fruits and vegetables – cancer
• Fibre-containing grain products, fruits, and vegetables – cancer
• Dietary sugar alcohols – dental caries (cavities)
• Wholegrain foods and other plant foods – heart disease and cancer
• Soya protein – reduced risk of coronary heart disease

The Ingredient List

Every food label carries a list of ingredients arranged in descending order by weight. Even standardized foods, such as mayonnaise and ice cream, have a list of ingredients. In addition, all FDA-certified colour additives must be listed by name. Another helpful requirement is that beverages that claim to contain juice must declare the total percentage of juice present: for example, 'Juice blend – 2 to 7 per cent juice.'

Sugar Is Sugar by Many Names

Some ingredients have many names, which makes deciphering food labels tricky. Corn syrup, high-fructose corn syrup, dextrose, glucose, corn sweetener, sucrose, sugar, brown sugar, fructose, maltose, sorbitol, mannitol, honey, and fruit-juice concentrate are all types of sweeteners.

There are also artificial sweeteners, sometimes called non-nutritive or non-caloric sweeteners, that are widely found in diet products: NutraSweet (the sweetener in Equal), saccharin (found in Sweet 'n Low and Sugar Twin), acesulfame K (found in Sweet One), and sucralose (found in Splenda). (See page 119 for information on using these products during pregnancy.)

Let's find out how looking at a food label can help you make a healthier food choice. To most people, jam is jam. You may look at the price per weight and pick up the cheapest. Or you may be partial to a particular brand and not look twice at the others. After all, jam is jam…right? Let's see.

Jam #1
Ingredients: High-fructose corn syrup, strawberries, pectin, natural flavouring.

Jam #2
Ingredients: Strawberries, high-fructose corn syrup, pectin, natural flavouring.

The better choice would be Jam #2, which gram for gram/ounce for ounce contains more strawberries than sugar.

Other Ingredients to Look For

Hey, what are all those funny words on food labels? You may have noticed there are many other things on ingredient lists besides food; these other ingredients are called food additives. An additive is a substance other than a basic foodstuff that is in food as a result of production, processing, storage, or packaging.

The media has given a lot of attention to food additives – so much that the word *additive* may have negative connotations to you. In truth, additives often protect our food from spoilage (and therefore keep us from getting ill) and bring clear benefits. For example, many foods are fortified with vitamins and minerals, which are considered additives. Many new fat-free products contain plant gums or seaweed derivatives that have been used safely for centuries. These are also considered additives.

Listed below are the main categories of additives and what they do.

Preservatives: Help give food a longer shelf life by retarding spoilage.

Antimicrobials: Prevent food spoilage from bacteria, mould, or fungus. For example, calcium propionate is used to keep bread from moulding.

Antioxidants: Prevent oil-containing foods from going rancid and also delay browning. Vitamin C (ascorbic acid) is commonly used in meats as an antioxidant.

Curing agents: Prevent spoilage in meats. Sodium nitrate is a curing agent often found in smoked meats.

Flavouring agents: Directly or indirectly add flavour to a product.

Sweeteners (including natural and artificial): Make foods taste sweeter.

Flavour enhancers: Enhance flavour without leaving flavours of their own. Monosodium glutamate (MSG) occurs naturally in food and is sometimes added to food to bring out natural flavours.

Artificial flavouring: Adds flavour lost in processing or increases natural flavour.

Colouring agents (natural, nature-identical, and synthetic): Most foods we eat have some added colouring – even Cheddar cheese!

Colour is often added to a product because consumers expect it to be a certain colour.

Texturizing Agents

Emulsifiers: Help evenly distribute tiny particles of liquid; keep oil and water mixed, as in creamy salad dressings.

Stabilizers or thickeners: Provide body or texture. Gums and other thickeners are used in fat-free salad dressings to give them the consistency of regular dressing.

Fat replacers or fat substitutes: Replace the properties of fat. They may be added to provide moisture or the taste or texture of fat. Fat replacers include natural plant substances, such as guar gum, xanthan gum, and carageenan, or they may be products developed specifically for replacing fat, such as Simplesse. Olestra a fat substitute used for frying, should be avoided during pregnancy.

Nutrients: Vitamins, minerals, and fibre are often added to replace nutrients lost in processing or to improve nutritional value.

Miscellaneous: Other types of additives include leavening agents, propellants, pH control agents, humectants, dough conditioners, and anticaking agents.

Are Food Additives Safe?

Yes, the vast majority of food additives are safe. Some are uniformly beneficial; others may cause reactions in sensitive individuals. Questionable additives continue to undergo evaluation. Keep in mind that overconsumption of any one food or food component can have consequences. Lack of variety in the diet causes an excess of some dietary elements and a deficit of others.

For example, sodium nitrate, which is found in cured meats, can be converted to nitrosamines, which may cause cancer. Vitamin C is often added with nitrates to prevent their conversion to nitrosamine. Sulfites, used as antibrowning agents, are another type of additive. They are most often found in dried fruits and in some beer and wine. Up to 10 percent of the population is sensitive to sulfites – particularly people with asthma. If a food contains sulfite, it is listed on the nutrition label.

If you have questions about food additives, below are some good places to begin searching for answers:

www.cfsan.fda.gov/~lrd/foodadd.html
www.cspi.org

If You Are Concerned about Food Additives

▶ **Make sure to eat a wide variety of foods.**

▶ **Eat as many 'whole foods' as possible, limiting mixes and convenience foods.**

▶ **Use fresh meat more often than cured or smoked meats.**

There has been some association between childhood cancer and eating cured meats during pregnancy.

▶ **Eat fresh fruits, vegetables, milk, and whole grains for snacks instead of packaged snack foods.**

▼

Eating on a Budget

Let's face it: Raising children is expensive. If you are pregnant with your first child, you may be discovering that just furnishing a nursery can cost a bundle! You may be looking for ways to cut costs on food. You *can* eat a nutritious diet and limit your food costs. But eating nutritiously on a budget does take some advance planning and investing in the long term.

Investing in the Long Term

Buy a Deep-Freeze

Deep-freezes aren't cheap, but owning one can allow you to buy food in bulk and stock up on sale items. A grocer in my city often has buy-one-get-one-free sales with no limit on the number of items one can buy. If one could buy enough chicken for six months and get it for half-price, that would be quite a bargain. If you live near a farm, you can invest in a side of beef (or split it with a friend) and get a great deal on very lean cuts of meat.

Try making a double pot of beans or lentil soup and freezing half. This ready-made meal will be wonderful on a cold winter night. You can also freeze leftovers instead of keeping them in the refrigerator and eventually throwing them away or feeding them to the dog when everyone is tired of them. Consider freezing small portions in microwaveable containers for homemade frozen dinners.

Buy Food in Bulk

This only works if you will actually use the food. If half of it spoils before you use it, bulk food is no bargain! A friend of mine makes homemade granola or muesli and lots of other homemade goods. She buys 25 kg or 50 pounds of oatmeal at a time from a health-food shop and saves lots of money.

Plant a Big Garden

Fresh produce can be expensive. Growing your own and preserving or freezing what you can't eat right away can save you a bushel of money, especially during the winter.

Plant Fruit Trees

Can you imagine stepping out in your back garden and picking a fresh grapefruit? My cousin in Florida does. Or how about some fresh apples to make a pie? Ask a local nursery which fruit trees grow well in your area.

Smart Shopping

▶ **Clip coupons and shop the sales.**

Many shops offer coupons. One Saturday I went to three stores, buying up all the great bargains. This storehopping was tiring, but I saved at least 30 per cent on my groceries that week!

▶ **Shop alone. Or if you must take children shopping with you, make sure they are not hungry or tired.**

Reducing distractions will help you concentrate on reading labels and comparing products. It'll also help you avoid buying extra treats to keep the kids happy.

▶ **Don't go shopping when you are tired or hungry.**

▶ **Always shop with a list.**

▶ **When using coupons, compare the discounted price of each food with the shop or generic brand.**

I often find that couponed items are still more expensive than other brands.

▶ **Go to farmers' markets.**

Farmers' market prices are often cheaper than supermarket prices. Again, if you can buy in bulk, you can save money. For example, we bought a large box of tomatoes for just five dollars and made homemade tomato sauce, which we then froze for future soups and sauces.

▶ **If you buy staples such as beans, cereals, dried fruit, and oats from bulk containers, you not only save money, but you also reduce packaging to help the environment.**

Ditto for buying large-size snack foods instead of single-serving packages.

▶ **Get the best per-weight value.**

Packaged fruit and vegetables are not always cheaper. Mushrooms and tomatoes are good examples of this. And packaged ready-to-eat produce such as salads are more expensive than the individual ingredients. However, if you don't have the time to make salads and the ingredients end up spoiling in your fridge, then buying packaged food is a much better value for your money and your body!

The Cost of Convenience

Westerners often want their food fast and easy, and they pay for it. When you compare the costs of homemade foods to various types of convenience foods, you may be shocked!

- Frozen pancakes are twice the price of pancakes made from a mix.
- By adding your own herbs and spices to oil and vinegar, you pay only about a third of the price for the same quantity of dressing.
- Packets of instant oatmeal cost three or four times the price of old-fashioned oatmeal, which offers the best nutrition – and that's for Quaker, a name brand.
- For the cost of one ready-to-eat muffin, you could feed the whole family with muffins from an easy-to-make muffin mix.

When Menu Planning

- Plan menus with your budget in mind. Make less-expensive foods like grains, beans, and vegetables the main course, with more expensive foods like meats as side dishes. Not only is a meatless or almost-meatless diet good for your food budget, it can save you the pain, anguish, and cost of having a diet-related chronic disease such as heart disease or cancer many years down the road. (See page 311 for vegetarian meal ideas.)
- Plan your menus around what's on sale at the store.
- When cooking, use powdered milk. You can double your calcium by using tinned

evaporated milk, which is cheaper than fresh milk.
- Fresh fruit may seem more expensive than a conventional dessert, but it's usually not!
- Plan your menus with leftovers in mind. Think of different menus you can do with one dish. For example, you could make beef fajitas the first night and fiesta salad with beans and beef strips the second night, or your could freeze the leftover fajita fixings in individual containers for future lunches or quick dinners. Most people end up throwing a lot of food away because they forget about it, get tired of it, or just don't like leftovers. (See page 307 for leftover menus.)
- Are you eating out or buying vending machine snacks often because of a busy schedule? Waffles or pancakes, though expensive, are still cheaper than a drive-through meal. Sandwiches are still cheaper than a burger meal. If you can plan ahead a bit and use leftovers for lunch, you'll probably see the greatest savings.

▼

Stocking the Kitchen Toolbox

To make tasty, nutritious meals with minimum hassle, you need to have the tools of the trade! I consider the following tools essential for a cook who wants to eat well but doesn't have lots of time to waste in the kitchen:

Essential Items

Blender or food processor. One of these is essential for making quick soups, low-fat cheese dips, stuffings, and meal-on-the-go drinks.

Meat thermometer. Using a meat thermometer is the most reliable method of determining whether your meat is cooked to the right temperature. If you like your meat rare, you definitely need a thermometer to make sure you have cooked your food enough to kill bacteria.

Microwave. I didn't realize how much I used mine until I started writing down the recipes for this book. Though most people use microwaves just for warming leftovers or heating water, using them for cooking can be a real timesaver. Microwave cooking can also preserve nutrients.

Non-stick pans. You don't have to add fat when you use non-stick cookware. I also like the fact that cleanup is a breeze.

Plastic cutting board. Use a plastic or acrylic cutting board instead of a wooden one (at least for raw meats). Wooden boards are harder to sterilize and can harbour bacteria from uncooked meats.

Microwave-safe cookware. Many people use leftover margarine containers for cooking in the microwave. This is risky because some of the chemicals in the plastic (also in plastic wrap) have been shown to migrate into food. Until further research is done on this, use Pyrex cookware or plastic containers made especially for the microwave.

Miscellaneous utensils. A few good-quality knives, nylon spatulas and spoons for non-stick cookware, measuring cups and spoons, and a wire whisk should be part of every kitchen. These few utensils will make life much easier for the cook!

Nice-to-Have Items

Minichopper. This little food processor holds only about 1 cup and is great for chopping onion, garlic, or other vegetables to a fine consistency. It's a great gadget for pregnant women who are sensitive to cooking smells in the first trimester. Another nice-to-have item is a hand-held slicer/chopper with several blades. With it you can chop an onion in about thirty seconds or slice a potato paper-thin in a minute.

Rotating platter for microwave. This item ensures that your food is cooked evenly to the correct temperature without having to be turned manually every few minutes.

Salad spinner. I love salad, but I hate washing and drying lettuce leaves. We received a salad spinner as a wedding gift, and now salad making is much easier.

Luxury Items

Add these to your wish list.

Ice-cream maker. This gadget is great for making frozen yogurts and sorbets that can satisfy your sweet tooth without a lot of fat.

Bread maker. Imagine waking up to fresh bread every morning! Making your own wholegrain bread may help you increase the fibre in your diet.

Hand-held blender. These are the type you see advertised on TV. Some of my clients have told me these gadgets really *do* whip skimmed milk and they really *can* mince meat, crush ice, and make milk shakes.

▼

Keeping the Vitamins in Your Vegetables

Which are better – frozen, tinned, or fresh vegetables? Nothing beats freshly picked food straight from your garden. However, in some cases, frozen vegetables can actually have a higher nutrient content than fresh.

Fresh vegetables may not be very fresh by the time you buy them, and they're even less fresh if they stay several days (or weeks) in your refrigerator. Recently, a University of Illinois researcher found that 'fresh' shop-bought beans had lost 50 per cent of their vitamin C since leaving the farm seven days earlier. After three days in a home refrigerator, they had lost 10 per cent more. However, frozen beans had lost only 30 per cent of their vitamin C after four months in the freezer. In this case, the frozen vegetables were a better choice.[3]

Tinned vegetables are not as nutritious as fresh vegetables, but eating tinned vegetables beats eating no vegetables at all! If you look in my cabinets, you will find a multitude of tinned beans, tuna, and tomato sauce. Because I rarely can (or want to) take the time to cook beans from scratch, buying tinned beans makes sense for me.

Caring for Vegetables

▶ **Store veggies in your refrigerator crisper in their bags.**

Ziploc makes special vegetable bags with air vents that let the right amount of moisture out to keep your veggies fresh.

▶ **To keep lettuce and other greens fresh, wrap in kitchen paper towels, then store in their bags.**

▶ **Don't cut, peel, or wash vegetables until you are ready to cook or eat them.**

An exception to this might be keeping carrot and celery sticks cleaned, cut, and ready to eat. Having them ready to eat will increase their chances of being eaten. Eating vegetables with reduced nutrient content is better than eating none at all!

▶ **If possible, avoid soaking vegetables to wash them; soaking depletes water-soluble vitamins.**

Healthiest Cooking Methods

1. No cooking

2. Steaming or microwaving

3. Stir-frying

4. Baking

5. Boiling

When foods are cooked to death, they taste bland, have the consistency of baby food, and lose water-soluble vitamins like B vitamins and vitamin C.

Cooking Tips for Healthy Vegetables

- To cook vegetables in the microwave, add 1 or 2 tablespoons of water and cover tightly. After the microwave cycle is finished, let the vegetables stand a few minutes while covered to continue cooking. This method is wonderful for cooking cubed potatoes, which wind up so moist, they taste great without any added fat. (See page 326 for variations on this recipe.)
- When stir-frying, put the more dense vegetables in the pan first. For example, start with onion, garlic, and spices for flavour, then add carrots, celery, cabbage, and broccoli. At the end, add softer vegetables such as peas, mushrooms, and greens.
- Steaming vegetables on a rack in a pressure cooker is almost too fast! Watch the time carefully to avoid overcooking.
- When boiling, use just enough water to prevent scorching. Some vegetables, such as potatoes, need to be covered with water. Cut large vegetables in pieces to shorten cooking time.

▼

The Essential Guide to Food Safety

You may be so busy cooking all the right foods, exercising, and preparing for your baby's arrival that you don't stop to think about making your kitchen safe. And I don't mean just making sure no pot handles are sticking out. Many other dangers lurk in kitchens, and they are related to how you select and handle your food.

The dangers I'm referring to usually can't be seen, smelled, or tasted. They are hidden in the forms of bacteria, fungi, and moulds. The US Centers for Disease Control and Prevention estimate that food-borne bacteria caused 76,000,000 illnesses; 325,000 hospitalizations; and 5,000 deaths in the United States in 1998. Pregnant women have more at risk; foetuses can be severely harmed by some bacteria. A bout of food poisoning reduces the mother's nutrition intake, which could also slow baby's growth.

Even if you don't read the rest of this chapter, make sure to read the summary on page 218.

Making Your Kitchen Safe

When You're Preparing Food

▶ **Wash your hands.**

Wash your hands in hot, soapy water before preparing food and after using the bathroom, blowing your nose, petting the dog, changing a nappy, and so on. This advice is common sense, of course, but hands are the most common spreaders of bacteria to food.

▶ **Keep raw meats and produce away from each other.**

Use a separate cutting board for raw meats and uncooked foods. Wash the meat board in the dishwasher after use. Use a plastic cutting board instead of a wooden one; wood can't be cleaned as well and may harbour bacteria. Use kitchen paper towels instead of a re-usable sponge or rag to wipe away juices from meat, fish, or poultry. Wash your hands well with soap after handling meat and before handling other foods, especially raw produce.

▶ **Wash sponges, towels, and kitchen cloths often.**

Bacteria can survive quite well in used sponges and fabrics. Wash sponges in the washing machine with bleach or in your dishwasher or soak them in a weak bleach solution daily. Replace sponges every few weeks.

▶ **Thaw food in the microwave or refrigerator – NOT ON THE KITCHEN COUNTER.**

When Eating Away from Home

▶ **Don't eat anything that has been sitting out for hours without proper refrigeration or heat.**

Cantaloupe melon once caused an outbreak of salmonella. The person who cut the cantaloupe did not wash the outside, and bacteria got onto the edible portion. After the cantaloupe was out of the refrigerator for a while, the bacteria multiplied enough to cause illness.

▶ **If meat, fish, or chicken doesn't look as though it is cooked well enough, ask to have it cooked more thoroughly.**

Be assertive. (Keep in mind that smoked foods will still look pink, even when they're done.)

▶ **If food that should be cold isn't, don't eat it.**

Recently, my husband and I ordered a piece of cream pie to share. After eating almost half of it, I realized that the pie wasn't cold at all and alerted the waitress. She found out that the refrigerator was broken, and no one had noticed it!

▶ **Avoid restaurants that don't practise good sanitation.**

People who handle food should wear hair coverings and should have clean hands. Employees who take money should not also be touching food. People who work with food must wash their hands after using the restroom, blowing their noses, smoking, or eating before they handle food again. Workers who don't follow these rules should be reported to your local health department.

Is It Still Good?

Do you find yourself asking this question often? On pages 211–216 you'll find guides about how long you can safely refrigerate and freeze various foods.

According to Dee Ann Whitmire, a registered dietitian and communications specialist with the Western Dairy Council, 'A good rule of thumb is that you can keep a dairy product one week after the date printed on the package. When in doubt, throw it out, since how you handle a product can affect its freshness.'[4]

When Is It Done?

Don't be impatient when you cook meats; thorough cooking is necessary to kill harmful bacteria, and cooking meat thoroughly takes time.

When checked visually, red meat is done when it's brown or grey inside; poultry is done when juices run clear; and fish is done when it becomes opaque and flakes with a fork.

If you're using a meat thermometer, cook beef, pork, and lamb to an internal temperature of 91°C (160°F), whole chicken or turkey to 82°C (180°F), and fin fish to 63°C (145°F) for at least five minutes. In general, fin fish should be cooked ten minutes per 25 mm (inch) of thickness.

Cook eggs until whites are firm and yolks are no longer runny. This reduces the likelihood that an egg is harbouring salmonella.

Microwave Cooking Tips[5]

▶ **Choose only microwave-safe containers.**

Chemicals from packaging and from containers not deemed microwave safe can leach into food at high temperatures.

▶ **Cover the dish with a lid, kitchen paper towel, or greaseproof paper. Avoid using cling film in the microwave unless it is labelled polyethylene.**

If you do use cling film, don't let it touch the food. The trapped steam will help regulate the food's temperature throughout.

▶ **Rotate the dish halfway through cooking time.**

Even if the dish is on a turntable, repositioning it is still a good idea. Turn over large food items. These practices help food cook more evenly and safely.

▶ **Let microwaved food stand for an additional third of the cooking time.**

Food continues cooking after being removed from the microwave. This helps equalize its temperature throughout.

▶ **Take care when cooking raw chicken or minced beef in the microwave.**

Even cooking is critical to killing food-borne bacteria in these vulnerable foods. It may be best to use an alternate cooking method. However, reheating these foods thoroughly in a microwave should be fine.

Other Hidden Risks in Your Food Supply

Recent research shows that exposure to some chemicals before and during pregnancy could be linked to infertility, spontaneous abortion, birth defects, and developmental problems.[6] While the verdict is still out on the specific chemicals and the amounts that could cause problems, it is prudent to learn what you can do to avoid being exposed to chemicals that could harm your baby. It's perfectly okay to be picky about what you eat; your baby will thank you for it! And it's especially important to eat a variety of foods to decrease your exposure to individual pollutants and pesticides and to increase your intake of a variety of nutrients.

Endocrine Disruptors

The scientific community has recently voiced concerns about environmental contaminants called endocrine disruptors. Endocrine disruptors are hormonally active agents that have been associated with reproductive and developmental problems in wildlife. It is known that exposure to high amounts of endocrine disruptors can affect humans as well as wildlife, but the effects of smaller exposures is debated. Scientists fear that endocrine disruptors do the most damage during times of rapid growth: the prenatal period, infancy, early childhood, and puberty. While further research is being conducted, you can try to avoid endocrine disruptors by following these tips:

Selection

Some pesticides – not only those found on food, but also the ones used on plants and in insecticides – are endocrine disruptors. Endocrine disruptors are also found in certain types of plastic, including cling film.[7] Environmental pollutants can be stored in the fat of meats, fish and poultry. Read the next few pages for more information on these topics.

Storage

Don't store high-fat food such as cheese, meat, pie, and cake in cling film. Some chemicals in cling film can migrate into high-fat foods. It's better to store such foods in plastic bags or microwave-safe plastic or glass containers. Plastic containers bearing a recycling code of '2' or '5' on the bottom are considered free of potential endocrine disruptors. If food is sold in plastic shrink-wrap, stretchy cling film, or a foam container, repackage it at home.

Cooking

Use microwave-safe plastic, glass, or ceramic to cook or reheat foods in the microwave. To cover food while microwaving, use greaseproof paper, kitchen paper towel, or cling film labelled 'polyethylene' and leave 25 mm or an inch between food and wrap. Avoid cling film labelled 'PVC' (polyvinyl chloride).

Pesticides

In 1996, the US Food Quality Protection Act was signed into law. Its purpose is to keep Americans safe from pesticide residues in food. The act takes special care in evaluating pesticides that infants and children might consume. The US Environmental Protection Agency (EPA) will probably be banning some harmful pesticides; however, it may take years to complete its evaluation. Because your unborn baby may be particularly vulnerable to some pesticides, it is best to be safe and follow the advice on the next few pages to decrease your pesticide exposure.

Consumers Union, an American non-profit group devoted to consumer product safety, has done toxicity testing on milk and common fruits and vegetables. It found that some products contained as many as twenty different pesticide residues, while others contained few.[8]

Fruits and Vegetables with Most Pesticide Residues

- Fresh peaches
- Frozen and fresh squash grown in the United States
- Domestic and imported apples, grapes, spinach and pears
- US-grown green beans

Among the foods listed above, U.S. peaches and frozen winter squash contained pesticide residues much higher than the other produce.

Fruits and Vegetables with Least Pesticide Residues

These foods contained the lowest amounts of pesticides:

- Frozen and tinned sweetcorn
- Milk
- US orange juice, broccoli, bananas, and tinned peaches

Other relatively 'clean' foods were:

- Frozen and tinned peas
- Apple juice
- Frozen winter squash from Mexico
- Tomatoes from Canada
- Brazilian orange juice
- US wheat

What's Organic?

Eleven US states now have standards for organic produce, and a national standard is coming soon. The Organic Foods Production Act of 1990 requires the establishment of national standards governing the marketing of certain agricultural products as organically produced. The National

Organic Program is now being formed to carry out the terms of the act. The programme would create national US standards for the organic production and handling of agricultural products, which would include a national list of synthetic substances approved for use in the production and handling of organically produced products.

According to a proposed rule,[9] an organic product is defined as one that:

- has been produced and handled without the use of synthetic chemicals;
- has not been produced on land to which any prohibited substances, including synthetic chemicals, have been applied during the three years immediately preceding the harvest of the products; and
- has been produced and handled in compliance with an organic plan agreed to by the producer and handler of the product and the certifying agent.

▼

How to Lower Your Risk

This section provides tips on selecting and handling foods so that you can eat the safest food possible.

Fruits, Vegetables, Grains, and Nuts

In recent years, bacteria that were once found mostly in animal products have made their way into fruits and vegetables. *Escherichia coli* (commonly known as E. coli), for example, has been found in alfalfa sprouts and unpasteurized apple cider. Because of this, you must be more careful about washing your produce well. Your risk of illness due to pesticide exposure is less than your risk of illness from inadequate fruit and vegetable intake, but you should still take steps to ensure the safety of the fruits and vegetables you eat.

Safety Tips

▶ **Grow your own produce without using pesticides.**

▶ **Consider buying organic produce.**

Consider buying organic produce or produce labelled 'no detectable residues' – especially when buying produce that is more likely to contain pesticide residues. (See page 208.) Remember that organic produce may not look as perfect as produce to which pesticides have been applied.

▶ **Buy locally grown produce.**

Such produce is fresher, picked closer to its peak ripeness, and probably isn't coated with wax or sprayed with post-harvest pesticides. Usually, a local farmers' market or roadside stand is a great source. But be inquisitive. Last summer when I asked where the produce came from at my local farmers' market, I found that some of it had been shipped from four states away!

▶ **Wash off pesticide residues.**
If you'd like a little help in removing pesticide residues, use a few drops of dish washer.

▶ **Buy domestically grown produce (this is also good for local farmers).**

▶ **Buy fruits and vegetables in season.**

If you live in the northern latitudes and buy a cantaloupe melon in the dead of winter, you can be sure it was grown pretty far south of you. That means it had to be picked early and was likely sprayed with post-harvest pesticides and wax to make sure it arrived at your shop looking just picked.

▶ **Exercise caution with nut products.**

The large brands of peanut butter probably have the highest quality standards in terms of aflatoxins, a naturally occurring carcinogen. Throw away any mouldy, discoloured, or shrivelled peanuts, pecans, walnuts, almonds, Brazil nuts, and pistachios – they can also contain aflatoxins.

▶ **Store potatoes in a cool, dark place.**

Trim away any green or damaged parts; they contain glycoalkaloids, toxins that can affect the nervous system.[10]

▶ **Avoid unpasteurized juices.**

▶ **Avoid eating sprouts, such as alfalfa and mung bean sprouts, unless you cook them first.**

Peeling and Washing Produce
To peel or not to peel? It's a toss up: Peeling does completely remove all surface pesticides (whereas washing might not), but peeling can also mean losing valuable fibre and nutrients. As a general rule, if your diet is otherwise rich in fibre, peel produce

– especially produce that is obviously waxed – to remove the wax and any other surface pesticides.

Always wash produce. Adding a few drops of dish washer to half a litre or a pint of water is more effective than plain water in removing many pesticides. Choose a soap that doesn't contain dyes and perfumes. Don't use salt water or vinegar; these won't help. Salt is something we get more than enough of in our diets. No evidence shows that specially formulated pesticide and wax washes are more effective than regular dish washer detergent – and they can cost up to eight times as much! Scrub with a vegetable brush, and be sure to rinse food completely.

Here are some tips for cleaning specific types of produce (instead of buying organic):[11]

▶ **For leafy vegetables such as lettuce and cabbage, discard outer leaves and wash inner leaves.**

▶ **Wash celery after trimming off the leaves and tops.**

▶ **For recipes that need grated peel, buy organic fruit if possible.**

▶ **Peel carrots. (You won't be losing fibre, since carrots contain fiber throughout.)**

Questions about Pesticides?

Contact the Pesticides Safety Directorate (PSD) at www.pesticides.gov.uk

▶ **Peel cucumbers if they're waxed.**

▶ **Wash aubergines, peppers, tomatoes, potatoes, green beans, cherries, grapes, and strawberries.**

▶ **Peel apples, peaches, and pears if you get plenty of fibre from other sources, since the peels of these fruits likely contain risky residues.**

▶ **Cut up cauliflower, broccoli, and spinach before you wash them, since pesticides may otherwise be hard to wash off.**

Dairy Products

The biggest potential risks from eating dairy products come from drinking raw or unpasteurized milk and from bacterial contamination due to improper handling.

Like all perishable foods, dairy products are very safe foods if handled properly. One issue that has gotten recent media attention is the use of the hormone bovine somatotropin (BST) on dairy cows.

Dairy cows produce this hormone naturally. Scientists have found a way to produce the hormone synthetically, and when given to cows, it can increase the cows' milk production by 10 to 30 per cent.

The US National Institutes of Health (NIH) have concluded that milk from BST-treated cows is safe for humans.[12] The medical community generally regards the use of supplemental BST as safe.[13]

So why all the fuss? Much of the controversy surrounding this issue is unrelated to human health. Some people feel that an

Dairy Products Storage Guide		
Food	Refrigerator at 4.4°C (40°F)	Freezer at -17°C (0°F)
Milk	8–20 days	Not recommended due to reduced quality of product after thawing
Buttermilk	2–3 weeks	
Eggnog	1–2 weeks	
Parmesan cheese	Almost indefinitely	
Soured cream	3–4 weeks	
Ultrapasteurized cream	6–8 weeks	
Yogurt	3–6 weeks	
Processed cheese food in jars, unopened	12 months	
Grated cheese in moisture-proof packaging, unopened	12 months	6–8 weeks
Swiss and Cheddar cheese	1 month	6–8 weeks

Note: Storage time begins at processing, not purchase.

Sources: *Newer Knowledge of Milk*, National Dairy Council, 1988, and *Newer Knowledge of Cheese*, National Dairy Council, 1986.

increased milk supply may take jobs away from dairy farmers. Some people are concerned that BST injections may adversely affect dairy cows. Others are just opposed to biotechnology in general.

Safety Tips

▶ **Buy only pasteurized milk products. Avoid any raw milk, including goat's milk.**

▶ **Avoid cheeses that have been known to have been contaminated with the dangerous listeria bacteria.**

These include Brie, Camembert, feta, blue cheese, and Mexican-style soft cheeses (queso blanco, queso fresco, queso de crema, and queso Asadero).

▶ **Keep your refrigerator at or below 4.4°C (40°F) and keep milk refrigerated.**

If you are accustomed to putting milk on the table for meals, don't keep it out long. Leaving milk out at room temperature, even briefly, can allow bacteria to grow and hasten spoilage.

▶ **Never return unused milk to its original container after it has been sitting out for a while.**

▶ **See chart above for storage times for dairy products.**

Eggs

The number-one food safety problem with eggs is salmonella bacteria. Though salmonella poisoning is rarely fatal, it is dangerous to people with weak immune systems, such as pregnant women, infants, children, people with chronic disease, and the elderly. Unfortunately, salmonella poisoning is on the rise. You don't have to entirely avoid eggs, which is fortunate because the protein in eggs is of very high quality. But do use the following tips to keep your eggs safe:

Safety Tips: Buying and Storing

▶ **Buy only eggs that have been refrigerated.**

▶ **Store eggs in their own container to keep them from cracking.**

▶ **Don't wash eggs; they are usually washed, sanitized, and coated with mineral oil to keep out bacteria.**

▶ **Buy eggs that aren't cracked; bacteria can seep through the cracks.**

Safety Tips: Eating

▶ **Avoid any food containing raw egg or egg white.**

According to Dr. Pat Kendall, Food Science Specialist with Colorado State University, most of the salmonella bacteria in an egg are found in the yolk.[14] When you eat out, you may want to avoid health shakes, caesar salad dressing, and cold mousses or soufflés, which may contain raw eggs. Also avoid unpasteurized eggnog and eggnog made with raw eggs, homemade ice cream, and lightly cooked egg products such as meringue and French toast.

▶ **Cook your eggs until yolk and white are firm or at least until yolk thickens.**
If you prefer your eggs runny, you might consider an egg substitute, which contains pasteurized eggs. Avoid the temptation to taste cake batter or biscuit dough that may contain raw eggs.

Beef and Pork

The food safety risks associated with eating beef and pork are bacterial contamination and the presence of parasites.

Eating raw and undercooked beef can increase your chances of getting toxoplasmosis, a disease caused by parasites. E. coli is a dangerous bacteria mostly associated with ground beef.

The danger of contracting trichinosis is much reduced from past generations. Trichinosis is an illness caused by eating raw or undercooked pork infected with a type of worm. It is completely destroyed at 59°C (138°F).[15]

The Facts about Drugs and Hormones

Drugs

One of the main concerns regarding consumption of animal meat is drug residues. About forty years ago we discovered that small, preventive doses of certain antibiotics improved livestock growth. The National Cattlemen's Association of America recommends against routine use of antibiotics in cattle feed, and most beef producers are following the recommendation. When antibiotics are used to treat illnesses in cows, the cow goes to the market only after a specified quarantine period.

Hormones

'Growth hormones have been used safely and successfully for almost thirty years to increase lean production and feed efficiency,' says Lowell L. Wilson, Animal Science

Department, Pennsylvania State University.[16]

Hormones improve animal growth. Beef cattle given a small amount of growth hormone grow faster, go to market sooner, and are leaner. According to the beef industry, if hormone implants were not used, the supply of beef would shrink and prices consumers pay would rise.

A Texas A & M University report concluded that the scientific community now agrees that the proper use of certain hormones is harmless to the consumer and may enhance animal growth performance by as much as 20 per cent.[17] The University of California Wellness Letter, March 1989, reported, 'At the prescribed dosages used in feedlots, these hormones have been certified safe by numerous scientific studies.'

Surprisingly, hormones are present in nearly all the plant and animal foods we eat. In fact, the estrogen in many common foods far exceeds the estrogen found in beef given supplemental estrogen. (See the chart below.)

Men, women, and children also produce estrogen in their bodies at levels thousands and millions of times greater than the levels found in beef. In the third trimester of pregnancy, your body will produce thirty-seven million times the amount of estrogen found in a 75-gram (3-ounce) serving of beef.

Poultry

The greatest risks from eating poultry are illnesses caused by the food-borne bacteria *Salmonella typhimurium, Salmonella enteritidis,* and *Campylobacter jejuni.*

Chicken is the most popular meat among my clients because it is a low-fat dish that can be prepared quickly. However, chicken is also a common carrier of campylobacter and salmonella bacteria. Campylobacter passes among chickens during processing. Salmonella is found in chicken faeces and spreads to other parts of chickens during processing. Improper handling of raw chicken in the kitchen adds to the risk of contracting salmonellosis and campylobacterosis.

Most people are aware of salmonellosis, but campylobacterosis is a different story. Because campylobacterosis symptoms (cramps, diarrhoea, and fever) are flu-like and can occur up to five days after eating

Estrogen Levels in Food		
Food	Serving Size	Estrogen (in nanograms*)
Beef, from a cow implanted with estrogen	75 g (3 oz)	1.85
Beef, from a cow not given estrogen	75 g (3 oz)	1.01
Egg	1	1,750
Cabbage	75 g (3 oz)	2,016

*One nanogram is one billionth of a gram. If a gram were a football field, a nanogram would be equal to one blade of grass.
Source: Inter-American Institute for Cooperation of Agriculture. *Report on Use of Hormonal Substances in Animals,* December 1986.

Eggs, Meat, and Poultry Storage Guide

Cooked

Food	Refrigerator at 4.4°C (40°F)	Freezer at -17°C (0°F)
Chicken, fried	3–4 days	4 months
Chicken nuggets	1–2 days	1–3 months
Chicken pieces, plain	3–4 days	4 months
Chicken pieces with stock or gravy	1–2 days	6 months
Corned beef (in pouch with pickling juice)	5–7 days	1 month drained and wrapped
Egg, chicken, tuna, ham, or macaroni salad (deli or homemade)	3–5 days	Don't freeze
Ham, tinned, unopened package	6–9 months	Don't freeze
Gravy and meat stock	1–2 days	2–3 months
Ham, cooked, half	3–5 days	1–2 months
Ham, cooked, slices	3–4 days	1–2 months
Ham, cooked, whole	7 days	1–2 months
Hard sausage (such as pepperoni)	2–3 weeks	1–2 months
Lunch meats, opened package	3–5 days	1–2 months in freezer wrap
Lunch meats, unopened package	2 weeks	1–2 months in freezer wrap
Meat and meat dishes, cooked	3–4 days	2–3 months
Pork and lamb chops, pre-stuffed, or chicken breast, stuffed	1 day	Don't freeze
Poultry dishes	3–4 days	4–6 months
Smoked sausage	1 week	1–2 months
Soups and stews (vegetable- or meat-based)	3–4 days	2–3 months
Store-cooked convenience foods (ready-to-eat)	1–2 days	Don't freeze
TV dinners, frozen casseroles		3–4 months
Bacon	1 week	1 month
Beef roast	3–5 days	6–12 months
Beef steaks	3–5 days	6–12 months
Chicken or turkey, pieces	1–2 days	9 months
Chicken or turkey, whole	1–2 days	1 year
Eggs, in shell	3 weeks	Don't freeze
Giblets	1–2 days	3–4 months
Hamburger and stew meats	1–2 days	3–4 months
Hot dogs, opened package	1 week	1–2 months in freezer wrap

a contaminated food, it is estimated that only one in a hundred cases is reported.

Sanitary kitchen procedures are your best defense against campylobacter and salmonella bacteria. Follow the safety tips below to protect your family:

Safety Tips

- Salmonella bacteria multiply at room temperature. Keep hot foods hot (above 160°C (40°F) and cold foods cold (below 4.4°C (40°F). Thaw poultry in the microwave instead of on the countertop. At a picnic or buffet dinner, keep cold poultry dishes in a coolbag or on ice.
- *Campylobacter* can live in your refrigerator for weeks! Clean up any juices that spill from a defrosting chicken. If juice falls on food that will be eaten raw, such as vegetables, fruit, or cheese, throw that food away.
- Because microwave ovens cook unevenly, they may not completely kill campylobacter or salmonella bacteria. Traditional methods like baking, grilling, or boiling are preferred for poultry.
- Research shows that most of the reported cases of campylobacterosis occur during barbecue season – a hint that perhaps people are undercooking their chicken! A combination of microwaving and grilling would ensure thorough and quick cooking. (An internal temperature of 82°C [180°F] ensures that chicken is thoroughly cooked.)
- Since campylobacter does not survive freezing, buy frozen chicken or freeze chicken for a few days before using.

Eggs, Meat, and Poultry Storage Guide (continued)		
Food	**Fresh** Refrigerator at 40°F	Freezer at 0°F
Hot dogs, unopened package	2 weeks	1–2 months in freezer wrap
Lamb chops	3–5 days	6–9 months
Lamb roast	3–5 days	6–9 months
Mayonnaise, commercial	2 months	Don't freeze
Minced turkey, veal, pork, or lamb	1–2 days	3–4 months
Offal (tongue, brain, kidney, liver, heart)	1–2 days	3–4 months
Pork chops	3–5 days	4–6 months
Pork and veal roast	3–5 days	4–6 months
Sausage, raw	1–2 days	1–2 months

Seafood Storage Guide

Food	Purchased Commercially Frozen for Freezer Storage	Purchased Fresh and Home-Frozen	Thawed, Never Frozen, or Previously Frozen and Home-Refrigerated at 0°C (32°F)
Fish Fillets/Steaks			
Lean:			
Cod, plaice, haddock, halibut	10–12 months	6–8 months	36 hours
Pollock, ocean perch, sea trout, rockfish (eg Bass, catfish), Pacific Ocean trout	8–9 months	4 months	36 hours
Fat:			
Mullet, smelt	6–8 months	N/A	36 hours
Salmon (cleaned)	7–9 months	N/A	36 hours
Shellfish			
Crabmeat, fresh	N/A	4 months	5–7 days
Crabmeat, pasteurized	N/A	N/A	6 months
Clams, shelled	N/A	N/A	5 days
Crab claws	N/A	4 months	5 days
Dungeness crab	6 months	6 months	5 days
King crab	12 months	9 months	7 days
Lobster, live	N/A	N/A	1–2 days
Lobster, tail meat	8 months	6 months	4–5 days
Oysters, shelled	N/A	N/A	4–7 days
Prawns	9 months	5 months	4 days
Snow crab	6 months	6 months	5 days
Surimi (imitation seafood)	10–12 months	9 months	2 weeks
Breaded Seafood			
Fish fingers	18 months	N/A	N/A
Portions	18 months	N/A	N/A
Scallops	16 months	10 months	N/A
Prawns	12 months	8 months	N/A
Smoked Fish			
Herring	N/A	2 months	3–4 days
Salmon, whitefish	N/A	2 months	5–8 days

Notes:
- *N/A–not applicable*
- *These storage guidelines indicate optimal shelf life for seafood refrigerated or frozen properly. Temperature fluctuations in home refrigerators will affect optimal shelf life, as will frequent opening and closing of refrigerator and freezer doors.*
- *Although the above storage times ensure a fresh product for maximum refrigeration storage life at 0°C (32°F), the consumer should plan on using seafood within 36 hours for optimal quality and freshness.*
- *To determine approximate storage time for species not listed, ask your retailer which category (lean, fat, shellfish, breaded, or smoked) they fall within and refer to the guide.*

Source: *National Fisheries Institute, 2000 M Street NW, Suite 580, Washington, D.C. 20036*

Seafood

Ben Franklin said, 'Fish and house guests begin to smell after three days.' He should have said 'two days' – at least for fish – because it's unwise to keep fresh fish longer than that.

People are eating more fish these days, probably because they are realizing how healthy it can be. It's low in fat and saturated fat and high in protein, and it contains significant amounts of omega-3 fats. Omega-3 fats can have very beneficial effects on your health. Research suggests that omega-3 fats may prevent blood platelets from sticking to the walls of arteries, thereby lowering the risk of atherosclerosis and heart attack.

The greatest potential risks from eating fish are food poisoning from bacteria or parasites and consumption of environmental pollutants. Proper handling and cooking can reduce or kill bacteria and parasites. If you are considering becoming pregnant, are already pregnant, or are breast-feeding, you should limit your tuna consumption to once or twice per week and your shark and swordfish intake to once a month.

Bacteria

Fish are among the most perishable foods; they have a shelf life of seven to twelve days once they're out of the water. Some fish stay on fishing boats for several days, so by the time they arrive in shops, they may have little shelf life left. If fish get warmer than 0°C (32°F), their shelf life decreases; at 5.5°C (42°F), the shelf life is cut in half. Fattier fish and cold-water fish spoil even faster. Poor sanitation practices, such as using unwashed knives and cutting boards and leaving fish at room temperature, can increase bacterial growth. So can some display procedures. For example, if a fish is kept under a hot light, it gets warm, and bacteria in it can multiply quickly. If raw fish is kept next to cooked fish, the cooked fish can be contaminated.

Pollutants

The environmental pollutants found in fish (as well as in other animal products) cannot be reduced or destroyed by cooking. You can, however, limit your risks by choosing fish with the least pollutants.

Organochlorines and dioxins are persistent organic pollutants (POPs), chemicals that persist in the environment. While you are pregnant, the POPs your baby is exposed to come mainly from what is already stored in your body (mostly in body fat). Large amounts of POPs accumulated in a pregnant woman's body are thought to affect neurological and cognitive development in a growing foetus.[18]

Mercury is a heavy metal that is a potent neurotoxin; it affects brain and nervous system development. Predatory fish generally have higher mercury content than bottom feeders. Fish with above-average mercury content include king mackerel, various bass, swordfish and freshwater fish from contaminated waters.[19] The FDA recommends limiting your consumption of shark and swordfish to once a month, due to its mercury content.

Since the body fat stored during pregnancy is used during breastfeeding, your diet during pregnancy can affect the amount of

---

Listeriosis and Toxoplasmosis: Bad Bugs for Babies

Listeria, a kind of food-borne bacteria, and *Toxoplasma gondii*, a parasite, can both be bad bugs for babies.

Listeria is most often found in soft cheeses, unpasteurized milk products, hot dogs, deli foods, and undercooked poultry, meat, and seafood. Listeriosis causes flu-like symptoms in pregnant women, but if listeria is passed on to a foetus, it can cause miscarriage, premature birth, blood poisoning, and birth defects. Listeriosis can be treated with antibiotics, but play it safe and avoid soft cheeses and unpasteurized milk products, cook ready-to-eat meat and seafood products, and cook raw meat, poultry, and seafood products thoroughly.

Toxoplasma gondii is carried by cats and can also contaminate food. Toxoplasmosis may cause mild flu-like symptoms in pregnant women, but if the parasite is passed on to a foetus, it can cause miscarriage, disability, and retardation. Toxoplasmosis can result from eating undercooked meat and poultry or unwashed fruits and vegetables, from cleaning a cat litter box, or from handling contaminated soil. Severity of the disease may be reduced with antibiotics, but prevention is best. Avoid cleaning cat litter boxes or wear gloves while doing so, wash fruits and vegetables well, and cook meat and poultry thoroughly.

For more information on these food-borne illnesses and their effects on pregnancy, contact:

March of Dimes Birth Defects Foundation
www.modimes.org

Food Standards Agency
www.foodstandards.gov.uk

Royal College of Obstetricians and Gynaecologists
www.acog.org.uk

Sources: Center for Science in the Public Interest. Protect Your Unborn Baby: Important Food Safety Information to Help Avoid Miscarriage.

U.S. Department of Agriculture Food Safety and Inspection Service. Expectant Mothers and Food-Borne Illness, revised May 1999.

U.S. Department of Agriculture Food Safety and Inspection Service. Listeriosis and Food Safety Tips. May 1999.

POPs your baby receives in breast milk. (See Chapter Eight for more information.)

Which Fish Are Safe for Pregnant and Breast-Feeding Women?

Given the complex and sometimes conflicting reports on environmental contaminants, this question isn't easy to answer. After consulting with toxicologists and government organizations and doing an extensive search of the literature, I advise the following:

- Limit consumption of shark and swordfish to once a month.
- Limit tuna consumption to twice a week.
- Choose smaller fish; they contain less stored pollutants.
- Avoid fish from polluted water. In general, fish caught the farthest from land have smaller amounts of POPs.
- Avoid recreationally caught fish, unless you know where they come from.
- Do not eat the fat or fatty parts of fish. Cook fish without the skin if possible. When making fish stock, remove the head and skin first.
- Remember, you should not avoid eating fish during pregnancy. On the contrary:

You should try to eat fish every week. Just limit or avoid the high-risk fish and eat a variety of others.

Did You Have Your Omega-3 Today?

Omega-3 fats, a type of oil found primarily in fish, shows great promise in controlling blood pressure, reducing heart disease, and improving the symptoms of rheumatoid arthritis. We also know that developing foetuses need omega-3 fats – especially docosahexanenoic acid (DHA) – for building brain tissue, for nerve growth, and for development of the retina. Omega-3 fats are so important that some scientists think that a lack of them could result in delays or deficiencies in nervous tissue development and possibly in impaired vision.[20] Before birth, your baby gets DHA from you – especially if you eat your share of fat-rich fish. After birth, your baby gets DHA from breast milk.

The omega-3 fats found in the foods below are particularly important for brain and retina development.

Fish

These fish are listed in descending order according to omega-3 content.[21]

- Atlantic salmon
- Anchovy
- Sablefish
- Salmon
- Mackerel
- Herring
- Tinned pink salmon
- Wild salmon
- Tuna (light, in water)
- Mussels
- Imitation crab made from surimi

Other Animal Products

- Eggs
- Meat (Although meat does not have a high content of omega-3 fats, it has been shown to be a significant source because of the popularity of meat in the diet.)[22]

Plant Products

These plant products contain omega-3 fats (linolenic acid) which can be converted to DHA and eicosapenaenoic acid (EPA) in small amounts.

- Flaxseed oil and flaxseed
- Canola oil
- Soya bean oil

While some physicians (such as those at the University of Michigan Multiples Clinic) recommend fish oil supplements, these should only be taken under close medical supervision. While there does not seem to be harm in fish oil supplementation, more research needs to be conducted before it can be recommended for pregnant women.[23]

Safety Tips: Buying Seafood

▶ **From a food safety standpoint, frozen fish is often the best choice.**

Frozen fish is usually quick-frozen (frozen right on the boat where it's caught), resulting in fish that is actually fresher than 'fresh'. Look for and avoid freezer burn, ice crystals, and broken wrappers. Don't buy fresh salmon, bluefish, or catfish and freeze it when you get home. According to Clare Vanderbeek of the US National Fisheries Institute, 'Fish with a higher fat content will deteriorate more quickly than low-fat fish. Consumers should buy those fish already commercially frozen, which will ensure a higher-quality product.'[24]

► If you choose to buy fresh fish, learn how to recognize freshness.

Fish gills should be bright red and moist, not brown and covered with mucus. Eyes should be bright, clear, and bulging. Avoid fish with cloudy or slime-covered eyes. The skin should have a translucent, varnished look. Fish with skin that is starting to dis-colour or has tears or blemishes should be left at the shop.

► Watch for troubling display habits.

Do not buy fish in supermarkets or shops where fish is stacked in large piles (harder to keep at coldest temperatures), where raw fish is displayed next to cooked fish, where you smell a strong fishy odour (means more bacteria), or where fish is displayed under bright, hot lights.

► Find out, if possible, where your fish came from – the farther from shore, the better.

You can also ask when the shellfish was caught and shipped. But be warned: This information may require some real 'fishing'.

► Avoid recreationally caught fish.

Fish caught recreationally are more likely to be from contaminated waters or handled improperly. It's also wise to avoid buying shellfish at roadside stands; they may be from polluted waters.

Good choices for pregnant women and women who breast-feed include plaice, cod, pollock, squid, clams, rockfish (eg bass, catfish, etc.), Alaskan salmon, shellfish, and sole.[25]

Variety is important!

Safety Tips: Storing and Handling Seafood

► Before refrigerating, remove fish from its package, rinse under cold water, and pat dry with kitchen paper towels.

To keep cleaned fin fish more than twenty-four hours, place the fish on a cake rack in a pan, fill with crushed ice, and cover tightly with cling film or tin foil. Rinse the fish daily, cleaning the rack and changing the ice.

► Keep fish stored at 0 to 3.3°C (32 to 38°F) or in the coldest part of your refrigerator and use within one day if possible.

Keep frozen fish at -17.7° C (0°F) and use within six months.

► Store live oysters, clams, and mussels in the refrigerator.

Keep live shellfish damp by covering them with a clean, damp cloth or moist kitchen paper towel. Do not place them on ice or allow fresh water to come in contact with them. Never store live shellfish in an air-tight container; this will kill them.

► Keep freshly shelled oysters, scallops, or clams in their shells and store them in the coldest part of the refrigerator, preferably packed with ice.

▶ **Keep live lobsters, crayfish, and crabs in the refrigerator in moist packages (use seaweed or damp paper strips), but not in airtight containers, fresh water, or salt water.**

Lobsters should remain alive for about twenty-four hours.

▶ **Be sure to discard any fish juices and marinade used for raw fish, and do not re-use sponges, utensils, or cutting boards used for raw fish.**

Don't forget to wash your hands well after handling raw seafood.

▶ **Throw out fish that smells fishy or like ammonia.**

▶ **Discard any shellfish that die during storage.**

Safety Tips: Cooking Seafood

▶ **Avoid raw and undercooked fish and shellfish at all times!**

▶ **Don't leave raw or cooked seafood out of the refrigerator for more than two hours (including preparation time and time on the table).**

▶ **Cooking fish well will destroy most or all bacteria present.**

Fish is done if the flesh is opaque and flakes easily when tested with a fork at its thickest part. You can also check doneness with a thermometer. Fish is ready when its internal temperature reaches 63°C (145°F).

Fin Fish

Although you don't want to undercook fish, overcooking it will make your fish less tasty.

National Seafood Educators suggest the following for perfectly cooked fish every time:

▶ **For baking (200–230°C/400–450°F/Gas mark 6–8), grilling, poaching, steaming, and sautéing, measure fish at its thickest part. Cook ten minutes per 25 mm (inch), turning halfway through cooking time.**

If the fish is stuffed, measure after it's stuffed. Pieces that are less than 12 mm (½ inch) thick don't need to be turned.

▶ **Add five minutes to cooking time if fish is cooked in tin foil or sauce.**

▶ **Double the cooking time for frozen fish that hasn't been thawed.**

Shellfish

▶ **450 grams (one pound) of medium prawn in the shell needs three to five minutes to boil or steam.**

▶ **Shelled oysters, clams, and mussels become plump and opaque when done.**

Overcooking causes them to shrink and toughen.

▶ **Oysters, clams, and mussels in the shell will open when cooked.**

Remove them one by one as they open.

▶ **Sea scallops take three to four minutes to cook through.**

Smaller scallops may take as little as thirty to sixty seconds.

▶ **Sautéed or deep-fried soft-shell crabs take about three minutes each.**

Steamed hard-shell crabs or rock crabs take about twenty-five to thirty minutes for a large pot.

▶ **If you poach or steam fish, let liquid come to the boil first, then add fish and cook as described above.**

Microwaving

▶ **Split-second timing is important when cooking fish in the microwave.**

Fish will continue cooking after it has been removed from the microwave, so take it out before it looks done – when the outer edges are opaque and the centre is still slightly translucent. Allow the fish to stand covered for a few minutes before serving.

▶ **Use a shallow microwave-safe dish.**

▶ **Arrange fillets with the thicker parts pointing outward and the thinner parts toward the centre of the dish.**

Rolled fillets cook more evenly than flat fillets.

▶ **Cover the dish with cling film and lift one corner to vent.**

▶ **Cook three to six minutes on high per 450 grams (pound) of boneless fish.**

▶ **Cook thawed, shelled shellfish two to three minutes per pound, stirring and rotating half a turn during cooking.**

Allow to stand for a third of the cooking time.

▶ **Place clams, mussels, or oysters in the shell in a single layer in a shallow dish.**

Cover with cling film, venting one corner. Cook two to three minutes on high. Check and remove shellfish as they open.

The above information comes from *Seafood: A Collection of Heart-Healthy Recipes* by Janis Harsila, R.D., and Evie Hansen, US National Seafood Educators.

Food Safety Reports: Who to Believe?

In 1989 two stories about food safety in the US hit the headlines, and people all over the country lingered at their plates, wondering whether anything was safe to eat. First there was the Alar scare. Alar is the brand name of the pesticide daminozide, which was banned by the EPA in 1989 because it was carcinogenic. It took Washington apple growers almost ten years to recover from this scare. Soon after the Alar scare, a story about two cyanide-tainted grapes made the news. As a result, the purchase of all imported foods from Chile dropped off, causing economic hardship in that country.

Food safety reports appeal to our emotions because they often imply that our families are in danger. But when we react with our hearts instead of our minds, our decisions are likely to be based on feelings, not facts.

Many activist groups are involved in food safety issues, and for the most part their claims are valid. However, scientific information is sometimes taken out of context and blown out of proportion to its real effect on our health, needlessly misleading, confusing, and frightening people.

Regardless of your position on a particular issue, you can probably find a scientific study to back you up. Frankly, we don't know all the answers about nutrition and health, which is why you may hear one story today and hear a completely different story tomorrow. When a nutrition or health report hits the headlines, you should ask yourself these questions:

1. *Who is reporting the information?*

Is it a neutral group or someone with something to gain from the information? For example, someone who is selling vitamin supplements may cite this or that convincing study. Though the facts may be true, they may be incomplete, or the person's opinions may be biased – so try to separate facts from opinion.

Keep in mind that large companies commonly fund research by well-respected universities. But don't assume this means the research is biased or of lower quality. Let's face it: Who else would want to put up millions of dollars for research on oatmeal?

2. *If the study is scientific, was it done on animals or humans?*

Though many effects are the same in animals and humans, you can't assume that this is always true.

3. *How large was the sample size?*

Research using a group of ten people won't be as reliable as research on a group of a thousand people.

4. *How many studies have been done on the subject?*

Many studies are usually necessary to prove a theory. However, in some cases one large, well-designed, multicentre study (such as the study that showed the benefits of folic acid) is enough to change the thinking of the scientific community.

5. *How old is the study?*

While some studies are still used as benchmarks of knowledge, others are outdated because of newer statistical methods or better study designs.

▼

Food Safety in a Nutshell

Choosing Foods

▶ **Choose a variety of foods.**

This limits your exposure to too much of one pesticide or pollutant.

▶ **Avoid raw or unpasteurized juices.**

Food labels should indicate whether juices are pasteurized.

▶ **Avoid raw sprouts such as, clover, or mung bean sprouts.**

▶ **Avoid eating deli food.**

▶ **Buy foods with as little pesticides as possible.**

Buy organic foods or foods with no detectable residues – especially those foods that tend to contain the largest amounts of residues.

▶ **Choose low-fat fish, meats, and milk.**

Pesticides, chemicals, and metals accumulate in fat.

▶ **Do not eat raw fish or shellfish.**

▶ **Avoid foods that may contain environmental pollutants.**

The FDA of the USA recommends that women of childbearing age limit eating shark and swordfish to once a month. These fish can be contaminated with heavy metals or chemicals that can harm a foetus. (See page 217 for more details.) While there is no official advisory regarding eating tinned tuna, it may be advisable to eat it no more than once or twice per week.

▶ **Avoid eating unpasteurized soft cheeses.**

These include Mexican-style cheeses (queso fresca, queso blanco, queso de crema and queso Asadero), feta, Brie, blue-veined cheeses, and Camembert.

▶ **Do not use water with high lead content for drinking or cooking.**

The only way to know for sure if your water contains lead is to have it tested. If you have lead pipes or lead-soldered pipes, let the water run for a few minutes before using it to decrease lead content. Avoid using warm tap water for drinking or cooking. (See page 40 for more information on lead exposure.)

If you are concerned about the quality of your tap water because of bacteria, lead, or other contaminants, consider getting a water purification system.

Kitchen Sanitation

▶ **Wash your hands often.**

Wash your hands before touching food and after blowing your nose, using the toilet, changing a nappy, or handling an animal. You should also wash your hands after handing raw meat or fish. To wash your hands thoroughly, scrub them with soap under running water for at least twenty seconds. Use gloves to change cat litter boxes and don't allow animals on food preparation areas.

▶ **Handle raw meat and fish with care.**

Use kitchen paper towels to wipe up juices from raw meat or fish on counters. Then follow with a kitchen paper towel soaked with a weak bleach solution (1 teaspoon bleach to 1 litre (1 quart) cool water), disinfectant, or antibacterial kitchen cleaner. Wash hands and utensils with hot, soapy water after contact with raw meats.

▶ **Clean your sink regularly with disinfectant or antibacterial kitchen cleaner.**

In a recent study, the kitchen sink was shown to harbour more bacteria than the toilet! You can also pour a weak bleach solution down the drain and garbage disposal unit to kill bacteria in your drainpipe.

Food Preparation

▶ **Wash fruits and vegetables well.**

Use water with a drop of dish washer detergent. Thorough washing removes bacteria as well as pesticide residues.

▶ **Keep raw and cooked foods separate.**

You should also use separate cutting boards and knives for each to prevent transfer of bacteria.

▶ **Remove skin, head, and inner organs of fish before making soups and stews.**

▶ **Use a meat thermometer to check the internal temperature of meat, fish, and egg dishes.**

This is the best way to know if food is safely cooked. Minimum internal temperatures:[26]
- Fresh minced beef, ham, veal, lamb, or pork: 71°C or 160°F
- Beef roast or steak: 63°C or 145°F for medium-rare (Cook to higher temperature for medium or medium-well.)
- Whole poultry: 82°C or 180°F
- Minced chicken or turkey: 74°C or 165°F
- Poultry breasts: 77°C or 170°F
- Fish: 63°C or 145°F
- Cooked ham, reheated: 60°C or 140°F
- Eggs: 63°C or 145°F
- Combination dishes, egg dishes, and leftovers: 74°C 165°F

▶ **Avoid raw or undercooked animal protein.**

Foods with uncooked or undercooked eggs include homemade Caesar salad dressing, eggnog, ice cream, and cold soufflés.

▶ **Do not consume marinade used for raw meat unless you boil it first.**

▶ **Reheat leftovers, deli foods, and ready-to-eat meat and seafood products like hot dogs, lunch meats, and smoked salmon until steaming hot.**

▶ **Keep hot foods at or above 60°C (140°F) and cold foods at or below 4.4°C (40°F).**

If you are serving food on a buffet, use a hot plate or Crock-Pot for hot foods and keep cold foods on ice. Foods should not be left at room temperature for more than two hours (one hour on hot days). Refrigerate or freeze leftovers as soon as possible.

Food Storage

▶ **When refrigerating large portions of leftover food, divide the food into smaller containers so it can cool more quickly.**

▶ **Clean your refrigerator regularly and keep its temperature between 1.5°C (35°F) and 4.4°C (40°)F.**

Listeria can grow in the refrigerator if it gets too dirty or too warm.

▶ **Store fresh fish and meats in the coldest part of the refrigerator and cook them within a day if possible.**

▶ **Don't store fruit juice or acidic foods in ceramic containers (especially imported ones) or crystal containers that may contain lead.**

The acid can cause lead to leach into the food or drink.

▶ **Don't drink hot liquids like coffee or tea from ceramic mugs that may contain leaded glaze.**

Hot, acidic beverages can cause small amounts of lead to leach from the glaze.

For information about food safety or food-borne illnesses call the Food Standards Agency (UK), Aviation House, 125 Kingsway, London WC2 8NH, telephone 020 7276 8100; or try their website at www.foodstandards.gov.uk.

CHAPTER TWELVE

Fast Foods: Eating In and Eating Out

What you will find in this chapter:

- *Tips for Choosing Convenience Foods*
- *Complete, Convenient Meals for One*
- *Convenience Foods for the Whole Family*
- *Healthy Convenience-Food Menus*
- *Last-Minute Meals from the Cupboard*
- *Fifty Quick-and-Easy Meals or Snacks*
- *Choosing Wisely at Restaurants*
- *Choosing Nutritious Fast Foods*
- *Healthy Fast-Food Menus for Pregnancy*

This chapter answers such questions as:

- *What can I add to a frozen entrée to make a quick, complete meal?*
- *Are there any fast foods that are high in iron?*
- *Which fast-food restaurants serve grilled chicken?*
- *Is it possible to eat out and have a low-fat meal?*
- *What can I keep at home to put together a quick meal?*

We live in a fast-paced society and often don't have time to cook. In America approximately forty cents of every food dollar is spent on food prepared away from home. You may be wondering whether you can eat out or prepare convenience foods and still have a balanced diet. The answer is yes – with a little planning.

Tips for Choosing Convenience Foods

Convenience foods such as frozen dinners are becoming more and more popular. Some are better than others. Consider these questions when choosing convenience foods:

- Does the product provide a balanced meal (including protein, starch, and vegetable and/or fruit)?
- How much fat does the product contain? Look for no more than 10 grams of fat per 300 calories.
- What is the sodium content? More than 800 milligrams per serving could be excessive. However, since you need more sodium during pregnancy, excess sodium should not be a concern unless you were following a low-sodium diet before pregnancy and your doctor has advised you to continue doing so. (See the next page for more on sodium.)
- Is the product a good value? One often pays for convenience. When checking the price of a convenience food, make sure to consider the cost of ingredients that you add, such as chicken or tuna.
- Does the product contain a lot of additives and preservatives?

Watching Your Sodium?

Although your need for sodium increases during pregnancy, you'll get more than enough in your food – especially if you eat any convenience foods. You can balance your daily sodium intake by limiting tinned or convenience foods to one serving per day.

If you had hypertension or kidney disease before you became pregnant, your doctor may ask you to moderate your salt intake. It will be important for you to read food labels for sodium content.

Most 'light' frozen meals and entrées contain 700 milligrams or less of sodium. That's much less than the usual frozen dinners, which can contain as much as 1,500 milligrams of sodium per serving! Tinned soups and entrées are also known for being high in sodium. An exceptions is Campbell's Select Soups.

Going Meatless?

If you prefer meatless meals, note that the convenience-food menus marked with asterisks on the following pages contain no meat. They may contain cheese and/or eggs.

▼

Complete, Convenient Meals for One

The following frozen dinners offer both convenience and good nutrition. I've also suggested what to add to the different types of convenience foods to create a balanced meal. Thousands of new products enter the market every year. Exclusion of an item from the list below does not imply that it is a bad choice. In addition, check at your local supermarket. Very often the larger supermarkets have their own brands of convenience foods. Read the labels on the packages to see exactly how many calories are in any one meal.

Low-Calorie Entrées

Healthy Choice Entrées
Weight Watchers Ultimate 200 Entrées
Lean Cuisine Entrées

For a complete meal, start with one of the entrées above and add:

250 ml (8 fl oz) milk or yogurt
1 serving fruit and/or raw veggies
(Consider buying a bag of oranges or apples to keep at work.)
1 piece of bread, bagel, bran or corn muffin, or roll

Then maybe add a dessert, and you have a complete meal!

Low-Calorie Dinners

These dinners offer more than an entrée but still contains only about 300 calories. For a complete meal, add milk or yogurt, a roll or piece of bread, and a fruit or vegetable.

Lean Cuisine

'Light' or lower-calorie meals are good choices because they are low in fat. Too much fat could give you heartburn and add too many extra calories. However, entrée-type meals don't always include a fruit or vegetable and can be too low in calories.

Doing Your Maths

Remember, the average pregnant woman needs about 2,200 calories. (Your calorie needs can range anywhere from a modest 2,000 calories to more than 3,000 calories, depending on your size and activity level.) You can count on about 400 calories for breakfast, 500 calories for lunch and dinner, and two 300-calorie snacks or three 200-calorie snacks. Most low-cal dinners have 300 calories. Adding milk, fruit, and starch makes 550 calories and a well-balanced meal for you and your baby.

Additional foods are necessary to make a balanced meal.

Reading nutrition labels can help you pick the healthiest meals. By studying labels, you can pick meals with lower fat, lower sodium, fewer additives, or more vitamin C. Scanning the percentage of vitamins A and C at the bottom of a label can help you determine the amount and quality of fruits and vegetables in a meal.

Meal Starters

These offer yet another choice for a quick, nutritious meal; they can be prepared in the microwave or on the stove top. Some include meat, others don't, so you can choose whether to add chicken, prawns, or beef or leave the meal meatless. One benefit of meal starters is that if you cook them as little as possible, the vegetables will retain more vitamins. These meals are especially nutritious because they include a lot of vegetables. You just need to add a starch, fruit, and milk for a complete, healthy meal.

Pot Pies, Frozen Pizza, Fried Chicken, Chicken Nuggets, Fish Fingers

These foods are usually less expensive than other frozen dinners, but they get 50 per cent or more of their calories from fat. However, many 'light' versions of these foods are now available. These are better (but more expensive) choices. If you are having a hard time gaining weight or don't have an appetite, you can eat the full-fat versions in moderation. Just watch out for indigestion due to their high fat content.

Shelf-Stable Foods

Don't have access to a refrigerator? Or are you stuck on bed rest? Shelf-stable foods don't need refrigerating until you open them. Good examples are microwaveable boxed meals, stews and soups in microwaveable containers, and Cup-of-Soup-type meals. Many tinned soups are also quick, healthy meals. These foods are truly fast; they can be ready to eat in under two minutes! To top off shelf-stable meals, keep dried fruit or individual servings of stewed apple, fruit, or pudding on hand.

Read the labels on the shelf-stable products; some of the smaller products are soups or side dishes, not entrées. Make sure to add milk or yogurt, fruit or a vegetable, and a starch to the entrées so that you get adequate calories and nutrients

Quick Extras to Add to Your Meal

Starches: Bulgur, instant brown rice, whole-wheat English muffin or bagel, bran muffin, bread sticks, canned legumes, corn, or peas.

Fruit: Any fresh fruit, frozen bananas or grapes, frozen melon balls, tinned pineapple, instant pudding with bananas, fruit shake, yogurt parfait, fresh fruit, or fruit juice.

Vegetables: Ready-to-make coleslaw or salad, pre-cut vegetable sticks, shelf-stable vegetables, tinned or frozen vegetables, or vegetable soup.

▼

Convenience Foods for the Whole Family

Frozen meals are fine for just one person, but how about when you need something quick for the whole family? Consider stocking some of these items in your freezer for days when you have no time to cook. (See page 234 for 'Fifty Quick-and-Easy Meals or Snacks.')

▼

Healthy Convenience-Food Menus

These menus can help you make complete, balanced meals starting with frozen dinners. Products marked with asterisks are meatless. All large supermarkets stock a range of similar convenience foods including their own brands. Read the labels on the packages for the nutrients in each meal and also for the calorie count in each meal.

Mexican/Southwestern

99% fat-free turkey chilli
2 wheat tortillas
25 grams (1 ounce) reduced-fat cheese
Orange

Chicken Enchiladas Suiza
Baked tortilla chips
Black beans
Tomato slices
Strawberries
Milk

Grilled Fajita-style Chicken
Vegetarian beans
Frozen melon balls and bananas
Milk

---

*Vegetarian Enchiladas
3-bean salad with tomato
Yogurt with peaches
Vegetable juice

---

*Weight Watchers Smart Ones Santa Fe
   Style Rice and Beans
Raw broccoli and carrots
Bran muffin
Watermelon
Milk

Italian

*Rigatoni with pomodoro sauce, broccoli,
   and olives
Wheat roll
Green beans in vinaigrette
Yogurt with blueberries

*Spinach Lasagna
Bread sticks
Spinach salad with artichoke hearts
Melon
Milk

Lean Cuisine Prawns with Angel Hair
    Pasta
Garlic toast
Tossed salad with green peppers
Grapefruit half

Italian Style Vegetables with White
    Chicken
Minestrone soup or Minute Minestrone
    (See page 284 for recipe.)
Wheat biscuits
Fresh peach
Milk

French Bread Pizza
Caesar salad
Strawberry sorbet
Milk

*Layered vegetable lasagna
French bread
Lemon sorbet with peaches
Milk

Linguine with seafood sauce
Peas and carrots
Canteloupe melon

*Tofu vegetable lasagna
Wheat toast
Apricots
Gingersnaps
Milk

American

*Lean Cuisine Roasted Potatoes with
    Broccoli and Cheddar Cheese Sauce
Tossed salad with kidney beans
Fresh apple
Vanilla pudding with banana
Milk

Weight Watchers Smart Ones Tuna
    Noodle Casserole
Spinach
Bran muffins
Fresh mango
Milk

Mesquite Beef with Barbecue Sauce
Coleslaw
Lemon yogurt with blueberries

*Veggie Loaf
Spinach salad with mandarin oranges
Mixed fruit
Biscuits
Milk

*Cheese Ziti Parmesano or Macaroni and
    Cheese Romano
Carrot-and-raisin salad
Cherries
Milk

Continental

Beef Pepper Steak with Rice
Cucumber and tomato slices
Dinner rolls
Tangerine
Milk

Rigatoni in Cream Sauce with Broccoli
and White Chicken
Wheat rolls
Vegetable soup
Mixed fruit salad
Yogurt

Lean Cuisine Honey Roasted Pork
Carrots
Bran muffin
Fresh strawberries with yogurt

Lean Cuisine Grilled Chicken
Tossed salad with carrot and bell pepper
strips
Fruit cocktail
Milk

Garlic Lemon Chicken with Rice
Courgette slices with dip
French bread
Apple slices
Milk

Chicken pesto with penne
Vegetable soup
Sourdough roll
Tropical fruit salad
Milk

Orange Glazed Chicken
Caesar salad
French bread
Frozen yogurt with raspberries

*Veggies au gratin
Half bagel
Strawberry yogurt with sliced banana

Asian

Sweet and Sour Chicken
Peach halves
Digestive biscuits
Milk

Chicken Fried Rice
Red peppers and cauliflower with dip
Wheat roll
Cinnamon stewed apple
Milk

Teriyaki Stir-Fry Vegetables
Roll
Grapes
Milk

Prawn lo mein
Wheat roll
Chocolate yogurt with raspberries

Mandarin Chicken
Cabbage with vinaigrette dressing
Honeydew melon
Milk

Garlic Chicken
Raw broccoli
Wheat roll
Yogurt with raisins and biscuit

Grab-and-Go Lunches

These sandwich-type meals are great to eat
at your desk while working.

Chicken Broccoli Supreme
Yogurt
Banana
Milk

*Vegetarian hotdogs
Baby carrots
Fresh apple
Milk

Chicken Fajita
Yogurt
V-8 juice

Pizza Burrito or Chicken Burrito
Tomato slices
Banana
Yogurt

French Bread Pizza
Baked tortilla chips
Salsa
Grapes
Milk

---

*Veggieburger on wheat bun with lettuce
 and tomato
Baby carrots
Fresh pear
Milk

---

*Spinach Feta in a Sandwich
Kiwi
Milk

Economy Frozen Meals

One often pays for the extra convenience of frozen meals, but there are exceptions. Some economy frozen meals are generally higher in fat. These can also fit into a healthy diet – just don't make a habit of eating them!

*Bean-and-cheese burrito
Shredded lettuce and tomato
Orange slices
Milk

Fish fingers
Microwave-baked sweet potatoes
Shredded cabbage with Italian dressing
Peach halves
Milk

Bacon Pizza
Tossed salad
Pineapple slices
Milk

Turkey Meal
Fresh apple
Milk

Macaroni and cheese
Carrot-and-pineapple salad
Tomato juice
Pudding

Last-Minute Meals from the Cupboard

The time is ten minutes to famished. You look in the cupboard and see a tin of tomato sauce, some olives, and a tin of salmon. What do you do? Improvise! If you think creatively, you can make a lot of great meals from the tins in your pantry. And by keeping a supply of staple ingredients on hand, you can avoid spending too much of your food budget on convenience foods or calling out for pizza!

Using the ingredients on the left side of the chart on page 235, you can make all the tasty dishes on the right.

▼

Fifty Quick-and-Easy Meals or Snacks

Some of my best meals are the kind thrown together in a hurry from what's available. On the following pages, you'll find lots of ideas for quick, healthy meals.

Pizzas

Crusts

English muffin
French bread
Pitta bread
Polenta bread baked in a round pan
Flour or corn tortilla
Refrigerated pizza dough
Pizza dough mix
Homemade crust
Frozen bread dough

Hot Toppings

Italian: Marinara sauce, cheese, and your choice of meat or veggies.

Mushroom: Cream-of-mushroom soup, mushrooms, onions, and mozzarella and Parmesan cheeses.

Spinach: Marinara sauce, cooked chopped spinach mixed with cream cheese, and mozzarella cheese.

Ratatouille: See page 332 for recipe.

California: Sun-dried tomatoes, cheese, marinara sauce, ham, mushrooms, and chopped fresh basil.

Chile con Queso: Beans with sauce of melted cheese and salsa over baked corn tortilla or English muffin.

All-White: White sauce, prawns, crab, mushrooms, and mozzarella cheese. (My version of the sauce is flour, margarine or butter, and milk; another is olive oil and garlic; or you can just skip the sauce altogether.)

Pepper and Olive: Using light creamy Italian or creamy garlic dressing, add a mix of red, yellow, and green peppers and black and green olives. Top with mozzarella cheese.

Hawaiian: Ham and crushed pineapple.

Mexican: For sauce, mix salsa and tomato sauce. For topping, use refried beans, Cheddar cheese, chilli or peppers, chopped tomatoes, and coriander or parsley.

Grilled Veggie: Marinara sauce with grilled aubergine, mushrooms, courgettes, and olives. Add grilled chicken pieces if desired.

Cold Toppings

Seafood: Cream cheese, cocktail sauce, and cooked prawns or crab.

Veggie: For sauce, use cream cheese and ranch dressing mix. Top with chopped broccoli, carrots, green onions, cauliflower, peppers, shredded cheese, and sliced black olives.

Layered Mexican: Start with a baked crust. Top with beans, guacamole, soured cream flavoured with taco seasoning, chopped tomatoes, shredded cheese, and sliced black olives. This can be made fat-free or full-fat. Also works well as a dip without crust.

Last-Minute Meals from the Cupboard

Ingredients

Pasta
Marinara sauce
Pizza crust, tinned biscuits,
    English muffin, or pitta bread
Tinned chicken
Tinned mushrooms
Capers
Artichoke hearts

Mozzarella cheese
Cottage cheese
Tuna
Salmon
Evaporated skimmed milk
Pasta
Parmesan cheese
Olives
Tinned peas
Mushroom soup
    (reduced-salt and reduced-fat)

Beans
Taco shells
Pineapple chunks
Instant brown rice
Mixed vegetables
Tinned tomatoes
Tinned chicken and vegetables
Potatoes
Black beans
Corn
Chicken stock
Fat-free dressing
Corn tortillas
Black bean soup

Baked beans
Polenta bread mix
Kidney beans
Rice or bulgur

Meals

Spaghetti with marinara sauce
Pizza with artichoke hearts
Chicken with mushrooms and
    capers over pasta with
    marinara sauce
Quick calzone (using biscuits)
Chicken tetrazzini

Fettuccine Alfredo with
    tuna or peas
Tuna casserole
Linguine, salmon, and
    Parmesan cheese toss
Macaroni and cheese

Bean tortillas
Chicken tacos
Chicken salad with pineapple
Baked potatoes with chicken topping
Black bean and chicken soup
Black bean tortillas
Black Bean and Corn Salad (page 254)
    with tortilla chips

Polenta bread and bean bake
Hoppin' John (See page 341 for recipe.)

Sandwiches

Tired of the same old peanut butter and jam on white bread? Try these ideas for a change of pace!

Breads

Rye
Wholemeal pitta
French bread
Flour tortilla
Digestive biscuits
Saltine crackers
Melba toast
Wheat bread
Sourdough bread
Oat bread
Hamburger bun

Warm Fillings

Leftover stir-fry vegetables (with or without chicken, pork, beef, or tofu) in pitta pocket or tortilla.

Light pastrami and sauerkraut with Swiss cheese on rye.

Grilled vegetables and cheese on crusty wholemeal French bread.

Beans and cheese in flour tortilla or on baked corn tortilla. Top with shredded lettuce and tomato.

Vegetarian burger found in frozen food section.

Salmon patties.

Cold prawns with melted mozzarella on top of tomato slice on an English muffin.

Grilled fish-fillet burger.

Sloppy joe with lean minced beef, minced turkey, or textured vegetable protein (TVP).

Spiced black beans with reduced-fat cheese and peppers in a folded tortilla.

Delightful Spinach (page 250) in a wholemeal tortilla.

Thinly sliced roast beef and microwave-steamed peppers on a French roll with beef stock for dipping on the side.

Cold Fillings

Chef salad stuffed in a pitta pocket with light Italian dressing on the side.

Cooked and chilled asparagus spears rolled up with ham and cheese in a wholewheat tortilla.

Chopped chicken with light mayonnaise, fat-free soured cream, curry powder, green onion, mango, and raisins stuffed in a pitta pocket or served as a salad over torn spinach leaves.

Boursin Cheese Spread (page 318) or light cream cheese, chopped parsley, sprouts, and thinly sliced cucumbers and tomatoes on thinly sliced bread.

Prawns or imitation crab in a sauce of light mayonnaise and ketchup over English muffin topped with chopped tomato and avocado.

Peanut butter with banana on digestive biscuits.

Light ricotta cheese on raisin English muffin topped with fruit of choice.

Cottage cheese with chopped carrots, broccoli, spring onion, and celery on English muffin.

Main-Dish Salads

These are great in the summer when no one feels like having a hot meal. To save time, keep chopped, cooked chicken in the freezer or use tinned, chopped white chicken meat.

Tortellini with ham, shredded cheese, tomatoes, artichoke hearts, and vinaigrette.

Rice or bulgur with corn, kidney beans, green beans, chopped red peppers, reduced-fat Cheddar cheese, and vinaigrette dressing.

Linguine with imitation crab, steamed carrots and broccoli, and creamy Italian dressing.

Mixed greens with grilled fish, walnuts, and cucumber dressing.

Black Bean and Corn Salad (See page 254 for recipe.)

Spaghetti with stir-fried chicken, mangetout, and red peppers with peanuts and teriyaki sauce.

Asian Salad with grilled chicken (See page 253 for recipe.)

Leaf lettuce, tinned tuna in brine, white beans, kidney beans, cherry tomatoes, cucumbers, olives, and spring onion with light ranch dressing.

Small shell pasta, prawns, chopped avocado, and tomato over bed of shredded cos lettuce with fat-free vinaigrette dressing.

Chicken-and-Spinach Salad (See page 256 for recipe.)

Chicken and pineapple chunks over shredded cabbage with Catalina dressing.

Mixed fresh fruit salad with fruit-flavoured yogurt and bran muffins.

Peas with light mayonnaise and cheese chunks over mixed greens garnished with tomato slices and yellow pepper rings.

Fajita salad: Grilled marinated chicken, beef, or prawns with peppers and onions over torn lettuce. Serve with baked flour tortilla triangles.

Rotini pasta with honey-dijon dressing, ham chunks, and 3-bean salad.

Taco salad with Baked Tostitos topped with shredded cos lettuce, tinned or leftover warmed chilli, reduced-fat cheese, chopped tomatoes or salsa, and fat-free soured cream.

▼

Choosing Wisely at Restaurants

Dining out offers many choices; which foods are best for the mother-to-be? If you eat out often, your diet will most likely be higher in fat and lower in nutrients like calcium, folacin, and vitamin C – unless you make your choices wisely! Following are some challenges for the pregnant diner:

- Large servings may tempt you to overeat. Take half your meal home in a doggie bag. Or order a half portion or an appetizer.
- High-fat foods and fried foods may cause heartburn. Foods you might think of as low-fat, such as Asian food, can sometimes surprise you.

- Servings of vegetables and fruits may be minimal, leaving your meal mostly meats and starches. Consider ordering a side salad, coleslaw, or an appetizer vegetable to round out your meal.
- Milk may not be available; this could be a problem if you dine out regularly.

Salad Bar Savvy

Most people think a trip to the salad bar means a healthy meal. It can be – but beware of the high-fat foods! Here are a few tips for making your trip to the salad bar a healthy one.

▶ Watch out for hidden fats.

Sunflower seeds, Chinese noodles, coconut, salad dressing, bacon bits, olives, marinated vegetables, puddings, mousses, and salads made with mayonnaise, such as potato salad, coleslaw, and egg salad, can all be high in fat. Also try to stay away from fried courgettes and potato skins.

▶ Make sure to eat enough protein foods.

Ham, turkey, cottage cheese, kidney beans, chickpeas, and Cheddar cheese are all good options.

At the Table

▶ **Try to avoid meals described with these words:** *butter, butter sauce, hollandaise, raw* **(as in seafood),** *au gratin, Alfredo, creamed, cream, sautéed, pan-fried,* **or** *fried.*

▶ **Choose wisely from the menu.**

You should be able to order a healthy entrée by looking for these key words: *marinara sauce, vegetarian, grilled, baked, poached, steamed, stir-fried, lean,* and *light.*

▶ Order a meal that contains one or two servings of vegetables.

You may need to order à la carte to get what you want. Pasta, potatoes, and brown or wild rice are good side dishes. Avoid fried potatoes.

▶ Order all salad dressings or sauces on the side.

▶ Are you tempted by the bread brought to your table before you order?

Eat a raw fruit on the way to the restaurant or before you leave home; you'll then be less likely to overindulge in before-dinner snacks. Or ask that bread not be brought to your table and request a salad to snack on.

Common Healthy Entrées

Mexican

   Chicken, beef, or prawn fajitas
   Chicken enchiladas
   Bean tostadas or burritos

Italian

   Pasta with marinara sauce
   Pasta primavera
   Tortellini or ravioli with marinara sauce
   Vegetable lasagna

Bistro

Grilled chicken sandwich

Chef salad

Chicken caesar salad

Grilled prawns with pasta

Steak House

Filet mignon

Seafood brochette

Grilled salmon

What's for Dessert?

Fresh fruit, sorbet, and low-fat yogurt are good choices. If you want to indulge in something heavier, split it with your dining partner.

▼

Choosing Nutritious Fast Foods

Which fast foods are healthiest? It depends on what you're looking for: low fat content? High vitamin C or A content? High fibre content? Every day the choices available at the drive-through seem to expand. You can now eat a healthy, balanced diet even when you eat fast food regularly. The key is to make the best choices and to round out your diet by snacking on fruits and vegetables that might not be available when you eat in the fast lane.

Tips for Making a Healthy Fast-Food Meal

▶ **Remember that having a food high in vitamin C with your meal will increase the amount of iron your body absorbs.**

Drink orange juice; eat a salad with high-vitamin-C veggies such as tomatoes, broccoli, or cauliflower; or choose fresh fruit or vegetables from the salad bar.

▶ **Cut the fat on sandwiches by asking for no mayonnaise or sauce.**

You can also ask for sauces on the side. Skipping the cheese will also cut the fat, but don't skip it if it's your primary source of calcium.

▶ **If you eat at the salad bar, balance your selections.**

Choose raw vegetables, like tomatoes, broccoli, cauliflower, carrot sticks, and fresh fruits. Have cottage cheese, beans, ham, or chopped eggs for a protein source. Be sure to have a source of starch, such as bread sticks or savoury biscuits. Go easy on the puddings, olives, and mayonnaise-based salads.

▶ **Bring along fresh fruit or vegetables to go with your meal or order a side-salad.**

▶ **If you are trying to keep your weight gain down, choose lower-calorie fare such as grilled chicken, fajitas, or bean burritos.**

Skip the additional toppings such as cheese, soured cream, and guacamole. Choose low-calorie or fat-free salad dressings.

► **If you have trouble with heartburn, avoid French fries, burgers, fried pies, and other fried foods.**

Fried foods are high in fat and will aggravate your heartburn.

Menus and Recipes for the First Trimester

What you will find in this chapter:

• About the Eating Expectantly Menus

• About the Eating Expectantly Recipes

• First-Trimester Menus
  – Don't Feel Like Eating Menus
  – Don't Feel Like Cooking Menus
  – Don't Feel Like Cooking or Eating Menu
  – Feel Like Staying in Bed but Can't Menu
  – Feel Great Menu
  – Blender Breakfasts (or Snacks to Go)
  – Snack Ideas
  – High-Energy Snack Ideas

• First-Trimester Recipes

About the Eating Expectantly Menus

Many people have trouble planning menus. Menu planning can be even tougher when you're dealing with the food moods of pregnancy. You know – when you're so hungry you could eat a horse, but nothing sounds good. Or when you'd rather stay in bed because you feel queasy, but you've got to get your kids ready for school. Or when you're exhausted, and you'd like to get dinner on the table in fifteen minutes or less. At the beginning of each chapter of recipes, I've tried to take some work out of menu planning by giving you lots of menu ideas. The types of menus in each chapter are listed at the beginning of each recipe chapter and at the ends of Chapters Three, Four, and Five.

Beverages are not included in all the menus. It is assumed that milk will be your choice at least twice per day. Other good choices include vegetable and tomato juice, fruit juice, soya milk, and sparkling water mixed with fruit juice. Of course, you should also try to drink plenty of water throughout the day.

Some menus include recipes found in this book. Page numbers are shown in parentheses following these recipes.

About the Eating Expectantly Recipes

When it comes to food, I have preferences like anyone else, and the recipes in this book reveal my own food biases. For example, you won't find any recipes that contain mustard greens or liver, because I don't care for these foods. You will find some French recipes and southern recipes, because my husband is French, and I am originally from Texas. The Eating Expectantly recipes were developed and chosen primarily for their taste, and then for nutritional value and ease of preparation. (After all, if food doesn't taste good, who would eat it even if it is nutritious?) Most recipes call for ingredients that are readily available. Vegetarian recipes may call for a few ingredients from a large health-food shop.

Nutrient Analysis

All recipes were analyzed using Nutritionist III Software Version 7.2 from N-Squared Computing. All numbers are rounded to the nearest whole number. When an alternate ingredient or serving amount is listed, the first listing is the one used for nutrient analysis.

Protein content is listed to help you compare each recipe to your total goal for protein intake. Fat content is listed because most people are interested in fat these days. Women who have heartburn will be especially interested in choosing the lowest-fat recipes. Carbohydrate content is listed to help diabetics and health professionals plan special diets. The fibre listed is dietary fibre. A recipe that contains less than 1 gram of fibre per serving will list no fibre.

Key Nutrients

I've compared the Eating Expectantly recipes to the Dietary Reference Intakes (DRIs) for pregnancy and listed each key nutrient as a percentage of the DRI. By looking at the key nutrients, you can pick foods high in important nutrients and compare the nutritional values of various dishes.

Diabetic Exchanges

Diabetic exchanges are included to help women who have diabetes or gestational diabetes plan meals. Exchanges are calculated according to the Exchange Lists for Meal Planning developed by the American Diabetes Association and the American Dietetic Association. Exchanges are rounded to the nearest half-exchange. If you have diabetes, consult with a registered dietitian to get an individualized meal plan based on your weight and activity level.

The diabetic exchanges are based on principles of good nutrition, so women who are not diabetic can also use them for keeping track of how many servings from the different food groups they are eating.

Diabetic Variations

A few of the recipes are high in sugar; a sugar-free variation follows each of these recipes. The diabetic variations use artificial sweetener. (See page 119 for information about the use of artificial sweeteners during pregnancy.) Use artificial sweeteners only with your doctor's approval. When a diabetic variation is listed, the exchanges that follow it refer to the diabetic variation.

▼

First-Trimester Menus

Keep in mind that during the first trimester, your priority is not to gain weight but to make your diet and health habits as high-quality as possible. Don't worry if you don't eat much for a while because of nausea. Lack of appetite should only become a concern if you begin losing weight.

Don't Feel Like Eating Menus

Many women find that drinking beverages between instead of with meals helps prevent nausea. Remember: Eating what you crave may help you get past nausea, so don't worry if a craving seems a little weird.

Cream-of-mushroom soup
Wheat toast
Peach slices

Chicken-noodle soup
Saltine crackers
Lime sorbet

Jelly with pears
Cottage cheese
Toast

Low-fat yogurt-and-banana shake
Digestive biscuits

Egg custard
Digestive biscuits

Granny Smith apple slices with peanut butter
Pretzels

Plain pasta
Stewed apple

Macaroni cheese
Grapes

Creamy Asparagus Soup (page 252)
Wheat savoury biscuits

Boursin Cheese Spread (page 318) or cream cheese on bagel
Pears

Don't Feel Like Cooking Menus

See 'Vegetarian Convenience-Food Choices' in Chapter Six and 'Using Leftovers with Flair' in Chapter Fifteen for more ideas.

Grilled cheese-and-tomato sandwich
Fresh apple

Black Bean and Corn Salad with Baked Tortilla Chips (page 254)
Strawberry sorbet

Taco with Basic Black Beans (page 287), cheese, lettuce, avocado, and tomato
Low-fat milk
Banana

Quick and Easy Lunches for Friends

Salmon Pâté (page 251) on crusty bread
Prawn-stuffed avocado with ranch
   dressing
Fresh pineapple slices

Tuna-and-pasta salad with artichoke
   hearts
Rye savoury biscuits
Cantaloupe melon quarters

Cold Sesame Beef (page 345) served
   warm over mixed greens
Marinated vegetables
Tropical Pudding (page 272)

Melted Boursin Cheese Spread (page
   318) on toast rounds over mixed
   greens and vegetables
Wheat roll
Berry Mousse Parfait (page 303)

Black Bean Enchilada Casserole
   (page 333)
Carrot-apple salad
Wheat roll
Watermelon

Aspen Black Bean Soup (page 321)
Muffin
Grilled grapefruit

Tabouli salad with cheese
French bread
Fresh fruit salad

Pasta with Quick Alfredo Sauce (page 260)
Peas
Tossed salad
Wheat rolls
Yogurt with strawberries

Light Lunch:

Thrive-on-Five Bread (page 265) with
   fat-free cream cheese
Apple Pie à la Mode Shake (page 266)

Don't Feel Like Cooking or Eating Menu

Breakfast
Frozen melon balls
Dry toast
Fruit spread or jam
Milk or juice (later)

Snack
Pretzels or baked crisps
Milk or vegetable juice

Lunch
Fresh fruit with cottage cheese
Vanilla wafers

Snack
Lemon-lime float with lime sorbet and
   lemon-lime soda

Dinner
Poached or scrambled eggs
Wheat toast
Milk

Snack
Peach Pops (page 268)
Milk

Feel Like Staying in Bed but Can't Menu

Before-Rising Snack
Saltine crackers or other salty snack
Ginger ale (later)

Breakfast

Jelly with peaches

Digestive biscuits

Snack

Lemonade

Lunch

Pasta with mozzarella cheese

Sliced tomatoes

Snack

Frozen fruit juice bars

Snack

Pretzels

Tomato juice

Dinner

Chicken or tuna salad

Vegetables in Vinaigrette (page 330)

Wheat biscuits

Apple slices

Bedtime Snack

Raspberry Surprise Shake (page 271)

Feel Great Menu

If you are lucky, you will feel almost normal and will want to eat that way. You may even feel especially hungry! Here's an example of a good day's diet:

Breakfast

Raisin bran

Blueberries

Pumpkin Muffin (page 263)

Milk

Snack

Dried figs or prunes

Lunch

Turkey-and-cheese sandwich

Fresh or tinned peaches

Raw broccoli and carrots with dip

Milk

Snack

Vegetable juice

Popcorn

Dinner

Asian Salad (page 253)

Grilled salmon steak

Roasted New Potatoes (page 329)

Carrots Antibes (page 257)

Snack

Tangy Salad (page 286)

Blender Breakfasts (or Snacks to Go)

Banana-Orange Flip (page 267)

Digestive biscuits

Piña Colada Frappé (page 270)

Bran toast

Very Berry Shake (page 273)

½ toasted wholemeal bagel

Raspberry Surprise Shake (page 271)

Bran muffin

Apple Pie à la Mode Shake (page 266)

Peanut butter on savoury biscuits

Peanut-Butter-Chocolate Shake (page 269)

Biscotti

Snack Ideas

Here are dozens of snack ideas for the first, second, and third trimesters to help you avoid between-meals boredom:

245

First Trimester

Rye crisp and cheese

Apple with peanut butter

Tangy Salad (page 286)

Cottage cheese and blueberries on
½ English muffin

Melba toast and reduced-fat cheese

Rice pudding with raisins

Bran flakes and granola or muesli
with milk

Dried figs and cheese

Apple-Date Bran Muffin (page 262)

Jelly with peaches

Creamy Asparagus Soup (page 252)

Digestive biscuits and milk

Stewed prunes

Favourite Snack Cake (page 351)

Pumpkin Muffins (page 263)

Pretzels

Second and Third Trimesters

Toasted cheese-and-tomato sandwich

Soft cheese, raisins, and cinnamon spread
on toasted English muffin

Devilled eggs and rye biscuits

Pear and cottage cheese

Thin-sliced turkey breast rolled up with
light cream cheese

Oven-Fried Courgettes (page 258) with
marinara sauce

Low-fat yogurt

Banana and peanut butter

Baked sweet potato

Apple slices with Caramel Dip (page 319)

Berry Mousse Parfait (page 303)

Corn cakes with cheese

½ pitta bread stuffed with salad, light
Cheddar cheese, and vinaigrette dressing

Popcorn

Tuna salad with apple and savoury
biscuits

Boiled eggs and crackers

Quick and Healthier Pancakes with fresh
fruit (page 282)

Chicken-and-Spinach Salad (page 256)

Beans with baked tortilla chips

Tropical Pudding (page 272)

Leek-and-Potato Soup (page 283) with
milk

Rocky Mountain Quesadillas (page 261)

Crisp wheat biscuits with spinach-
cottage-cheese dip

Cheerios with peaches and milk

Figs stuffed with light cream cheese

Yogurt with fresh strawberries and
blueberries

Toasted English muffin and yogurt

Fibre bar and milk

Leftover pizza and vegetable juice

Nachos

Raw vegetables, ranch dressing, and
savoury biscuits

Orange juice with soda and yogurt with
Grape Nuts and raisins

Strawberry Bread (page 264) and milk

Hot apple cider and Thrive-on-Five
Bread (page 265)

Ham and cheese in wheat tortilla

Chicken salad on ½ bagel or bagel crisps
(baked)

Corn muffin with spicy cheese and
tomato juice

Orange, cheese on celery, and carrots and cucumbers

Fruit kebab with strawberries, kiwi fruit, pineapple, and cheese

High-Energy Snack Ideas

Peanut-Butter-Chocolate Shake (page 269)

Egg custard and gingersnaps

Oven-baked potato crisps with Parmesan cheese and Italian seasoning

Delightful Spinach (page 250) in a flour tortilla and milk

Macho Nachos (Corn tortilla toasted and served with melted Cheddar cheese, vegetarian beans, pepper strips, lettuce, tomato, light soured cream, and avocado)

Egg-and-olive salad on rye with tomato juice

Mocha Java Cake (page 304) with strawberries and vanilla yogurt

Tortellini salad with ham

Peanut-butter biscuits and vanilla yogurt

English muffin with melted part-skimmed mozzarella cheese, sun-dried tomatoes, and marinated artichoke hearts

Fruit Pizza for a Crowd (page 353)

Fruit Crisp (page 352) with vanilla yogurt

Fat-free chocolate yogurt with strawberries and granola or muesli

Old-fashioned banana pudding with vanilla wafers

Raspberry Surprise Shake (page 271) and granola or muesli bar

Beans, cheese, and baked tortilla chips with vegetable juice

Low-fat cheesecake with fresh peaches and blueberries

Pound cake topped with peaches and raspberry yogurt and milk

Favourite Snack Cake (page 351) with cream cheese

Avocado-and-prawn salad with hard rolls

First-Trimester Recipes

Dips and Spreads
Delightful Spinach, 250
Salmon Pâté, 251

Soups
Creamy Asparagus Soup, 252

Salads
Asian Salad, 253
Black Bean and Corn Salad with
  Baked Tortilla Chips and Yogurt
  Sauce, 254
Bridget's Garden Salad, 255
Chicken-and-Spinach Salad, 256

Side Dishes
Carrots Antibes, 257
Oven-Fried Courgette Sticks, 258
Spring Vegetables in Cream Sauce,
  259

Entrées
Pasta with Quick Alfredo Sauce, 260
Rocky Mountain Quesadillas, 261

Breads and Muffins
Apple-Date Bran Muffins, 262
Pumpkin Muffins, 263
Strawberry Bread, 264
Thrive-on-Five Bread, 265

Sweets
Apple Pie à la Mode Shake, 266
Banana-Orange Flip, 267
Peach Pops, 268
Peanut-Butter-Chocolate Shake, 269
Piña Colada Frappé, 270
Raspberry Surprise Shake, 271
Tropical Pudding, 272
Very Berry Shake, 273

Delightful Spinach

Do you groan at the thought of eating greens? This simple recipe will tempt you to ask for seconds! The creamy sauce boosts calcium and protein content. This delightful dish can be used as a side dish or a dip.

Makes: 3 servings

1 275-g (10-oz) package frozen spinach, chopped

100–125 g (4 oz) fat-free or low-fat cream cheese

½ teaspoon mixed herbs

Salt and pepper to taste

2 drops Tabasco sauce (optional)

1. Cook spinach (or thaw completely) and squeeze out all its water; place in small saucepan over low heat.

2. Add remaining ingredients and stir until well blended.

Variations

You can prepare this recipe using Swiss chard, kale, mustard greens, or any greens – even cooked lettuce.

Nutrient Analysis per Serving

44 calories
4 grams carbohydrate
7 grams protein
less than 1 gram fat
1 gram fibre

Key Nutrients

61% vitamin A
15% folic acid
15% magnesium
8% vitamin B₁₂

Diabetic Exchanges

1 very lean meat
1 vegetable

Salmon Pâté

This creamy spread can be used as a dip or a sandwich filling. It tastes so good you won't believe its low fat content!

Makes: 20 servings

225 g (8 oz) fat-free cream cheese or 225 g (8 oz) low-fat cottage cheese

1 410-g (15½-oz) tin salmon with skin removed

2½ tbsp grated onion

1½ teaspoons white horseradish

2 tbsp lemon juice

1 teaspoon dry dill or 1 tablespoon fresh dill

2 teaspoons dry parsley or 2 tablespoons fresh parsley, chopped

1. Place cheese in food processor and blend until smooth.

2. Add remaining ingredients and blend until smooth. When you taste it you shouldn't feel any bones.

Variations

Serve on rye biscuits, toasted pitta bread, or on a sandwich with thinly sliced cucumbers. For appetizers, stuff cherry tomatoes or mushroom caps, or spread on crackers.

Nutrient Analysis per Serving

50 calories
1 gram carbohydrate
7 grams protein
2 grams fat

Key Nutrients

41% vitamin B_{12}
22% selenium
5% calcium

Diabetic Exchanges

1 very lean meat

Creamy Asparagus Soup

If you like home-made soup but don't have much time to cook, this is the recipe for you. Pre-cooking the asparagus in the microwave preserves its important nutrients.

Makes: 3 servings

1 275-g (10-oz) package frozen
asparagus

4 tbsp each onion and celery,
finely chopped, or 1
tablespoon dehydrated onion
flakes and a few pinches
celery salt

1 to 2 garlic cloves, chopped, or
garlic powder to taste

1 chicken bouillon cube or 1
heaping teaspoon stock mix

125 ml (4 fl oz) hot water

1 350-g (12-oz) can skim
evaporated milk

1½ tbsp flour

½ teaspoon seasoned salt or
garlic salt

⅛ teaspoon pepper or to taste

1. Place asparagus, onion, celery, and garlic in bottom of microwave-safe dish. Add 1 tablespoon water, cover, and cook on high in microwave for 2 minutes. Rearrange spears and cook 3 minutes more, or until tender. Leave covered several minutes to cool and cut into 25-mm (1-inch) pieces.

2. Meanwhile, dissolve 1 bouillon cube (or enough to make 250 ml [8 fl oz] stock) in hot water. Pour into blender pitcher. Add milk and flour. Blend on low speed; then on high, until well blended.

3. Pour mixture into large saucepan, leaving about 200 ml (6½ fl oz) in blender. Add asparagus and blend until asparagus is well puréed.

4. Add asparagus mixture to saucepan. Cook over medium-low heat, stirring well until it reaches the desired thickness. Add seasoned salt and pepper.

5. Serve with Bridget's Garden Salad (page 255) and bran muffins.

Variation

Use a 275-g (10-oz) package of frozen broccoli instead of asparagus for a creamy broccoli soup.

Nutrient Analysis per Serving

150 calories
23 grams carbohydrate
14 grams protein
1 gram fat
2 grams fibre

Key Nutrients

33% vitamin C
21% folic acid
36% calcium
26% vitamin A

Diabetic Exchanges

1 skimmed milk
1 vegetable
½ starch

Asian Salad

Makes: 6 servings

Salad

275 g (10 oz) romaine lettuce, shredded

1 celery stalk, finely chopped

1 or 2 spring onions, sliced

8 tbsp sliced water chestnuts, rinsed

1 250-g (10-oz) package frozen mangetout, thawed or steamed; then cooled

1 teaspoon toasted sesame seeds

8 tbsp mung bean sprouts

1 300-g (11-oz) tin mandarin oranges (optional)

Dressing

200 ml (6.5 fl oz) white wine vinegar

4 tbsp sugar

½ teaspoon sesame oil

1 teaspoon soy sauce

¼ teaspoon pepper

1. Toss salad ingredients in large salad bowl.

2. Combine dressing ingredients and toss with salad.
(If you are accustomed to having more oil in your salad dressing, add a few extra teaspoons of vegetable oil.)

Nutrient Analysis per Serving

76 calories
12 grams carbohydrate
1 gram protein
3 grams fat

Key Nutrients

16% vitamin C
11% folic acid
14% vitamin A

Diabetic Exchanges

1 vegetable
½ fat
½ starch

Black Bean and Corn Salad with Baked Tortilla Chips and Yogurt Sauce

This easy-to-make dish is chock-full of important nutrients for you and your baby! You can prepare it for a light meal or eat a smaller portion as a snack.

Makes: 4 servings

Salad

225 g (8 oz) tinned sweetcorn, drained

1 450-g (16-oz) tin black beans, drained

8 tbsp fat-free Italian dressing

275 g (10 oz) cos or soft leaf lettuce leaves, torn

100–125 g (4 oz) reduced-fat Cheddar cheese

2 tomatoes

Yogurt Sauce

8 tbsp natural non-fat yogurt

½ teaspoon cumin

⅛ teaspoon garlic powder

Tortilla Chips

6 corn tortillas

Cooking spray

1. Mix corn, beans, and dressing. Marinate in refrigerator at least 30 minutes.

2. Spoon corn and bean mixture over lettuce. Sprinkle 25 g (1 oz) of cheese on each serving. Garnish with 2 tomato quarters.

3. Mix yogurt with cumin and garlic powder.

4. Serve with homemade tortilla chips and yogurt sauce.

Baked Tortilla Chips

1. Preheat oven to 190°C/350°F/Gas mark 5. Cut each tortilla into 6 pieces, spray with cooking spray, and sprinkle with salt and/or spices.

2. Bake on baking sheet for 20 to 30 minutes, turning once.

Nutrient Analysis per Serving

350 calories
52 grams carbohydrate
21 grams protein
8 grams fat
12 grams fibre

Key Nutrients

32% vitamin C
24% chromium
13% folic acid

Diabetic Exchanges

3 starches
1½ medium-fat meats
1 vegetable

Bridget's Garden Salad

I often create meals from my refrigerator leftovers or from my garden. Many of my creations work – and my family lets me know when they don't. I created this salad one summer when it seemed as though our garden was producing only green beans.

Makes: 4 servings

275 g (10 oz) soft leaf or cos lettuce, torn

250 g (9 oz) green beans, cooked

50 g (2 oz) purple cabbage, shredded

4 large mushrooms, sliced

2 tomatoes, coarsely chopped

100–125 g (4 oz) smoked turkey, cubed

8 tbsp kidney beans, drained

50 g (2 oz) reduced-fat cheese, grated

8 tbsp fat-free Italian dressing

2 tbsp low-fat soured cream

Sesame seeds, sunflower seeds, or pine nuts (optional)

1. Toss all ingredients except cheese, dressing, and soured cream.

2. Mix soured cream and dressing in small bowl.

3. Toss salad with dressing. Sprinkle cheese on top. Garnish with toasted sesame seeds or sunflower seeds, if desired.

Variation

Substitute 675 g (1½ lb) of cooked pasta (rotini or shells) for lettuce. Increase fibre content by using wholemeal pasta.

Nutrient Analysis per Serving

177 calories

16 grams carbohydrate

17 grams protein

6 grams fat

5 grams fibre

Key Nutrients

50% vitamin C

26% vitamin A

22% vitamin B_6

10% zinc

Diabetic Exchanges

2 lean meats

2 vegetables

½ starch

Chicken-and-Spinach Salad

This dish makes a wonderful summertime lunch. Substitute other fruit if fresh strawberries are not available. Try using leftover grilled chicken and pre-washed spinach for an especially quick meal.

Makes: 7 servings

Salad

175 g (6 oz) fresh spinach

2 oranges, peeled and cut into chunks

275 g (10 oz) chicken, cooked and cubed

275 g (10 oz) sliced strawberries

Dressing

3 tbsp red wine vinegar

3 tbsp orange juice

1½ tbsp corn oil

¼ teaspoon dry mustard

⅓ teaspoon poppy seeds

1. Mix dressing ingredients in a bowl and refrigerate.

2. Wash spinach and tear into bite-size pieces into a large bowl.

3. Add oranges, chicken, and strawberries.

4. Serve with dressing.

Source: Reprinted with permission from *Quick and Healthy Recipes and Ideas* by Brenda J. Ponichtera, R.D. (ScaleDown Publishing, Inc.).

Nutrient Analysis per Serving

152 calories
9 grams carbohydrate
14 grams protein
7 grams fat

Key Nutrients

88% vitamin C
39% niacin
27% vitamin A
23% selenium
13% folic acid

Diabetic Exchanges

1½ lean meats
1 fruit
1 vegetable (free)

Carrots Antibes

While visiting my husband's family in France, I ate this dish in a restaurant on the Mediterranean coast. Europeans love puréed vegetables, and once you try Carrots Antibes, you'll know why! This is my version of the dish, which even kids will love!

Makes: 4 servings

8 carrots (about 450 g/1 lb), peeled and sliced

8 tbsp water

1 egg

½ teaspoon sugar

¼ teaspoon nutmeg

1. Place carrots and water in microwave-safe dish. Cover and cook 10 minutes in microwave on high, turning halfway once during cooking. Drain liquid.

2. Place carrots in blender or food processor with egg and spices. Blend until well puréed.

3. Return mixture to microwave dish and cook 4 minutes, rotating once.

4. Serve as a side dish or as a snack with crackers.

Nutrient Analysis per Serving

82 calories
15 grams carbohydrate
3 grams protein
2 grams fat
5 grams fibre

Key Nutrients

509% vitamin A
24% potassium
19% vitamin C

Diabetic Exchanges

3 vegetables

Oven-Fried Courgette Sticks

What a great way to eat vegetables; they taste almost too good to be healthy!

Makes: 4 servings

8 tbsp Italian bread crumbs

2 tbsp Parmesan cheese, freshly grated or tinned

¼ teaspoon garlic powder

3 medium courgettes

Water or milk

250 ml (8 fl oz) fat-free or low-fat spaghetti sauce

Cooking spray

1. Preheat oven to 230°C/450°F/Gas mark 8. Spray baking sheet with cooking spray.

2. Place bread crumbs, cheese, and garlic powder in a Ziploc bag and shake well to combine all ingredients. Set aside.

3. Cut each courgette in half horizontally. Then cut each half lengthwise into 8 pieces. Fill a pie plate with water or milk. Dip each courgette stick in water or milk, then drop into crumb mixture. Shake until courgette stick is coated on all sides. Place on baking sheet. Repeat with rest of sticks.

4. Bake on baking sheet for 10 to 15 minutes or until brown and tender. Serve with warm spaghetti sauce.

Variation

Use 1 medium peeled aubergine, sliced into thin rounds, instead of courgettes.

Nutrient Analysis per Serving

107 calories

17 grams carbohydrate

5 grams protein

2 grams fat

Key Nutrients

Small amounts of all nutrients

Diabetic Exchanges

2 vegetables

½ starch

½ fat

Spring Vegetables in Cream Sauce

This recipe is very versatile; it can be a side dish, a light meal over angel hair pasta, or a filling for crêpes. You can also add cooked chicken breast, prawns, crab, or white beans for a complete meal.

Makes: 4 servings

Sauce

375 ml (12 fl oz) fat-free chicken stock

250 ml (8 fl oz) skimmed milk

3 tbsp cornflour

½ teaspoon tarragon

¼ teaspoon each dill and basil

½ teaspoon onion powder

½ teaspoon garlic salt

1 teaspoon lemon pepper

1 teaspoon lemon juice

Vegetables

1 450-g (1-lb) package Green Giant Vegetables (cauliflower, carrots, asparagus) or other frozen mixed vegetables

1 200- or 400-g (7- or 14-oz) tin artichoke hearts, quartered

½ red pepper, sliced thinly

1. Put chicken stock, milk, and cornflour in blender. Blend on high until well mixed.

2. Pour mixture into large saucepan and add rest of sauce ingredients.

3. Cook over medium heat, stirring often until thickened.

4. Meanwhile, steam vegetables or cook in microwave.

5. Add steamed vegetables to thickened sauce and serve.

Nutrient Analysis per Serving

103 calories
22 grams carbohydrate
6 grams protein
0 grams fat
4 grams fibre

Key Nutrients

124% vitamin A
56% vitamin C
13% folic acid

Diabetic Exchanges

1 starch
2 vegetables

Pasta with Quick Alfredo Sauce

Do you love alfredo sauce, but hate its rich ingredients? Try this delicious, healthier version.

Makes: 4 servings

250 ml (8 fl oz) low-fat cottage cheese

4 tbsp Parmesan cheese, preferably freshly grated

¼ teaspoon garlic salt

4–6 tbsp skimmed evaporated milk or fresh milk

2 dashes nutmeg

150 g (5 oz) frozen peas, thawed or lightly cooked

675 g (1½ lb) cooked pasta

1. Purée all ingredients except peas and pasta in food processor or blender.

2. Pour into microwave-safe container and cook on medium-high for 2 minutes. Or place in saucepan and cook on a low flame until warm.

3. Toss pasta with peas.

4. Pour sauce over pasta. Garnish with more Parmesan cheese.

Variation

Use tinned mushroom pieces instead of peas. Add two or three tablespoons of chopped lean ham.

Nutrient Analysis per Serving

313 calories
46 grams carbohydrate
20 grams protein
5 grams fat

Key Nutrients

20% vitamin B$_{12}$
19% calcium
7% folic acid

Diabetic Exchanges

3 starches
1½ lean meats

Rocky Mountain Quesadillas

These can be served as a snack, an appetizer, or a light meal. The figs give this dish a real nutritional boost!

Makes: 1 serving

4 figs

1 small wholemeal flour tortilla

26 g (1 oz) Cheddar cheese, grated or sliced

1. Cut figs in half. Arrange them on one half of flour tortilla.

2. Top with cheese.

3. Grill until cheese is just melting; then fold over.
OR
Fold over tortilla and cook in microwave on medium-high for 45 seconds to 1 minute.

Nutrient Analysis per Serving

268 calories

44 grams carbohydrate

10 grams protein

7 grams fat

4 grams fibre

Key Nutrients

28% calcium

15% potassium

10% magnesium

Diabetic Exchanges

2 fruits

1 lean meat

1 starch

Apple-Date Bran Muffins

This recipe was developed by Deborah Compton, who loves to cook. Muffins can be baked and served fresh or kept as ready-to-bake dough in the refrigerator for up to one week.

Makes: 24 muffins

50 g (2 oz) oat flake cereal

100 g (4 oz) 100% bran cereal

250 ml (8 fl oz) low-fat buttermilk, scalded, or natural non-fat yogurt, heated

2 large eggs or 8 tbsp egg substitute

8 tbsp margarine, at room temperature

300 g (11 oz) brown sugar, packed

250 ml (8 fl oz) low-fat buttermilk or natural non-fat yogurt

250 ml (8 fl oz) unsweetened applesauce (see page 264)

225 g (8 oz) plain flour

8 tbsp wholemeal flour

2½ teaspoons baking soda

¼ teaspoon salt

150 g (5½ oz) chopped dates

Cooking spray, margarine, or muffin liners

1. Preheat oven to 200°C/400°F/Gas mark 6. In a large bowl, combine oat and bran cereals; pour scalding buttermilk over the cereal mixture and stir.

2. Add eggs, margarine, sugar, the second cup of buttermilk, and applesauce; mix to blend.

3. Mix flour, soda, and salt in a separate bowl and then stir into cereal mixture until moistened.

4. Fold in dates.

5. Grease muffin tins, spray with cooking spray, or line with paper. Fill muffin tins ⅔ full. Bake 20 to 25 minutes.

Diabetic Variation

Reduce brown sugar to 8 tbsp and substitute 8 tbsp thawed apple juice concentrate.

Nutrient Analysis per Serving

147 calories
27 grams carbohydrate
3 grams protein
4 grams fat
2 grams fibre

Key Nutrients

Small amounts of all nutrients

Nutrient Analysis per Serving
(Diabetic Variation)

134 calories
24 grams carbohydrate
3 grams protein
4 grams fat
2 grams fibre

Diabetic Exchanges

1½ starches
1 fat

Pumpkin Muffins

Makes: 12 muffins

2 egg whites or 1 egg

1 tbsp light margarine or
  1½ teaspoons margarine +
  1½ teaspoons water

175 g (6 oz) + 2 tablespoons
  tinned unsweetened pumpkin

130 g (4½ oz) brown sugar

200 ml (6.5 fl oz) skimmed milk

225 g (8 oz) flour

2 teaspoons baking powder

½ teaspoon baking soda

½ teaspoon salt

¼ teaspoon ground ginger

½ teaspoon each ground
  cinnamon and nutmeg

8 tbsp raisins (optional)

Cooking spray

1. Preheat oven to 200°C/400°F/Gas mark 6. In large bowl, combine egg whites, margarine, pumpkin, sugar, and milk.

2. In small bowl, combine remaining ingredients.

3. Fold the wet ingredients into the dry ingredients until blended. Fold in raisins, if desired.

4. Spray muffin pan with cooking spray. Pour batter into pan and bake for 20 to 25 minutes.

5. Remove from pan and cool on wire rack.

Serving Suggestion

Serve with creamy orange spread: Mix fat-free cream cheese, orange marmalade, and icing sugar to taste.

**Nutrient Analysis
per Serving**

169 calories

36 grams carbohydrate

4 grams protein

1 gram fat

Key Nutrients

50% vitamin A

17% thiamin

12% iron

Diabetic Exchanges

2½ starches

Strawberry Bread

My friend, Peggy Conner, made and served this bread at a baby shower for me. Serve with fat-free cream cheese that's been whipped with strawberry fruit spread.

Makes: 16 pieces

175 g (6 oz) sifted flour

8 tbsp wholemeal flour

8 tbsp old-fashioned rolled oats

2 tbsp wheatgerm

½ teaspoon baking soda

2 teaspoons baking powder

½ teaspoon salt

2½ teaspoons cinnamon

4 tbsp sugar

2 tbsp vegetable oil

2 275-g (10-oz) packages frozen, sliced, sweetened strawberries, thawed and drained

8 tbsp unsweetened applesauce

2 eggs

8 tbsp chopped pecans (optional)

Cooking spray or margarine

1. Preheat oven to 160°C/325°F/Gas mark 3.

2. Combine first 8 ingredients. Mix well.

3. Add remaining ingredients and mix until moistened. Gently fold in nuts, if desired.

4. Pour into 200-by-200-mm (8-by-8-inch) pan that has been sprayed with cooking spray or lightly greased and bake for 45 to 55 minutes.

Quick Tip

No applesauce in the house? Peel a medium-size apple, place in a microwave-safe dish, cover, and cook in microwave 5 minutes. When cool, remove core and mash with fork. One cooked apple makes about 8 tbsp applesauce.

Nutrient Analysis per Serving

131 calories

24 grams carbohydrate

3 grams protein

3 grams fat

3 grams fibre

Key Nutrients

17% manganese

16% vitamin C

Small amounts of many other nutrients

Diabetic Exchanges

1½ starches

½ fat

Thrive-on-Five Bread

Experimenting with a basic courgette bread recipe, I added ingredients until I came up with a bread that contained five different fruits and vegetables.

Makes: 1 15-slice loaf

8 tbsp each wholemeal flour, plain flour, and wheatgerm

2 teaspoons baking soda

1 teaspoon baking powder

½ teaspoon cinnamon

¼ teaspoon cloves

¼ teaspoon ginger

4 tbsp vegetable oil

1 egg

4 tbsp brown sugar

6 tbsp molasses

8 tbsp crushed pineapple in juice, drained well

8 tbsp applesauce (see page 264)

250 ml (8 fl oz) each grated carrot and grated courgettes

8 tbsp raisins

Cooking spray or margarine

1. Preheat oven to 180°C/350°F/Gas mark 4.

2. Mix together in a bowl all dry ingredients except sugar and set aside. In a separate bowl, mix together oil, egg, brown sugar, and molasses. Add vegetables and fruits.

3. Gradually add dry ingredients to sugar mixture. Mix until moistened.

4. Pour mixture into 225-by-125-mm (9-by-5-inch) loaf pan that is lightly greased or sprayed with cooking spray. Bake 50 to 60 minutes.

Nutrient Analysis per Serving

136 calories
23 grams carbohydrate
3 grams protein
5 grams fat
2 grams fibre

Key Nutrients

24% manganese
17% vitamin A
7% iron

Diabetic Exchanges

1½ starches
1 fat
A tiny portion each of fruit and vegetable

Apple Pie à la Mode Shake

All the shakes in this chapter can be made with either natural yogurt or milk. Yogurt adds a little tanginess and makes the shake very thick.

Makes: 2 servings

8 tbsp applesauce, frozen (see page 264)

2 tbsp brown sugar

250 ml (8 fl oz) skimmed milk or natural non-fat yogurt

½ teaspoon cinnamon or apple pie spice

½ teaspoon vanilla extract

Ice as needed

1. Blend all ingredients in blender and serve.

2. Add ice if needed.

Diabetic Variation

Instead of brown sugar, use approved artificial sweetener to taste.

Nutrient Analysis per Serving

120 calories
26 grams carbohydrate
4 grams protein
0 grams fat
1 gram fibre

Key Nutrients

18% vitamin B$_{12}$
15% potassium
16% calcium

Nutrient Analysis per Serving
(Diabetic Variation)

86 calories
17 grams carbohydrate
4 grams protein
0 grams fat
1 gram fibre

Diabetic Exchanges

⅔ fruit
½ skimmed milk

Banana-Orange Flip

Makes: 2 servings

*8 tbsp skimmed milk or natural
  non-fat yogurt*

8 tbsp orange juice

1 frozen banana

1. Blend all ingredients in a blender and serve in tall glasses.

2. Add ice if needed.

**Nutrient Analysis
per Serving**

100 calories
22 grams carbohydrate
3 grams protein
0 grams fat

Key Nutrients

38% vitamin C
21% potassium
11% riboflavin

Diabetic Exchanges

1¼ fruits
¼ skimmed milk

Peach Pops

This recipe may be just the trick for morning sickness. It also makes a great warm-weather snack. If you like chunky treats, experiment with adding a few fresh blueberries, grape halves, or other small pieces of fruit to fruit purée before pouring into freezer-pop moulds.

Makes: 8 servings

1 450-g (16-oz) tin sliced peaches with juice

2 tablespoons sugar

1. In a blender, mix the ingredients until smooth.

2. Pour into freezer-pop moulds and freeze about 3 to 5 hours until firm.

Diabetic Variation

Omit sugar or use approved artificial sweetener.

Source: Reprinted with permission from *Quick and Healthy, Volume II* by Brenda J. Ponichtera, R.D. (ScaleDown Publishing, Inc.).

Nutrient Analysis per Serving

36 calories
10 grams carbohydrate
0 grams protein
0 grams fat

Key Nutrients

Small amounts of many nutrients

Diabetic Exchanges

⅔ fruit

Peanut-Butter-Chocolate Shake

This shake is filling. Drink it when you're really hungry, trying to gain weight, or don't feel like preparing or eating an entire meal.

Makes: 1 serving

250 ml (8 fl oz) natural non-fat yogurt or skimmed milk

1 package chocolate instant meal mix

2 tablespoons smooth peanut butter

Ice as needed

1. Blend all ingredients in blender and serve in tall glasses.

Variations

Chocolate-Mint: Omit peanut butter and substitute ½ teaspoon peppermint flavouring.

Vanilla-Fruit: Use vanilla instant meal mix and substitute frozen unsweetened berries, frozen pineapple and banana, or peaches for peanut butter.

Mocha: Dissolve 1 teaspoon of instant decaffeinated coffee in milk before blending.

Note: This recipe is high in sugar. If you are watching your sugar intake, use sugar-free hot cocoa mix or sugar-free instant meal mix.

This recipe's high nutrient content is due to the instant meal mix, which is vitamin-fortified. If you eat more than one fortified food in a day, such as instant breakfast and a fortified cereal, plus your prenatal vitamin, you will be getting more than your daily requirements of some vitamins and minerals.

Nutrient Analysis per Serving

351 calories
43 grams carbohydrate
24 grams protein
9 grams fat

Key Nutrients

66% vitamin A
55% calcium
42% magnesium
41% vitamin C
37% zinc

Piña Colada Frappé

Makes: 2 servings

8 tbsp frozen pineapple

½ frozen banana

250 ml (8 fl oz) natural non-fat yogurt

½ teaspoon coconut extract

2 teaspoons of sugar or equivalent approved artificial sweetener (optional)

1. Blend all ingredients in a blender and serve in tall glasses.

Nutrient Analysis per Serving

127 calories
25 grams carbohydrate
7 grams protein
0 grams fat
1 gram fibre

Key Nutrients

24% calcium
23% potassium
14% vitamin C

Diabetic Exchanges

1 fruit
¾ skimmed milk

Raspberry Surprise Shake

Makes: 2 servings

250 ml (8 fl oz) natural non-fat yogurt or skimmed milk

2 fresh peaches or nectarines, peeled, sliced, and frozen

150 g (5 oz) frozen sweetened raspberries

1. Blend all ingredients in a blender and serve in tall glasses.

Variation

Use frozen strawberries instead of raspberries.

Diabetic Variation

Use unsweetened fruit and add approved artificial sweetener to taste.

Nutrient Analysis per Serving

174 calories
36 grams carbohydrate
8 grams protein
0 grams fat
3 grams fibre

Key Nutrients

27% potassium
26% vitamin B_{12}
26% vitamin C

Nutrient Analysis per Serving
(Diabetic Variation)

135 calories
26 grams carbohydrate
8 grams protein
3 grams fibre
0 grams fat

Diabetic Exchanges

1½ fruits
½ milk

Tropical Pudding

Women who are lactose intolerant will enjoy this dessert.

Makes: 4 servings

1 package vanilla instant pudding

8 tbsp orange juice

250 ml (8 fl oz) natural non-fat yogurt

8 tbsp crushed pineapple, well drained

½ teaspoon coconut extract

1. Mix juice into pudding mix using wire whisk.

2. Stir in yogurt and coconut extract. Follow package directions.

3. Stir in pineapple.

4. Chill at least 30 minutes.

5. Garnish with pineapple slice.

Diabetic Variation

Substitute sugar-free instant pudding for instant pudding.

Nutrient Analysis per Serving

157 calories
36 grams carbohydrate
4 grams protein
0 grams fat

Key Nutrients for Regular and Diabetic Variations

30% vitamin B$_{12}$
22% vitamin C
12% calcium

Nutrient Analysis per Serving
(Diabetic Variation)

86 calories
18 grams carbohydrate
4 grams protein
0 grams fat

Diabetic Exchanges

½ fruit
½ starch

Very Berry Shake

This is my favourite shake. If you have children at home, they will love its pretty purple colour.

Makes: 2 servings

250 ml (8 fl oz) unsweetened frozen strawberries and blueberries, or any combination of berries

250 ml (8 fl oz) vanilla non-fat yogurt or skimmed milk plus 1 teaspoon vanilla and sugar to taste

1. Blend all ingredients in a blender and serve in tall glasses.

Diabetic Variation

Use vanilla sugar-free non-fat yogurt.

Nutrient Analysis per Serving

112 calories
23 grams carbohydrate
6 grams protein
0 grams fat
2 grams fibre

Key Nutrients

60% vitamin C
20% calcium
18% potassium

Diabetic Exchanges

1 fruit
½ skimmed milk

Menus and Recipes for the Second Trimester

What you will find in this chapter:

• *Second-Trimester Menus*

   – *A Month of Breakfast Ideas*

   – *Menus for a Hungry Appetite*

   – *I Could Cook All Day Menus*

   – *Company's Coming! Menus*

• *Second-Trimester Recipes*

Second-Trimester Menus

A Month of Breakfast Ideas

Do you get tired of eating the same breakfast day in and day out? Here is a whole month's worth of meal ideas to help relieve your breakfast boredom:

• Peanut butter on toast with banana
• Frozen waffles topped with blueberries
• Vanilla yogurt with granola and bran muffin
• Oat bran cereal with strawberries
• Country Brunch Casserole (page 339), oat toast, and milk
• Apple-Date Bran Muffin (page 262), mixed fresh fruit salad, and milk
• Orange slices and English muffin with farmhouse cheese
• Strawberry Bread (page 264) with light or fat-free cream cheese, mango slices, and milk
• French French Toast (page 280), grilled grapefruit, and milk
• Microwaved scrambled eggs with low-fat cheese, mushrooms, and tomato slices, toast, and milk
• Cantaloupe melon and cottage cheese with blueberry bagel
• Bran cereal with mixed dried fruit and milk
• Oatmeal with raisins, peanut butter on digestive biscuits, and milk
• Poached egg and ham on English muffin, tangerine, and milk

- Mixed fresh fruit salad, Quick and Healthier Pancakes (page 278), and yogurt
- Bran muffin, honeydew melon, and milk
- Thrive-on-Five Bread (page 265) with fat-free cream cheese and hot cocoa
- Breakfast Pancakes with Raspberry Sauce (page 281) and milk
- Hot wheat cereal with chopped dried figs and milk
- Berry Mousse Parfait (page 303), cinnamon toast triangles, and milk
- Melted Swiss cheese on rye bread, apple pieces, and milk
- Cantaloupe melon, wheat toast with peanut butter, and milk
- Vegetable juice, boiled eggs, wheat bagel, and milk
- Cheerios, banana, and milk
- Corn muffins, refried beans with cheese, fresh pear, and milk
- Vegetarian Breakfast Tacos (page 350), kiwi fruit, and milk
- Peanut butter and honey on wholemeal bread, kiwi fruit, peaches, and milk
- Banana-Orange Flip (page 267) and oat bran toast
- Leftover Broccoli Quiche (page 334), watermelon cubes, and milk
- Cinnamon bread with Caramel Dip (page 319)
- Raspberry Surprise Shake (page 271) and poppy-seed muffin
- Very Berry Shake (page 273) and bran muffin

Menus for a Hungry Appetite

Mixed green salad
Stuffed Aubergine Creole (page 300)
Wheat baguette
Yogurt with berries

Vegetable juice
French French Toast (page 280)
Mixed fruit salad

Leek-and-Potato Soup (page 283)
Chicken Roll-Ups (page 291)
Carrots Antibes (page 257)
Wheat rolls
Fruit Crisp (page 252)

Salad with grated carrot, red cabbage, chickpeas, and corn
Pasta with Quick Alfredo Sauce (page 260)
Garlic bread
Tropical Pudding (page 272)

Raw veggies with Boursin Cheese Spread (page 318)
Tortellini with Creamy Pesto Sauce (page 293)
Wheat rolls
Mocha Java Cake (page 304) with strawberries

Caesar salad
Spinach-Stuffed Shells (page 346)
Carrots, courgettes, and yellow squash
Hard rolls
Frozen melon balls

Coleslaw with pineapple
Vegetarian Chilli (page 324)
Baked Tortilla Chips (page 254)
Yogurt with blueberries
Biscuits

Chicken and Prawn with Fruit Salsa
(page 336–337)
Broccoli-and-carrot stir-fry
Roasted New Potatoes (page 329)
Strawberry Bread (page 264)

Piña Colada Frappé (page 270)
Breakfast Pancakes with Raspberry Sauce
(page 281)
Turkey sausage slices
Milk

Creamy Broccoli Soup (page 252)
Greek Island Pitta Pockets (page 296)
Banana pudding

I Could Cook All Day Menus

Sesame Beef (page 345)
Asian noodles
Stir-fried vegetables
Tangy Salad (page 286)

Vegetables in Vinaigrette (page 330)
Turkey Pot Pie (page 301)
Mocha Java Cake (page 304)

Mushroom-and-Barley Soup (page 285)
Grilled pork loin chops
Ratatouille (page 328) over rice or bulgur
Yogurt with fresh fruit

Orange-glazed Cornish hens
Thanksgiving Sweet Potatoes (page 290)
Green beans with almonds
Pumpkin Roll (page 305)

3-bean salad
Crab Marinara over angel hair pasta
(page 340)
Herbed dinner rolls
Sunshine Sorbet (page 354)

Homemade cream-of-tomato soup
Hoppin' John (page 341)
Cheese corn bread rolls
Lime sorbet with blueberries

Company's Coming! Menus

Brunch

Watermelon and cantaloupe melon balls
Country Brunch Casserole (page 339)
Apple-Date Bran Muffins (page 262)
Steamed milk with amaretto flavouring

Asian Salad (page 253)
Broccoli Quiche (page 334)
Strawberry Bread (page 264)

Very Berry Shake (page 273)
Breakfast Pancakes with Raspberry Sauce
(page 281)
Vegetarian breakfast sausage

Creamy Broccoli Soup (page 252)
Chicken-and-Spinach Salad (page 256)
French bread
Apple slices with Caramel Dip
(page 339)

Pineapple-orange juice spritzers
Crêpes with various fillings
(pages 294–295)
Grilled bacon

Berry Mousse Parfait (page 303)
Strawberry Bread (page 264) and
Pumpkin Muffins (page 263)
Lite or fat-free cream cheese whipped
with orange marmalade and icing sugar
Cinnamon-orange herb tea

Lunch or Dinner

Boursin Cheese Spread (page 318) with
fresh vegetables and French bread
Cranberry juice and sparkling water
spritzers
Company Fondue (page 292)
Fruit Pizza for a Crowd (page 353)

Spinach-Stuffed Shells (page 346)
Garlic bread sticks
Tossed salad
Blueberry yogurt with raspberries

Mushroom-and-Barley Soup (page 285)
Chicken with Dijon Sauce (page 320)
Bulgur-and-Veggie Mix (page 325)
Wheat rolls
Blueberry Cobbler (page 306)

Apricot-Glazed Chicken (page 331)
Steamed asparagus with lemon
Rice wheat-berry pilaf
Mixed fruit salad
Apple-Date Bran Muffin (page 262)

Mixed green salad
Corn muffins
Spanish Steak Roll with Sautéed
Vegetables (page 299)
Potatoes Marie Louise (page 289)
Raspberry sorbet

Salmon en Papillote with julienne
vege-tables (page 298)
Spaghetti squash with warm tarragon
vinaigrette
Country sourdough bread
Peaches and blueberries topped with
lemon yogurt

Sliced tomatoes and cucumbers in
vinaigrette dressing
Spring Vegetables in Cream Sauce
(page 259) over linguine
Peach Cobbler (page 306)

Coleslaw
Quick Grilled Fish (page 344)
Carrots Antibes (page 257)
Wild rice pilaf
Mocha Java Cake (page 304) with
strawberries and Lite Cool Whip

Minute Minestrone (page 284)
Crêpes (pages 294–295)

Oven-Fried Courgettes (page 258) with
ranch dip
Crab Marinara (page 340)
Sunshine Sorbet (page 354)

Vegetables in Vinaigrette (page 330)
Veal Piccata with Roasted Red Pepper
and Cream Sauce (page 259)
Spinach pasta with vegetables
Apple tart

Tossed salad
Cheese-Topped Fish (page 335)
French-style green beans and corn
Roasted New Potatoes (page 329)
Fresh melon

Mexican Kale-and-Pork Soup (page 323)
Stuffed Aubergine Creole (page 300)
Low-fat cheesecake with raspberries

Second-Trimester Recipes

These recipes were developed for your second-trimester eating moods. Most women feel their best during these months, so the recipes are hearty and require a bit more preparation time than recipes for the other trimesters.

Breakfast Foods
French French Toast, 280
Pancakes with Raspberry Sauce, 281
Quick and Healthier Pancakes, 282

Soups
Leek-and-Potato Soup, 283
Minute Minestrone, 284
Mushroom-and-Barley Soup, 285

Salad
Tangy Salad, 286

Side Dishes
Basic Black Beans, 287
Beans 101, 288
Potatoes Marie Louise, 289
Thanksgiving Sweet Potatoes, 290

Entrées
Chicken Roll-Ups, 291
Company Fondue, 292
Creamy Pesto Pasta, 293
Crepe Dinner, 294–295
Greek Island Pitta Pockets with
    Cucumber Yogurt Sauce, 296
Leg of Lamb, 297
Salmon en Papillote, 298
Spanish Steak Roll with Sautéed
    Vegetables, 299
Stuffed Aubergine Creole, 300
Turkey Pot Pie, 301
Turkey with Hoisin Sauce, 302

Sweets
Berry Mousse Parfait, 303
Mocha Java Cake, 304
Pumpkin Roll, 305
Quick and Easy Blueberry Cobbler,
    306

French French Toast

When you're married to someone from another country, you find out which ethnic foods are authentic. The American version of French toast doesn't exist in France, but my mother-in-law remembers eating French French Toast as a child. This dish is great for those with a hearty appetite or those who need to gain more weight.

Makes: 2 servings

2 large eggs or 4 egg whites

3 tbsp skimmed or low-fat milk

Salt and pepper to taste

6 slices stale French loaf or 4 slices bread

Cooking spray

50 g (2 oz) ham

40 g (1½ oz) Swiss cheese

1. Mix eggs, milk, salt, and pepper. Soak bread slices in egg mixture. Spray pan with cooking spray.

2. Place bread in pan and cook over medium heat for several minutes.

3. Turn bread slices over and add ham and cheese to each piece. Cook several more minutes, and remove when cheese is melted.

Nutrient Analysis per Serving

347 calories

29 grams carbohydrate

24 grams protein

14 grams fat

1 gram fibre

Key Nutrients

80% selenium

30% calcium

23% chromium

Diabetic Exchanges

2½ medium–fat meats

2 starches

½ fat

Pancakes with Raspberry Sauce

With this dish, Margo Marrow won first place in the bread category of the Delicious and Nutritious Recipe Contest in the US. Margo has a special interest in nutrition because she works for the Women, Infants, and Children (WIC) nutrition programme. Her recipe shows her love of good food and nutrition. The variety of grains boosts the recipe's nutrient and fibre content, and the raspberry sauce is high in vitamin C.

Makes: 3 servings

Pancakes

3 egg whites

200 ml (6.5 fl oz) skimmed evaporated milk or skimmed milk

4 tbsp soya flour and 8 tbsp wheat flour

4 tbsp each cornmeal, oatmeal, and white flour

8 tbsp orange juice

Margarine, canola oil, or cooking spray

Raspberry Sauce

1 275-g (10-oz) package frozen raspberries (unsweetened) or 275 g (10 oz) fresh berries

1 tbsp cornflour

6 tbsp any juice (orange, apple, or cranberry)

3 tbsp sugar

1 teaspoon vanilla

Pancakes

1. Lightly beat egg whites. Add milk, flours, and orange juice. Spray pan with cooking spray or using kitchen paper towel, lightly grease pan with oil.

2. Pour 75-mm (3-inch) pancakes using 1 full tablespoon for each.

3. Serve on plates kept hot in the oven.

Raspberry Sauce

1. Strain thawed berries, reserving juice. Heat raspberry juice in saucepan until it simmers.

2. Dissolve cornflour in cold juice. Add with sugar to simmering raspberry juice. Stir occasionally to prevent sticking.

3. Cook until slightly thick and clear. Add vanilla and berries.

4. Serve warm over pancakes.

Diabetic Variation

Omit sugar and use 6 tbsp diluted frozen juice concentrate instead of regular juice in sauce.

Diabetic Exchanges

2 starches
1 fruit
½ skimmed milk
½ fat

Nutrient Analysis per Serving

298 calories
58 grams carbohydrate
12 grams protein
2 grams fat
5 grams fibre

Key Nutrients

32% vitamin C
20% magnesium
13% calcium

Nutrient Analysis
(Diabetic Variation)

292 calories
55 grams carbohydrate
13 grams protein
2 grams fat
5 grams fibre

Key Nutrients
(Diabetic Variation)

90% vitamin C
31% potassium
20% folic acid

Quick and Healthier Pancakes

I developed this recipe for those who aren't quite ready for 100-per cent wholegrain pancakes but want something healthier than 'all-white' pancakes.

Makes: 4 servings

250 ml (8 fl oz) reduced-fat Bisquick mix

8 tbsp old-fashioned oatmeal

8 tbsp wheatgerm

4 tbsp molasses

8 tbsp skimmed or semi-skimmed milk (or low-fat yogurt)

1 teaspoon cinnamon

1 egg or 2 egg whites

Cooking spray or oil

1. Mix all ingredients together until blended.

2. Spray pan with cooking spray or grease it with a small amount of oil. Pour about 6 tbsp of batter for each pancake.

3. Cook over medium heat until bubbles form on top and batter looks set.

4. Flip pancakes and cook briefly until golden brown.

Variation

After pouring batter, add raisins and/or thinly sliced bananas on top of batter. Gently push into batter. Cook as usual. Fruit makes the pancakes sweet, so you can reduce or omit the syrup. The leftovers also make a good snack.

Nutrient Analysis per Serving

279 calories

47 grams carbohydrate

10 grams protein

5 grams fat

2 grams fibre

Key Nutrients

38% selenium

19% zinc

19% calcium

17% iron

Diabetic Exchanges

3 starches

1 fat

Leek-and-Potato Soup

When you taste this soup, you may swear it has ham in it. It doesn't! This soup is great on an autumn or winter's day with cheese toast and fresh fruit. Spinach, leftover green vegetables, or mixed vegetables can be substituted for the carrots and leeks.

Makes: 16 servings

8 potatoes

4 medium carrots

900 g (2 lb) leeks

500 ml (17 fl oz) evaporated skimmed milk

Salt and pepper to taste

1. Peel potatoes and carrots. Trim ends off leeks, then cut lengthwise and rinse thoroughly. Cut all vegetables into 25-to-50-mm (1-to-2-inch) pieces.

2. Place all vegetables in large pot of hot water. Bring to the boil and simmer, covered, for 45 minutes, or until potatoes and carrots are tender. (Since carrots take longer to cook, you may want to give them a head start in the pot.)

3. Drain 90 per cent of water. Purée in batches in blender, adding small amount of milk to each batch.

4. Place all puréed batches in large bowl. Stir well, adding additional milk if needed. Add salt and pepper to taste.

Nutrient Analysis per Serving

141 calories

30 grams carbohydrate

6 grams protein

0 grams fat

3 grams fibre

Key Nutrients

74% vitamin A

28% vitamin B_6

17% vitamin C

11% folic acid

Diabetic Exchanges

2 vegetables

1 starch

$^{1}/_{2}$ skimmed milk

Minute Minestrone

This hearty vegetable soup can't be beaten for a quick, nutritious meal on a cold night.

Makes: 4 servings

150 g (5 oz) frozen spinach, thawed or cooked and not drained

1 225-g (8-oz) tin tomato sauce

1 410-g (14½-oz) tin diced tomatoes

130 g (4½ oz) green beans

190 g (6½ oz) chickpeas or kidney beans

100–125 g (4 oz) pasta, cooked

250 ml (8 fl oz) water

½ teaspoon onion powder

½ teaspoon garlic powder

1 teaspoon Italian spices

½ teaspoon basil, dried

Parsley, 1 teaspoon dried or 2 teaspoons fresh

1. Combine all ingredients in 1½-litre (2½ pt) saucepan.

2. Simmer 10 to 15 minutes, until heated. Add more water for thinner soup.

Variation

Omit green beans and spinach and add 1 275-g (10-oz) package frozen mixed vegetables to soup. Cook until vegetables are done.

Nutrient Analysis per Serving

182 calories
36 grams carbohydrate
9 grams protein
2 grams fat

Key Nutrients

51% vitamin A
46% vitamin C
41% potassium
15% iron

Diabetic Exchanges

3 vegetables
1½ starches
½ fat

Mushroom-and-Barley Soup

You can make this a main dish by adding about 350 g (12 oz) cooked chicken or white beans.

8 tbsp pearl barley, uncooked

1.25 l (2 pt) water

1 medium onion, chopped

2 medium cloves garlic, crushed

450 g (1 lb) mushrooms, sliced

1 to 2 tbsp dry sherry

750 ml (1¼ pt) fat-free chicken stock

Freshly ground black pepper

Makes: 6 servings

1. Place barley and 2½ cups water in large saucepan. Bring to the boil, cover, and simmer until barley is tender (20 to 30 minutes).

2. Meanwhile, heat 1 to 2 tablespoons water in a pan. Add onions and sauté for about 5 minutes over medium heat; add garlic and mushrooms. Cover and cook, stirring occasionally, until everything is very tender (about 10 to 12 minutes).

3. Add sauté with all its liquid to cooked barley, along with remaining water, sherry, and stock. Grind in generous amount of black pepper and simmer, partially covered, another 20 minutes over very low heat. Season to taste and serve.

Nutrient Analysis per Serving

87 calories
17 grams carbohydrate
3 grams protein
0 grams fat
3 grams fibre

Key Nutrients

14% selenium
13% niacin
10% potassium

Diabetic Exchanges

1 starch
½ vegetable

Tangy Salad

Gwen Shaw often serves this to her family. Even picky children should enjoy this salad. It tastes like a Waldorf salad, but yummier!

Makes: 4 servings

Salad

4 large leaves lettuce

1 green apple, peeled and chopped

1 large carrot, peeled and thinly sliced

1 celery stalk, chopped

1 medium orange, peeled, seeded, and sectioned (or use 1 300-g [11-oz tin] mandarin oranges, drained)

4 tbsp raisins

2 tbsp walnuts, chopped

Dressing

200 ml (6½ fl oz) natural non-fat or low-fat yogurt

1½ tbsp honey

1 tbsp lemon juice

¼ teaspoon each cinnamon and nutmeg

Fresh mint or orange twists for garnish

1. Combine ingredients for dressing in small bowl. Set aside.

2. Wash and drain lettuce. Line each plate with 1 whole lettuce leaf.

3. Combine fruits and vegetables and toss with dressing. Divide into equal portions on plates. Garnish each with orange slice and/or mint sprig.

Diabetic Variation

Substitute 2 packets of approved artificial sweetener for honey.

Nutrient Analysis per Serving

170 calories
30 grams carbohydrate
5 grams protein
3 grams fat
3 grams fibre

Nutrient Analysis (Diabetic Variation)

145 calories
23 grams carbohydrate
5 grams protein
3 grams fat
3 grams fibre

Key Nutrients

67% vitamin A
37% vitamin C
19% potassium

Diabetic Exchanges

1 fruit
1 vegetable
½ fat

Basic Black Beans

Black beans often satisfy my craving for something creamy and rich that sticks to my ribs. I often eat them for lunch topped with fresh tomatoes and melted cheese. Or I make a soft taco or tostado. If you don't have time to cook beans from scratch, keep a stock of tinned beans on hand. This recipe can easily be turned into soup or a dip.

Makes: 10 servings

450 g (1 lb) dry black beans or any dry bean

4 cloves garlic

3 medium shallots or 1 onion, chopped

1 teaspoon each cumin and chilli powder

½ teaspoon pepper

2 to 3 pieces bacon or ham (optional)

1. Soak beans overnight or use the quick-soak method. (See next page.) Discard soaking water.

2. Combine all ingredients in large pot. Add enough water to cover.

3. Cook 4 to 6 hours, or until beans are tender.

Variations

'Refried' Black Beans: To 500 ml (17 fl oz) cooked beans, add 1 to 2 cloves crushed garlic or garlic powder, cumin, and salt to taste. Mash by hand or in food processor or blender.

Quick Soup: Blend cooked beans and chicken stock in blender to desired consistency. Add onion and garlic powder, cumin, and chilli powder to taste. (See Aspen Black Bean Soup, page 321.)

Dip: Place 375 ml (13 oz) cooked beans in food processor. Add 1 tablespoon vinegar, 1 to 2 cloves crushed garlic, and ½ teaspoon salt (or use garlic salt to taste in place of garlic and salt). Process until smooth. Serve with baked tortilla chips.

Nutrient Analysis per ⅔-Cup Serving

201 calories
34 grams carbohydrate
14 grams protein
1 gram fat
6 grams fibre

Key Nutrients

43% folic acid
34% magnesium
12% zinc and iron

Diabetic Exchanges

2½ starches
1 very lean meat

Beans 101

Soaking

Quick Soak

Add 1.5 to 2 l (2½ to 3½ pt) hot water to 450 g (1 lb) beans. Bring to boil and boil for 2 minutes; set aside and cover. Let soak 1 hour. Drain and rinse before cooking.

Overnight Soak

Add 1.5 l (2½ pt) cold water to 450 g (1 lb) dry beans. Let soak overnight or at least 6 hours in cool place; do not refrigerate. Drain and rinse before cooking.

Cooking

Standard Method

Place beans in large pot with 1.5 l (2½ pt) hot water. Boil gently, with lid tilted, to desired tenderness.

Savoury Method

Place beans in large pot with 750 ml (1¼ pt) hot water. Add:

  2 teaspoons onion salt
  ¼ teaspoon garlic salt
  ¼ teaspoon white pepper
  1 tablespoon chicken-stock base or 3 bouillon cubes.

Boil gently, with lid tilted, to desired tenderness. Add water as needed to keep beans covered.

Source: *Favorite Recipes of Four Generations, Featuring California's Large Lima Beans,* by the Large Lima Council of the California Dry Bean Advisory Board.

Helpful Hints

- Simmer beans slowly; cooking too fast and stirring frequently breaks skins.
- Add 1 to 2 tablespoons oil to prevent foaming.
- Acid slows down cooking. Add tomatoes, vinegar, and other acidic foods last.
- At high altitudes, beans take longer to cook.
- When cooking in hard water, add ⅛ to ¼ teaspoon baking soda (no more) per 450 grams (pound) of beans to shorten cooking time.
- When cooking beans for casseroles and stews, avoid overcooking. (Beans should not be falling apart.) To purée or mash, cook until very soft.
- Some old recipes call for cooking unsoaked beans with meats, vegetables, and so on. This is acceptable. However, soaking, draining, and rinsing beans improves their flavour and digestibility and shortens their cooking time. Nutrient loss from soaking is minimal.
- Long, slow cooking in water is essential for rehydration and digestibility of dry beans.
- Microwave ovens can be used for reheating cooked or canned beans.

Bean Maths

1 450-g (1-lb) package
    = 450 g (1 lb) dry beans
    = 1.125 kg (2½ lb) soaked beans
1 440-g (15½-oz) tin
    = 365 g (¾ lb) beans

Potatoes Marie Louise

This is a favourite dish in our home. It's a great way to sneak more vegetables into your diet, and picky children will gobble it up! Vary the amount of carrots for a different flavour and colour.

Makes: 18 servings

10 medium potatoes (about 200 g [7 oz] each), peeled and cubed

5 medium carrots, peeled and sliced

250 to 375 ml (8 to 12 fl oz) evaporated skimmed milk

2 tbsp soft margarine

Salt and pepper to taste

1. Place potatoes and carrots in large pot; cover with water. Cook 45 minutes to 1 hour, or until both are tender.

2. Drain; place vegetables in large bowl. Whip with electric beater, adding milk, margarine, and seasoning. Add more milk until desired consistency is reached.

Variation

Add 3 75 g (3 oz) light cream cheese while beating for a richer, creamier dish.

Nutrient Analysis per Serving

127 calories
26 grams carbohydrate
3 grams protein
1 gram fat
2 grams fibre

Key Nutrients

70% vitamin A
23% potassium
12% vitamin C

Diabetic Exchanges

1½ starches
1 vegetable

Thanksgiving Sweet Potatoes

Have Thanksgiving anytime with this variation of a classic French dish!

Makes: 6 servings

*3 medium sweet potatoes,
   peeled and thinly sliced*

2 tbsp margarine, melted

2 tbsp brown sugar

*1 teaspoon ginger root, grated or
   in a jar (prepared)*

Cooking spray

1. Preheat oven to 200°C/400°F/Gas mark 6.

2. Spray a 230-mm (9-inch) glass pie plate with cooking spray.

3. Toss potatoes with 1 tablespoon melted margarine, sugar, and ginger.

4. Line bottom and sides of pie plate with a layer of overlapping potato slices.

5. Brush the remaining melted margarine on the potatoes. Cover with tin foil and place another pie plate upside down on top.

6. Bake on the bottom rack for 30 minutes. Remove tin foil and top pie plate and bake another 30 minutes or until potatoes are brown and caramelized.

Nutrient Analysis per Serving

126 calories
18 grams carbohydrate
1 gram protein
2 grams fibre

Key Nutrients

158% vitamin A
20% vitamin C

Diabetic Exchanges

1 starch
1 fat

Chicken Roll-Ups

This can be an elegant meal for company or just a casual meal for family.

Makes: 4 servings

*4 skinless, boneless chicken
  breast halves*

*3 tbsp light or fat-free cream
  cheese*

*2 teaspoons fresh parsley, finely
  chopped*

6 tbsp Italian-style bread crumbs

1 teaspoon lemon pepper

½ teaspoon garlic salt

½ teaspoon basil

1 tbsp grated Parmesan cheese

*50 g (2 oz) lean ham, thinly
  sliced*

1 egg plus 1 tbsp milk, beaten

*Fresh parsley and lemon wedges
  for garnish*

Cooking spray

1. Preheat oven to 180°C/350°F/Gas mark 4. Place all chicken breast halves between greaseproof paper or cling film and pound flat until they're almost 6 mm (¼-inch) thick.

2. In a small bowl, combine cream cheese with parsley. In a shallow dish, mix bread crumbs, spices, and Parmesan cheese.

3. Lay out 1 chicken breast half on a clean surface. Place 1 slice ham 12 g (½ oz) on top. Spread ½ tablespoon cream cheese mixture evenly over ham.

4. Roll up chicken breast, starting with small end. Secure with toothpicks, if necessary.

5. Beat 1 egg and 1 tablespoon milk in a shallow bowl. Dip rolled chicken breast in egg mixture and roll in crumb mixture. Place in small baking dish coated with cooking spray.

6. Repeat steps 3 to 5 with remaining chicken halves.

7. Bake uncovered for 30 minutes or until tender. Increase oven heat to grill last 2 to 3 minutes of cooking. Remove toothpicks before serving.

8. Serve with fresh chopped parsley and lemon wedges.

**Nutrient Analysis
per Serving**

270 calories
38 grams protein
8 grams carbohydrate
8 grams fat

Key Nutrients

79% niacin
60% selenium
35% vitamin B$_6$
21% chromium

Diabetic Exchanges

4½ very lean meats
½ starch

Company Fondue

The first time I ate this dish was at a gathering of co-workers. It was great fun because everyone brought a small portion of the meal, so the host didn't have much to prepare. For a last-minute company meal, I can't think of a faster meal to cook and serve.

Makes: 8 servings

Fondue

1.75 kg (4 lb) any combination of beef, chicken, shellfish, or tofu

1.35 l (2½ pt) chicken or beef stock

450 g (1 lb) fresh spinach, washed and trimmed

900 g (2 lb) fresh mushrooms, washed and trimmed

Dipping Sauces

Teriyaki sauce

Dijon cream sauce:
Mix 8 tbsp natural non-fat yogurt with 8 tbsp low-fat soured cream and 1 or 2 tbsp Dijon mustard to taste.

Sweet and sour sauce:
Heat 8 tbsp fruit spread (apricot or plum) with 1 tablespoon soy sauce and 1 or 2 teaspoons vinegar to taste.

Horseradish mayonnaise:
Mix 1 tablespoon white horseradish with 8 tbsp low-fat or fat-free mayonnaise.

Honey-mustard sauce

Steak sauce

Barbecue sauce

1. Cut meat and chicken into 25-mm (1-inch) pieces.

2. Heat stock to boiling. Pour into fondue pot or Crock-Pot.

3. Arrange meats and vegetables on separate platters.

4. Using fondue forks, guests cook meat and vegetables to desired doneness and dip in sauces.

5. When everyone is finished eating, add dash of sherry or sherry vinegar into stock, divide it among guests, and pass out soup spoons.

Variation

Serve fondue with noodles or brown rice and tossed green salad.

Nutrient Analysis per Serving (not including stock or sauces)	**Key Nutrients**	**Diabetic Exchanges**
259 calories	23% vitamin B$_6$	5½ lean meats
3 grams carbohydrate	20% zinc	½ vegetable
41 grams protein	17% iron	
9 grams fat	11% folic acid	

Creamy Pesto Pasta

If you like a lot of flavour without a lot of fat, you'll love this recipe. Try the sauce over fettuccine or small shells.

Makes: 4 servings

250 ml (8 fl oz) low-fat cottage cheese

4 tbsp Parmesan cheese (preferably freshly grated)

4 tbsp prepared pesto sauce

2 teaspoons tarragon vinegar

Freshly ground pepper

Salt

250 ml (8 fl oz) natural non-fat yogurt

1. Combine all ingredients except yogurt in food processor or blender.

2. Blend until smooth, adding yogurt to desired consistency.

3. Pour into microwave-safe bowl and heat 2 minutes on medium-high. Or cook slowly, stirring frequently, on stove until hot.

Nutrient Analysis per Serving

179 calories
8 grams carbohydrate
15 grams protein
9 grams fat

Key Nutrients

30% vitamin B$_{12}$
24% calcium
14% potassium

Diabetic Exchanges

1½ lean meats
1 fat
½ skimmed milk

Crêpe Dinner

Crêpes are another family favourite. They're so versatile; you can have them for breakfast, lunch, dinner, dessert, or a leftover snack. Consider hosting a make-your-own-crêpes party!

Makes: 10 to 12 servings

Batter

1 whole egg or 2 egg whites

2 teaspoons corn or vegetable oil

¼ teaspoon salt

225 g (8 oz) flour

250 ml (8 fl oz) skimmed or evaporated skimmed milk

250 ml (8 fl oz) plus 2 tbsp water

Cooking spray

For dessert crepes add:
  1 teaspoon vanilla
  2 tablespoons sugar

1. In large bowl, beat eggs, oil, and salt. Gradually stir in flour, milk, and water. Add vanilla and sugar for dessert crepes. Beat until smooth. Let stand several minutes.

2. Using ladle, pour 2 to 3 tablespoons of batter into heated 250-mm (10-inch) non-stick pan sprayed with cooking spray. It is essential to use a pan with no nicks or scratches. After pouring batter into pan, quickly rotate pan so that batter completely covers bottom of pan.

3. Cook over medium to medium-high heat until 1 side starts browning. Turn crêpe over and cook briefly on other side.

4. Fill immediately with one of the fillings listed below (or use your own filling) or place between pieces of greaseproof paper or tin foil to refrigerate or freeze.

5. Unused batter may be kept several days in refrigerator. Before using, let batter sit at room temperature a few minutes; then beat well.

Fillings

Breakfast
Peanut butter and banana
Berries and strawberry fruit spread or icing sugar
Ham and cheese
Margarine and sugar or honey
Applesauce and cinnamon
Fresh fruit and yogurt

(continued on next page)

Crêpe Dinner
(continued)

Lunch or Dinner

Spinach filling from Spinach-Stuffed Shells (page 346)

Ham and Swiss cheese, topped with Dijon Sauce (page 320)

Chicken and mushrooms topped with thick cream-of-mushroom soup

Ratatouille (page 328) and mozzarella cheese

Salmon Pâté (page 251) with Cucumber Yogurt Sauce (page 296)

Sautéed or steamed prawns and scallops with white sauce

Boursin Cheese Spread (page 318)

Dessert

Peaches with Caramel Dip (page 319)

Fresh fruit with vanilla yogurt

Chocolate yogurt topped with raspberries

Margarine and sugar or honey

Vanilla yogurt and blueberries with heated strawberry all-fruit spread

Vanilla yogurt with bananas cooked in orange juice and brown sugar

Nutrient Analysis per Serving
(2 unfilled crepes)

120 calories
22 grams carbohydrate
5 grams protein
1 gram fat

Key Nutrients

Small amounts of all nutrients. Depending upon the fillings you choose, your crepes can be chock-full of nutrients.

Diabetic Exchanges

1 starch
½ fat

Greek Island Pitta Pockets
with Cucumber Yogurt Sauce

Makes: 4 servings

Pitta Stuffing

**450 g (1 lb) boneless pork loin
or loin chops**

1 clove garlic, crushed

8 tbsp lemon juice

1 teaspoon dry oregano

1 tbsp Dijon mustard

Cooking spray

4 pieces wholemeal pitta bread

1 tomato, chopped

Soft leaf or cos lettuce, shredded

Cucumber Yogurt Sauce

8 tbsp natural low-fat yogurt

**½ small clove garlic (Use less if
you can't tolerate garlic. You
may want to use only a few
dashes of garlic powder.)**

¼ teaspoon oregano

1 teaspoon lemon juice

½ cucumber, peeled and chopped

⅛ teaspoon salt

1. Cut pork into 6-mm (¼-inch) strips.

2. Mix together garlic, lemon juice, and spices in Ziploc bag or glass container. Add pork and marinate in refrigerator at least 1 hour.

3. Spray pan with cooking spray. Over medium-high heat, stir-fry pork 6 to 8 minutes until it is no longer pink and is thoroughly cooked. Stuff meat, lettuce, and tomato inside pitta bread.

4. To make sauce, place all sauce ingredients in food processor or blender and blend until cucumbers are finely chopped but not puréed. Or chop cucumber finely by hand and mix with all other ingredients.

5. Top stuffed pitta with Cucumber Yogurt Sauce.

Nutrient Analysis per Serving	**Key Nutrients**	**Diabetic Exchanges**
417 calories	*88% thiamin*	*4½ lean meats*
26 grams carbohydrate	*43% niacin*	*1½ starches*
38 grams protein	*28% vitamin B₆*	*½ vegetable*
15 grams fat	*19% zinc*	
2 grams fibre		

Leg of Lamb

If not for my husband, I may never have had the joy of discovering leg of lamb. The French usually eat it with *flagolet*, green beans, and some type of potato. The leftovers are good served cold with Dijon mustard or as a sandwich on an onion roll. *Bon appétit!*

1 leg of lamb, with or without bone

4 to 6 garlic cloves, peeled and sliced into 2 or 3 pieces

1½ teaspoons each rosemary, oregano, thyme, and marjoram

OR

3 to 4 teaspoons Herbes de Provence

1. Preheat oven to 230°C/450°F/Gas mark 8.

2. Cut small slits in leg. Insert garlic clove pieces as deep as possible into slits.

3. Sprinkle outside of leg with herbs.

4. Reduce oven heat to 160°C/325°F/Gas mark 3.

5. Bake 30 minutes per 450 g (lb). If you prefer pink or rare meat, reduce cooking time to 15 or 20 minutes per 450 g (lb). Internal temperature of meat should be 80°C to 82°C (175°F to 180°F) for well-done and 71°C to 74°C (160°F to 165°F) for medium-rare.

6. Serve with pan juices or mint jelly.

Nutrient Analysis per 4-Ounce Serving

217 calories
0 grams carbohydrate
32 grams protein
9 grams fat

Key Nutrients

46% zinc
16% iron
9% folic acid

Diabetic Exchanges

4 lean meats

Salmon en Papillote

The beauty of fish is that it cooks so quickly. This recipe is based on the 'dash of this and a dash of that' principle – so use your imagination! This dish is traditionally cooked in parchment paper; I use tin foil. Some people like to add a teaspoon of dry white wine or tarragon vinegar for flavour. Salmon is a good source of omega-3 fatty acid, which is important for the development of your baby's nervous system and brain.

Makes: 4 servings

**4 pieces salmon steak
    (about 450 g/1 lb)**

Lemon pepper

Dill, preferably fresh

Spring onion and garlic, chopped

Basil, fresh

Lemon juice (fresh or bottled)

Wine, soy sauce, or vinegar

Tomatoes, chopped

Garlic powder

**Courgettes and carrots,
    cut julienne-style (optional)**

Lemon slices

1. Preheat oven to 200°C/400°F/Gas mark 6. Place each piece of fish on top of piece of tin foil or parchment paper big enough to wrap the fish in.

2. Top each piece of fish with herbs, lemon juice, and dash of wine, soy sauce, or vinegar. Add or delete any spices according to your tastes. Add herbs and vegetables. Top with several very thin lemon slices.

3. Bring together edges of paper above fish and fold sides and ends of paper so that fish is enclosed in an almost airtight package.

4. Place on baking sheet and bake for 10 minutes per each 25 mm (inch) of thickness of fish. Or cook on medium-hot grill for 15 to 20 minutes.

5. Serve fish still wrapped in its baking package, so your guests can open their packages and enjoy the aroma.

Nutrient Analysis per Serving

210 calories
0 grams carbohydrate
31 grams protein
9 grams fat

Key Nutrients

53% niacin
53% selenium
12% magnesium

Diabetic Exchanges

4 lean meats

Spanish Steak Roll with Sautéed Vegetables

Sandy Collins won first place with this recipe in a National Beef Cookoff in the US. I'm sure you'll agree that this dish is delicious! Omit the chillies if you can't tolerate spicy foods.

Makes: 6 servings

675 g (1½ lb) boneless 1-inch-thick beef sirloin steak

¼ teaspoon black pepper, freshly ground

1 teaspoon garlic powder

1 teaspoon butter

2 teaspoons vegetable oil

¾ teaspoon salt

1 red and 1 green pepper, cut lengthwise into strips

1 small white onion, thinly sliced

75 g (3 oz) fresh mushrooms, sliced

6 tbsp walnuts, chopped

¼ teaspoon chilli powder

1 tbsp soured cream or low-fat yogurt

1 110-g (4-oz) tin green chillies, chopped

Lemon slices

Coriander sprigs

1. Pound boneless beef sirloin steak to about 6-mm (¼-in) thickness. Sprinkle with pepper and ½ teaspoon garlic powder.

2. Heat butter and 1 teaspoon oil in 300-mm (12-in) heavy frying pan over medium-high heat until hot.

3. Pan-fry steak 5 to 7 minutes for medium-rare, turning once.

4. Remove steak to heated platter and sprinkle with ½ teaspoon salt. Keep warm.

5. Add remaining 1 teaspoon oil to frying pan. Add red and green peppers, onion, mushrooms, and walnuts. Cook 2 minutes, stirring frequently.

6. Add remaining ½ teaspoon garlic powder, ¼ teaspoon salt, and chilli powder; continue cooking 2 minutes, stirring frequently.

7. Spread steak with soured cream and top with chillies.

8. Starting at long side of steak, roll up and secure with 6 wooden picks. Place vegetables around steak roll; garnish with lemon slices and coriander sprigs. To serve, slice steak roll between wooden picks, then remove and discard picks.

Reprinted with permission, 1991 National Beef Cookoff.

Nutrient Analysis per Serving

320 calories
7 grams carbohydrate
37 grams protein
16 grams fat
2 grams fibre

Key Nutrients

58% vitamin C
52% zinc
16% magnesium
15% iron

Diabetic Exchanges

5 lean meats
1 vegetable

Stuffed Aubergine Creole

This recipe is pretty mild, so most pregnant women should be able to tolerate it. Add more Tabasco sauce if you like it hot!

Makes: 4 servings

2 small aubergine (450 g/1 lb each)

1 tbsp vegetable oil

1 clove garlic, crushed

450 g (1 lb) prawns, minced beef, or tofu (or a combination)

4 tbsp each finely chopped onion, green pepper, and celery

1 410-g (14½-oz) tin tomatoes, undrained

¼ teaspoon dried thyme

½ teaspoon salt

Dash of Tabasco sauce or cayenne pepper (optional)

160 g (5½ oz) seasoned or unseasoned dry breadcrumbs

8 tbsp low-fat soured cream

1. Preheat oven to 190°C/375°F/Gas mark 5.

2. Wash aubergine; cut in half lengthwise. Place in large pan and cover with water. Bring to the boil, cover, and simmer 15 minutes. Drain and cool.

3. Scoop out pulp from aubergine, taking care to leave shell 6-mm (¼-in) thick.

4. In pan, heat vegetable oil. Sauté garlic with either beef, seafood, or tofu.

5. Add raw vegetables and cook 5 minutes over low flame, stirring occasionally.

6. Stir in tomatoes, thyme, salt, and dash of Tabasco or cayenne pepper, if desired.

7. Add half the breadcrumbs. Add aubergine pulp and soured cream. Stir.

8. Stuff mixture back into 4 aubergine shells and top with remaining breadcrumbs.

9. Place in baking dish and bake 30 minutes.

Nutrient Analysis per Serving

347 calories
37 grams carbohydrate
29 grams protein
9 grams fat
6 grams fibre

Key Nutrients

35% vitamin C
23% magnesium
19% iron
15% zinc

Diabetic Exchanges

3 lean meats
3 vegetables
1½ starches

Turkey Pot Pie

This recipe is a great way to use holiday leftovers. Divide leftovers into individual microwave/freezer containers for pot pies.

Makes: 4 servings

Filling

4 medium carrots, peeled and sliced

2 spring onions, thinly sliced

1 clove garlic, minced

1 teaspoon oil

4 tbsp hot water

2 tbsp cornflour

200 ml (6.5 fl oz) chicken stock

8 tbsp evaporated skimmed milk

500 ml (17 fl oz) white turkey meat, skin removed, diced

8 tbsp frozen peas, thawed

2 tbsp parsley, chopped

¼ teaspoon each thyme, salt, and pepper

Topping

1 tin prepared biscuit dough

1. Preheat oven to 190°C/375°F/Gas mark 5.

2. Place carrots, spring onions, garlic, and oil in microwave-safe dish; add 4 tbsp hot water and cover. Cook 5 to 8 minutes on high. Drain (reserving liquid) and set aside.

3. Mix cornflour with 4 tbsp stock. Stir in rest of stock, cooking liquid from carrots, and evaporated skimmed milk. Cook, stirring constantly, until thickened (about 5 minutes).

4. Stir in remaining ingredients. Pour into pie pan or baking dish.

5. Arrange 8 round pieces of biscuit dough over mixture. Bake 15 to 20 minutes or until browned.

Nutrient Analysis per Serving

326 calories
39 grams carbohydrate
29 grams protein
6 grams fat

Key Nutrients

247% vitamin A
32% vitamin B₆
15% zinc
10% iron

Diabetic Exchanges

3 lean meats
2 starches
1½ vegetables

Turkey with Hoisin Sauce

I've discovered that turkey breast is even more versatile than chicken breast. It's larger, so you can cook it as a 'roast', slice it into 'fillets' or 'scallopini' (as in veal), or slice it thin for stir-fry dishes. Also, turkey is often less expensive than boneless chicken breast!

Makes: 4 servings

2 teaspoons corn/vegetable oil

1 clove garlic, minced

450 g (1 lb) turkey cutlets or turkey tenderloin, sliced into 12-mm (½-in) slices

2 spring onions, chopped

1 teaspoon cornflour

8 tbsp water

2 tbsp frozen orange juice concentrate, thawed

2 tbsp soy sauce

1 tbsp hoisin sauce

1. Heat oil in non-stick pan over medium-high heat.

2. Add garlic. Sauté for 1 to 2 minutes.

3. Add turkey and sauté for 2 to 3 minutes on each side. Remove and keep warm.

4. Add spring onions to pan and sauté briefly.

5. In small bowl, mix cornflour with 8 tbsp water. Add mixture to pan along with orange juice, soy sauce, and hoisin sauce. Bring to the boil and cook until slightly thickened.

6. Pour sauce over turkey and serve.

Serving Suggestions

Serve with brown rice and stir-fried vegetables.

Nutrient Analysis per Serving

197 calories

3 grams carbohydrate

34 grams protein

4 grams fat

Key Nutrients

47% niacin

34% vitamin B_6

17% vitamin B_{12}

Diabetic Exchanges

5 very lean meats

Berry Mousse Parfait

This delicious dish can be a dessert or a snack. You can vary the types of yogurt and fruit.

Makes: 4 servings

2 225-g (8-oz) containers fat-free or low-fat blueberry yogurt

500 ml (17 fl oz) strawberries and blueberries, sliced

Sprig of mint

1. In 4 parfait or wineglasses, layer yogurt, then berries, then yogurt.

3. Garnish with a few berries and a sprig of mint.

Diabetic Variation

Use sugar-free yogurt instead.

Nutrient Analysis per Serving

152 calories
31 grams carbohydrate
5 grams protein
2 grams fat
2 grams fibre

Key Nutrients

52% vitamin C
19% potassium
18% calcium

Nutrient Analysis per Serving
(Diabetic Variation)

106 calories
19 grams carbohydrate
5 grams protein
2 grams fat
2 grams fibre

Diabetic Exchanges

1 fruit
½ skimmed milk

Mocha Java Cake

Just because you're pregnant doesn't mean you need to give up chocolate – just make it a little healthier! This cake is so moist, it reminds me of chocolate cheesecake; just a small piece should be enough to satisfy your craving.

Makes: 15 servings

200 g (7 oz) flour

8 tbsp brown sugar, packed

4 tbsp vegetable/corn oil

200 ml (6.5 fl oz) evaporated skimmed milk

4 tbsp cocoa powder

8 tbsp applesauce

250 ml (8 fl oz) strong decaffeinated coffee

1 teaspoon baking powder

1 teaspoon baking soda

1 teaspoon vanilla

Margarine and flour (for greasing)

1. Preheat oven to 190°C/375°F/Gas mark 5.

2. Mix all ingredients until well blended, about 1 to 2 minutes with electric mixer.

3. Pour into 200-by-200-mm (8-by-8-in) or 225-mm (9-in) round cake tin that has been lightly greased and floured.

4. Bake 35 to 40 minutes.

5. Sprinkle cake with icing sugar and serve with low-fat yogurt and strawberries for a special treat!

Nutrient Analysis per Serving

155 calories

26 grams carbohydrate

3 grams protein

4 grams fat

Key Nutrients

11% potassium

11% thiamin

7% calcium

Diabetic Exchanges

2 starches

1 fat

Pumpkin Roll

Although this recipe may look complicated, it's actually easy to prepare. It makes an elegant (and healthy) dessert for company or a potluck.

Makes: 12 servings

Cake

3 eggs (or 2 eggs and 2 egg whites)

150 g (5 oz) unsweetened pumpkin

175 g (6 oz) sugar

75 g (3 oz) wholemeal or white flour

1 teaspoon baking soda

1½ teaspoons cinnamon

Icing sugar

Filling

1 225-g (8-oz) package any type cream cheese (fat-free, light, or full-fat)

8 tbsp icing sugar

1 teaspoon vanilla

1. Preheat oven to 190°C/375°F/Gas mark 5. In bowl, beat together eggs, pumpkin, and sugar.

2. In separate bowl, mix together flour, baking soda, and cinnamon; then add to pumpkin mixture. Spread on Swiss roll pan (375-by-250-by-25-mm/15-by-10-by-1-in) that has been covered with greaseproof paper, well coated with cooking spray, or greased. Bake 15 minutes.

3. Sift generous amount of icing sugar onto clean tea towel.

4. Turn hot cake onto towel and roll up towel with cake Swiss-roll fashion. Refrigerate at least 1 hour.

5. In bowl, beat together cream cheese, sugar, and vanilla.

6. Unroll cake. Spread filling onto cake, roll up cake without towel, wrap in tin foil, and keep chilled until ready to serve. Freezes well.

7. When you're ready to serve, sprinkle again with icing sugar.

Nutrient Analysis per Serving

141 calories
28 grams carbohydrate
5 grams protein
1 gram fat

Key Nutrients

40% vitamin A
9% manganese
9% selenium

Diabetic Exchanges

2 starches

Quick and Easy Blueberry Cobbler

If you like cobbler, you'll find this one worth the small effort.

Makes: 6 servings

Cooking spray

100–125 g (4 oz) flour

175 g (6 oz) sugar

1½ teaspoons baking powder

½ teaspoon salt

1 teaspoon almond extract

200 ml (6.5 fl oz) tinned evaporated skimmed milk

1 600-g (21-oz tin blueberry pie filling

Slivered almonds (optional)

1. Preheat oven to 180°C/350°F/Gas mark 4.

2. Spray 2-l (3½ pt) casserole with cooking spray.

3. Mix together flour, sugar, baking powder, salt, almond extract, and milk. Pour into casserole.

4. Spoon pie filling on top.

5. Bake for 35 to 40 minutes or until golden brown. If desired, sprinkle almonds on top of cobbler during last 10 minutes of baking.

Variation

Use peach pie filling instead of blueberry to make a Peach Cobbler.

Note: This recipe is high in simple sugar. Diabetic mothers should eat only a small amount or none at all.

Nutrient Analysis per Serving

275 calories

64 grams carbohydrate

5 grams protein

0 grams fat

Key Nutrients

15% riboflavin

12% calcium

Diabetic Exchanges

3½ starches

½ fruit

CHAPTER FIFTEEN

Menus and Recipes for the Third Trimester

Third-Trimester Menus

Using Leftovers with Flair

Day 1

　Tossed salad

　Grilled chicken

　Rotini pasta

　Steamed courgette and yellow squash

Day 2

　Colorado Stuffed Peppers (page 338)

　　(Cook black beans in Crock-Pot during the day.)

　Corn bread

　Fresh fruit salad

Day 3

　Grilled chicken (from Day 1) in pitta pocket with lettuce,
　　tomatoes, and vinaigrette dressing

　OR

　Chicken-and-Spinach Salad (page 256)

Day 4

　Bridget's Garden Salad (page 255)

　　(Use rotini pasta and leftover veggies from Day 1.)

　Strawberries and vanilla yogurt

**What you will find
in this chapter:**

- *Third-Trimester Menus*
  - *Using Leftovers
    with Flair*
  - *Meals in Minutes*
  - *Feel Full Meals*
  - *Best Bite Snacks*
  - *Vegetarian Budget
    Menus*
- *The Bean Routine*
- *Third-Trimester Recipes*

Day 5

Black bean soup with cheese (Use beans
  from Day 2.)
Corn bread
Tomato and avocado slices with fat-free
  Italian dressing

Day 6

Fajitas with chicken, beef, or prawns
Guacamole dip (Use tomato and avocado
  from Day 5.)
Lettuce, tomato, and reduced-fat cheese

Day 7

Salmon en Papillote (page 298)
Steamed asparagus
Easy Microwave Potatoes (page 326)
Sorbet

Day 8

Tossed salad with leftover fajita strips
  (from Day 6), tinned kidney beans,
  tomatoes, carrots, and cheese
Aspen Black Bean Soup (Use black beans
  from Day 5.)
Baked Tortilla Chips (page 254)

Day 9

Linguine with salmon, tinned artichoke
  hearts, and Parmesan cheese (Use fish
  from Day 7.)
Delightful Spinach (page 250)
Crusty wholemeal French bread
Coleslaw
Fruit salad

Day 10

Creamy Asparagus Soup (page 252)
  (Use asparagus from Day 7.)
Baked chicken
Potatoes Marie Louise (page 289)
Green beans
Tangerine

Day 11

Spinach, mushroom, and cheese quesadillas with tomatoes (Use spinach
  from Day 9.)
OR
Curried chicken salad and cos lettuce in
  pitta pocket (Use chicken from Day 10.)
Fresh melon

Day 12

Grilled fish with grilled pineapple
Grilled vegetable shish kebabs:
  courgettes, mushrooms, aubergine,
  tomatoes
Bulgur or brown rice pilaf

Day 13

Fish on a Kaiser roll
Tossed salad with vinaigrette dressing
Black Bean and Corn Salad (page 254)
Apple slices with Caramel Dip (page 319)

Day 14

Tangy Salad (page 286)
Vegetable tacos with courgettes, mushrooms, aubergine, tomatoes, and
  cheese (Use vegetables from Day 12.)
Roasted New Potatoes/Home Fries
  (page 329)

Day 15

    Ratatouille (page 328)

    Brown rice (from Day 12) with poached
       egg

    Kiwi fruit and peaches over angel food
       cake

Day 16

    Chicken with Dijon Sauce (page 320)

    Pasta with steamed vegetables

    Fruit Crisp (page 352)

Day 17

    Ratatouille (from Day 15) and cheese on
       Wholemeal bread

    Tossed salad

    Frozen melon balls

Day 18

    Crêpes (pages 294–295) with chicken
       and Dijon Sauce (from Day 16)

    Black Bean and Corn Salad (from Day
       13)

    Vanilla yogurt with Fruit Crisp (from
       Day 16) as topping

Day 19

    Vegetarian Chilli (page 324)

    Coleslaw

    Sunshine Sorbet (page 354)

Day 20

    Vegetarian tacos or taco salad (Use chilli
       from Day 19.)

    Tossed salad

    Berry Mousse Parfait (303)

Meals in Minutes

Cup of soup
Turkey with Hoisin Sauce (page 302)
Instant brown rice with snow peas
Banana

Split-pea soup
Microwaved grilled cheese sandwich
Tomato slices
Fresh fruit

Bean tostadas with lettuce and tomato
Yogurt with strawberries
Scallop-and-prawn stir-fry with frozen
    veggie mix
Angel hair pasta
Fresh peach

Salad with smoked turkey, cherry toma-
    toes, and cos lettuce
Bread sticks
Fresh orange

Hoppin' John (page 341)
Steamed broccoli
Strawberries and banana slices

Minute steak on wheat bun
Spinach salad (in a bag)
Banana pudding

Minute Minestrone (page 284)
Turkey breast and cheese quesadilla in
    wholemeal tortilla
Apple

Turkey with Hoisin Sauce (page 302)
Kids' Carrots (page 327)
Spinach pasta twists

Tomato soup
Cheese-Topped Fish (page 335)
Bulgur-and-Veggie Mix (page 325)
Mixed fruit salad

Raw vegetables with ranch dip
Hoppin' John (page 341)
Very Berry Shake (page 273)

Apricot-Glazed Chicken (page 331)
Easy Microwave Potatoes with Italian
    seasoning (page 326)
Delightful Spinach (page 250)

Quick Grilled Fish (page 344) with
    grilled vegetables
Angel hair pasta, fresh
Tropical Pudding (page 272)

Caesar salad (in a bag)
Prawn cocktail
Garlic French bread with melted low-fat
    cheese
Grapes
Biscuits

European-style salad (in a bag)
Aspen Black Bean Soup (page 321)
Baked Tortilla Chips (page 254) with
    salsa
Fresh pineapple rings

Salad with leftover grilled chicken, cos
    lettuce, corn, and tomato
Bread sticks
Cantaloupe melon chunks
Strawberry ice milk

Bean tostada
Sliced tomatoes and cucumbers
Frozen fruit salad (peaches, raspberries,
    grapes)

Tossed salad
Crab Marinara (page 340) over linguini
Lemon sorbet with fresh raspberries

Feel Full Meals

These menus give you the very most nutrition per bite when you can't eat much!

Crab Marinara (page 340)
Tossed cos salad
Cantaloupe melon slices

Spanish Steak Roll (page 299)
Delightful Spinach (page 250)
Bulgur pilaf

Leg of Lamb (page 297)
Green beans and flageolets
Potatoes Marie Louise (page 289)
Raspberries

Sesame Beef (page 345)
Stir-fried peppers and tomatoes
Brown rice or bulgur pilaf
Berry Mousse Parfait (page 303)

Black Bean and Corn Salad (page 254)
Baked Tortilla Chips (page 254)
Fresh orange

Asian Salad (page 253)
Cheese-Topped Orange Fish (page 335)
Steamed broccoli
Mango slices

Stuffed Aubergine Creole (page 300)
Brown rice or quinoa
Sunshine Sorbet (page 354)

Country Brunch Casserole (page 339)
Very Berry Shake (page 273)

Raw veggies with Boursin Cheese Spread
  (page 318)
Spinach-Stuffed Shells (page 346)
Bread sticks
Watermelon balls

Chicken and Prawns with Fruit Salsa
  (pages 336–337)
Carrots Antibes (page 257)
Barley pilaf

Veal Piccata with Roasted Red Pepper
  Sauce (page 348)
Wholemeal pasta
Strawberry and banana slices

Broccoli Quiche (page 334)
Tomato slices
Wheat baguette
Fruit Crisp (page 352)

Spanish Steak Roll with Sautéed
  Vegetables (page 299)
Roasted New Potatoes (page 329)
Cantaloupe melon

Apricot-Glazed Chicken (page 331)
Cos lettuce salad
Piña Colada Frappé (page 270)

Vegetables in Vinaigrette (page 330)
Black Bean Enchilada Casserole
  (page 333)
Tangy Salad (page 286)

Best Bite Snacks

These snacks have the most nutrients per calorie:

  Boursin Cheese Spread (page 318)
  Favourite Snack Cake (page 351)
  Spiced refried beans with Baked Tortilla
    Chips (page 254)
  Very Berry Shake (page 273)
  Raspberry Surprise Shake (page 271)
  Stuffed Figs (page 51)
  Berry Mousse Parfait (page 303)
  Pumpkin Muffins (page 263)
  Thrive-on-Five Bread (page 265)
  Layered Mexican Dip (page 234)
  Tropical Pudding (page 272)
  Tangy Salad (page 286)
  Oven-Fried Courgette or Aubergine
    (page 258)
  Aspen Black Bean Soup (page 321)
  Peach Pops (page 268)

Vegetarian Budget Menus

The following two weeks' worth of sample menus can help if you are becoming vegetarian or are just looking for ways to cut food costs. Meatless meals can be very affordable and very healthy! The Week 1 menus require ingredients found in most kitchens and little preparation. Week 2 introduces meals using some common recipes. These menus do include milk and eggs. If you are vegan, you can use egg substitute, soya milk, or soya cheese instead.

These menus use semi-skimmed milk and may contain fats like margarine, butter, or oil added while cooking. The menus average 2,200 calories and assume serving sizes such as 375 ml (12 fl oz) cereal or soup, 125 ml (4 fl oz) fruit, 125 ml (4 fl oz) vegetables, 2 tablespoons peanut butter, 250 ml (8 fl oz) milk, and so on. Unlike other menus in this book, these vegetarian menus include beverages because beverages have been used to calculate calories and nutrients.

A recommended vegetarian cookbook for busy people is *Meatless Meals for Working People: Quick and Easy Vegetarian Recipes,* available from the Vegetarian Resource Group at www.vrg.org.

Week 1

Monday

Breakfast

Quick and Healthier Pancakes (page 282) with sliced peaches

Semi-skimmed milk

Lunch

Tomato soup

Grilled cheese sandwich with wholemeal bread

Apple

Dinner

Vegetarian Chilli (page 324)

Corn muffins

Coleslaw

Watermelon

Semi-skimmed milk

Snacks

Savoury biscuits with peanut butter and semi-skimmed milk

Tortilla chips with bean dip and tomato juice

Tuesday

Breakfast

Raisin Bran

Banana

Semi-skimmed milk

Lunch

Sloppy joes made with textured vegetable protein (TVP)

Carrot-and-raisin salad

Semi-skimmed milk

Dinner

Broccoli Quiche (page 334) (a good way to use leftovers)

Wheat toast

Grilled tomato halves

Roasted New Potatoes/Home Fries (page 329)

Snacks

Digestive biscuits with semi-skimmed milk

Tinned pineapple with cottage cheese and fruit juice

Wednesday

Breakfast

Oatmeal with raisins and molasses

Banana bread

Semi-skimmed milk

Lunch

Black Bean and Corn Salad (page 254)

Baked corn tortillas with cheese

Fruit Crisp (page 352)

Dinner

Hoppin' John (without ham – page 341)

Corn bread

Greens or spinach

Carrot sticks

Grapes

Snacks
  Popcorn and semi-skimmed milk
  Piña Colada Frappé (page 270) and
    gingersnaps

Thursday

Breakfast
  Poached eggs on wheat toast
  Grapefruit
  Semi-skimmed milk

Lunch
  Macaroni and cheese
  Tossed salad with kidney beans and
    tomato slices
  Kiwi fruit

Dinner
  Vegetables in Vinaigrette (page 330)
  Colorado Stuffed Peppers (page 338)
  Fresh cantaloupe melon slices
  Semi-skimmed milk

Snacks
  Cheese and biscuits
  Pumpkin Muffins (page 263) and semi-
    skimmed milk

Friday

Breakfast
  Hot wheat cereal
  Peanut butter and banana on toast
  Semi-skimmed milk

Lunch
  Bean and brown rice burritos
  Spinach salad with orange pieces
  Apple

Dinner
  Tossed salad with chickpeas
  Wholemeal pasta with marinara sauce
    and cheese
  Wheat rolls
  Cinnamon grilled peach halves

Snacks
  Oatmeal biscuits and semi-skimmed milk
  Brown rice pudding with raisins

Saturday

Breakfast
  Cheese toast
  Apple-and-pear salad
  Semi-skimmed milk

Lunch
  Lentil Soup (page 322)
  Celery and carrot sticks
  Strawberries with yogurt
  Semi-skimmed milk

Dinner
  Wholemeal couscous with mushrooms,
    courgettes, tomato sauce, and
    Parmesan cheese
  Kids' Carrots (page 327)
  Garlic bread
  Fruit salad
  Semi-skimmed milk

Snacks
  Hot cocoa
  Fig bars
  Very Berry Shake (page 273)
  Favourite Snack Cake (page 351)

Sunday

Breakfast
  Vegetarian Breakfast Tacos (page 350)
  Mango slices
  Semi-skimmed milk

Lunch
   Grilled vegetable-and-cheese sandwich
      on rye toast
   Banana
   Semi-skimmed milk

Dinner
   Cabbage salad
   Tofu Loaf (page 347)
   Steamed courgettes
   Strawberry Bread (page 264) with light
      cream cheese
   Fresh orange

Snacks
   Yogurt sundae
   Granola or muesli bar and semi-skimmed
      milk

Week 2

Monday

Breakfast
   French toast with strawberries
   Semi-skimmed milk

Lunch
   Leek-and-Potato Soup (page 283)
   Wholemeal English muffins
   Celery with low-fat cream cheese
   Grapes
   Semi-skimmed milk

Dinner
   Ratatouille (page 328) over brown rice
      or bulgur
   Macaroni, black beans, and corn
   Kiwi fruit slices

Snacks
   Digestive biscuits with peanut butter
   Semi-skimmed milk
   Thrive-on-Five Bread (page 265)

Tuesday

Breakfast
   Oatmeal with raisins
   Fresh orange
   Apple-Date Bran Muffin (page 262)
   Semi-skimmed milk

Lunch
   Grilled Swiss cheese and sauerkraut on
      rye bread
   Potato salad
   Fresh apple

Dinner
   Oat-Nut Burgers (page 343)
   Thanksgiving Sweet Potatoes (page 290)
   Wheat rolls
   Fruit cocktail
   Semi-skimmed milk

Snacks
   Bran muffin and semi-skimmed milk
   Fat-free cream cheese dip, cauliflower
      and carrot sticks, and wheat biscuits

Wednesday

Breakfast
   Muesli
   Cantaloupe melon
   Wheat toast

Lunch
   Boursin Cheese Spread (page 318) on
      wheat roll with lettuce, cucumber,
      tomato, and sprouts
   Carrot-and-pineapple salad
   Biscuits

Dinner
Tomatoes in vinaigrette
Black Bean Enchilada Casserole (page 333)
Wheat garlic toast
Fresh fruit salad
Semi-skimmed milk

Snacks
Tangerine and cheese
Leftover veggies, beans, and cheese in
wheat tortilla with semi-skimmed milk

Thursday

Breakfast
Wholegrain cereal
Sliced banana
Semi-skimmed milk

Lunch
Sliced avocado, cheese, tomato, and
lettuce on wheat bread
Salad
Plums
Semi-skimmed milk

Dinner
Bean and Corn Bread Bake (page 332)
Coleslaw
Strawberries over angel food cake
Semi-skimmed milk

Snacks
Yogurt with fruit
Vegetarian beans and homemade tortilla
chips or toasted pitta bread triangles

Friday

Breakfast
Poached eggs
Cinnamon-raisin bagels
Apple juice
Semi-skimmed milk

Lunch
Minute Minestrone (page 284)
Cottage cheese with raw vegetables
Corn bread
Grapes

Dinner
Asian Salad (page 253)
Vegetable-and-Tofu Stir-Fry (page 349)
Chinese noodles or brown rice
Pineapple slices

Snacks
Savoury biscuits and peanut butter with
semi-skimmed milk
Granola or muesli bar and semi-skimmed
milk

Saturday

Breakfast
Country Brunch Casserole (page 339)
Raisins or prunes
Toast
Semi-skimmed milk

Lunch
Oven-Fried Aubergine Slices (page 258)
with marinara sauce and cheese
Crusty French bread
Watermelon
Semi-skimmed milk

Dinner
Spring Vegetables in Cream Sauce
(page 259)
Spinach salad
Garlic bread
Semi-skimmed milk

Snacks
Berry Mousse Parfait (page 303)
Vegetarian nachos made with Baked
Tortilla Chips (page 254) and orange
juice

Sunday

Breakfast
  Frozen waffles
  Strawberries
  Semi-skimmed milk

Lunch
  Aspen Black Bean Soup (page 321)
  Savoury biscuits
  Carrot and celery sticks
  Apple slices with Caramel Dip (page 319)
  Semi-skimmed milk

Dinner
  Spinach-Stuffed Shells (page 346)
  3-bean salad with cherry tomatoes
  Melon

Snacks
  Popcorn and tomato juice
  Banana, peanut butter, and semi-
    skimmed milk

▼

The Bean Routine

Dry beans are a nutritional gold mine for today's mother-to-be! They are high in protein, complex carbohydrate, and fibre; low in fat; and full of important nutrients. They make a great main dish when you can't tolerate meat. Beans will save you money on your food budget, and you can save time by using tinned beans.

A 250 ml (8 fl oz) cup of cooked dried beans provides 27 per cent of a pregnant woman's daily need for protein, 25 per cent of her requirement for manganese, 18 per cent of her requirement for iron, and 31 per cent of her requirement for folic acid. Plus, beans provide about 9 grams of fibre. Pregnant women should eat 20 to 35 grams of fibre per day.

Beating Bean Bloat

One common concern about beans is that they can cause wind. A University of California-Berkeley study reported greater intestinal tolerance after three weeks of eating beans regularly. Here are some tips for adjusting to the bean routine.[1]

1. Build up your body's tolerance. Eat small servings at first; then increase your intake slowly over a period of weeks.

2. Soak beans overnight, cook your beans properly, and always pour off the soaking water and add fresh water for cooking. Proper cooking can break down starches, making the beans more digestible.

3. Chew well and slowly. This assists in digestion and can minimize your bloating problem.

4. Drink enough fluids. Sufficient fluid intake helps your digestive system handle the increased dietary fibre.

Third-Trimester Recipes

Dips, Sauces, and Spreads
Boursin Cheese Spread, 318
Caramel Dip, 319
Dijon Sauce, 320

Soups
Aspen Black Bean Soup, 321
Lentil Soup, 322
Mexican Kale-and-Pork Soup, 323
Vegetarian Chilli, 324

Side Dishes
Bulgur-and-Veggie Mix, 325
Easy Microwave Potatoes, 326
Kids' Carrots, 327
Ratatouille, 328
Roasted New Potatoes/Home Fries,
  329
Vegetables in Vinaigrette, 330

Entrées
Apricot-Glazed Chicken, 331
Bean and Corn Bread Bake, 332
Black Bean Enchilada Casserole, 333
Broccoli Quiche, 334

Cheese-Topped Fish, 335
Chicken and Shrimp with Fruit Salsa,
  336–337
Colorado Stuffed Peppers, 338
Country Brunch Casserole, 339
Crab Marinara, 340
Hoppin' John, 341
Mock Egg Foo Yung, 342
Oat-Nut Burgers, 343
Quick Grilled Fish, 344
Sesame Beef, 345
Spinach-Stuffed Shells, 346
Tofu Loaf, 347
Veal Piccata with Roasted Red
  Pepper Sauce, 348
Vegetable-and-Tofu Stir-Fry, 349
Vegetarian Breakfast Tacos, 350

Sweets
Favourite Snack Cake, 351
Fruit Crisp, 352
Fruit Pizza for a Crowd, 353
Sunshine Sorbet, 354

Boursin Cheese Spread

This recipe is from *More Low-Fat Favorites* by Ceacy Thatcher. Try it with pitta bread crisps, savoury biscuits, raw vegetables, or in crêpes with veggies. Or thin it with a little skimmed milk to make a sauce for pasta or vegetables or to use as salad dressing.

Makes: 12 servings

225 g (8 oz) fat-free margarine

450 g (16 oz) fat-free cream cheese

2 cloves fresh garlic, crushed, or 1 teaspoon chopped garlic from jar

½ teaspoon dried oregano

¼ teaspoon dried marjoram

¼ teaspoon dried thyme

¼ teaspoon dried basil

¼ teaspoon dried dill

¼ teaspoon white pepper

1. Using a hand mixer or spoon, mix all ingredients until well blended.

2. Chill 1 hour before serving.

Nutrient Analysis per Serving

40 calories
3 grams carbohydrate
5 grams protein
1 gram fat
373 milligrams sodium

Key Nutrients

Small amounts of all nutrients

Diabetic Exchanges

½ very lean meat
¼ milk

Caramel Dip

This is Cindy McKee's recipe, and you won't believe it's fat-free! Serve it with apple slices or digestive biscuits.

225 g (8 oz) fat-free cream cheese, softened

6 tbsp brown sugar

1 teaspoon caramel flavour

1 teaspoon vanilla

1. Beat all ingredients with mixer.

Variation

Caramel Sauce: Over very low heat, thin mixture with small amount of milk until desired consistency is reached. Serve over crêpes, fruit, or sorbet.

Diabetic Variation

Instead of brown sugar, use approved artificial sweetener to taste.

Nutrient Analysis per Serving

57 calories
11 grams carbohydrate
4 grams protein
0 grams fat

Key Nutrients

Small amounts of many nutrients

Nutrient Analysis per Serving
(Diabetic Variation)

23 calories
2 grams carbohydrate
4 grams protein
0 fat

Diabetic Exchanges

1 very lean meat

Dijon Sauce

In France, this sauce is made with crème fraîche and makes any meat taste divine! This healthy version goes well with chicken breast, pork tenderloin chops, or new potatoes.

Makes: 4 servings

8 tbsp low-fat or fat-free soured cream or crème fraîche

8 tbsp natural non-fat yogurt

1 to 2 tbsp Dijon mustard

Salt, pepper, and garlic powder to taste

1. Mix all ingredients in saucepan.

2. If you are serving with meat, blend sauce with pan juices. Heat until very warm.

Nutrient Analysis per Serving

52 calories
6 grams carbohydrate
3 grams protein
2 grams fat

Key Nutrients

Small amounts of all nutrients

Diabetic Exchanges

½ skim milk

Aspen Black Bean Soup

Serve this hearty, delicious soup after your morning walk.

Makes: 6 servings

Soup

1 medium onion, chopped

3 cloves garlic or 3 teaspoons chopped garlic in jar

1 teaspoon dried whole oregano

½ teaspoon dried whole thyme

½ teaspoon cumin

¼ teaspoon cayenne pepper (optional)

2 435-g (15-oz) tins black beans, drained and rinsed

750 ml (1¼ pt) fat-free chicken stock

Cooking spray

Garnish

2 tomatoes, chopped

1 onion, finely chopped (optional)

8 tbsp part-skimmed mozzarella cheese

1. Spray pan with cooking spray. Cook onion and garlic until tender (about 5 minutes); add water if needed.

2. Stir in herbs and spices; cook 2 to 3 minutes.

3. Place half of beans in blender and purée until smooth, adding stock as needed to help make it smooth.

4. Add puréed beans, remaining stock, and remaining beans to onion mixture. Bring to the boil and then lower to medium heat and simmer 20 to 30 minutes.

5. Serve garnished with chopped tomatoes, onions, and cheese.

Serving Suggestion

For a complete meal, add a salad, fruit, and corn bread, or a grilled vegetable sandwich.

Nutritional Analysis per Serving

240 calories
37 grams carbohydrate
15 grams protein
4 grams fat
8 grams fibre

Key Nutrients

25% folic acid
21% magnesium
18% zinc
15% chromium

Diabetic Exchanges

2 starches
1 lean meat
1 vegetable

Lentil Soup

Lentils cook quickly and don't need to be soaked before cooking. They are also delicious!

Makes: 6 servings

2 medium onions, chopped

6 large garlic cloves, crushed

2 stalks celery, chopped

450 g (1 lb) dry lentils

1.75 l (3 pt) water

250 ml (8 fl oz) chicken stock

½ teaspoon basil

1½ teaspoons each thyme
    and oregano

1 bay leaf

1 to 2 teaspoons salt

2 to 3 medium carrots, sliced

Freshly ground black pepper
    to taste

Cooking spray

Garnish

Red wine vinegar

Tomatoes, chopped

1. Brown onions, garlic, and celery in pan sprayed with cooking spray, adding 1 tablespoon water as needed.

2. Place lentils, water, chicken stock, herbs, and salt in large saucepan. Bring to the boil, lower heat to very slow simmer, and cook covered for 20 to 30 minutes.

3. Add carrots and black pepper. Cover and let simmer another 30 to 45 minutes, stirring occasionally. Remove bay leaf.

4. Serve hot, with sprinkle of red wine vinegar and chopped tomatoes on top of each bowl.

**Nutrient Analysis
per Serving**

182 calories

33 grams carbohydrate

13 grams protein

1 gram fat

9 grams fibre

Key Nutrients

41% folic acid

38% vitamin A

16% magnesium

Diabetic Exchanges

2 starches

1 very lean meat

Mexican Kale-and-Pork Soup

This recipe offers an interesting combination of flavours and textures.

Makes: 8 servings

1 teaspoon corn/vegetable oil

1 medium onion, chopped

1 clove garlic, crushed

450 g (15 oz) pork loin or loin chops, trimmed of all fat and cut into 25-mm (1-in) cubes

1.25 l (2 pt) water

1 bunch fresh kale, trimmed and cut into 25-mm (1-in) pieces

1 450-g (16-oz) tin whole peeled tomatoes

5 tomatoes, halved and sliced, or 3 medium tomatoes, chopped

1½ teaspoons ground cumin

¾ teaspoon chilli powder

1 425-g (15-oz) tin corn

½ tin tomato paste

Salt, pepper, and hot pepper sauce to taste

1. In saucepan, heat oil over medium heat. Add onion, garlic, and pork. Cook about 10 minutes, stirring occasionally.

2. Place pork in large microwave-safe dish. Add water. Cook 5 minutes on high.

3. Add kale. Cook 5 minutes on high.

4. Add tinned and fresh tomatoes, spices, corn, and tomato paste. Cook 15 minutes on high, or until kale reaches desired tenderness. Add more tomato paste for thicker soup.

Serving Suggestion

Serve with homemade corn chips and guacamole.

Vegetarian Variation

Substitute tofu or pinto beans for pork.

Nutrient Analysis per Serving

229 calories

19 grams carbohydrate

19 grams protein

9 grams fat

4 grams fiber

Key Nutrients

49% vitamin C

43% thiamin

40% vitamin A

21% vitamin B_6

Diabetic Exchanges

2 medium-fat meats

2 vegetables

½ starch

Vegetarian Chilli

This hearty chilli is chock full of nutrients and makes a great potluck dish or casual dinner.

Makes: 6 servings

1 medium onion, chopped

2 large cloves garlic, crushed

1 medium courgette or 1 medium pepper, chopped

1 750-g (28-oz) tin chopped tomatoes in purée

1 425-g (15-oz) tin tomato sauce

2 425-g (15-oz) tins kidney beans, drained

2 to 4 teaspoons chilli powder

2 teaspoons cumin

½ teaspoon oregano

4 tbsp uncooked bulgur

Cayenne or black pepper to taste

Garnish

Parsley

Tomato, fresh, chopped

Onion, finely chopped

1. Heat small amount of water in non-stick pot. Add onion and garlic. Sauté over medium heat about 5 to 10 minutes.

2. Add courgette or pepper and sauté until all vegetables are tender.

3. Add tomatoes, tomato sauce, beans, spices, and bulgur. Simmer over lowest heat, stirring occasionally, for 15 minutes.

4. Season to taste and serve hot, topped with parsley, chopped fresh tomato, and onion.

Variations

• Spooned over baked tortilla chips and topped with fat-free Cheddar cheese.
• Rolled up in a flour tortilla.
• Stuffed in a pepper.

Nutrient Analysis per Serving

220 calories
44 grams carbohydrate
12 grams protein
1 gram fat
11 grams fibre

Key Nutrients

53% vitamin B_6
28% vitamin C
22% iron
12% folic acid

Diabetic Exchanges

2½ starches
1½ vegetables
1 very lean meat

Bulgur-and-Veggie Mix

Bulgur is a quick and healthy alternative to rice. It is also very versatile.

Makes: 5 servings

500 ml (17 fl oz) fat-free chicken stock or water

¼ teaspoon salt (optional)

600 g (1¼ lb) broccoli, chopped, or other vegetable in season

175 g (6 oz) dry bulgur

½ teaspoon thyme

1. In saucepan, bring stock or water to boil. Add salt and broccoli. Simmer 5 minutes.

2. Place bulgur in heatproof serving bowl. Pour water and broccoli over bulgur and add the thyme.

3. Cover and let sit until most of water is absorbed.

4. Pour off excess water and fluff with fork.

Variation

Substitute any vegetable, or vegetable combinations, fresh or frozen, for broccoli.

Nutritional Analysis per Serving

103 calories
22 grams carbohydrate
6 grams protein
0 grams fat
6 grams fibre

Key Nutrients

103% vitamin C
16% vitamin A
15% magnesium
14% chromium

Diabetic Exchanges

1 starch
1 vegetable

Easy Microwave Potatoes

With the help of a microwave, the potato can be a quick and nutritious side dish.

Potatoes, any amount, peeled or unpeeled, cut into 25-mm (1-in) pieces

2 to 3 tablespoons water

Salt and pepper to taste

1. Cook potatoes in water and seasoning in covered microwave-safe dish on high for 5 minutes.

2. Rotate dish. Cook 5 more minutes on high. Continue cooking until fork can easily pierce potatoes.

Variations

Italian: Add Italian spices before cooking and top potatoes with Parmesan cheese the last few minutes of cooking.

German: Add sautéed onions and bacon bits or ham to potatoes the last few minutes of cooking. Sprinkle with vinegar and toss.

Nutrient Analysis per Serving
(1 medium potato)

178 calories
41 grams carbohydrate
4 grams protein
0 grams fat
2 grams fibre

Key Nutrients

38% potassium
36% vitamin C
30% vitamin B_6

Diabetic Exchanges
(per ½-cup serving)

1 starch

Kids' Carrots

You're never too young to be in the kitchen! That philosophy paid off for twelve-year-old Andy Hawk, who placed third in the vegetable category of the Delicious and Nutritious Recipe Contest in the US.

Makes: 5 servings

1 450-g (1-lb) package frozen baby carrots

2 tbsp honey

Mint, 1 tbsp chopped fresh or 1½ teaspoons dried

1. Cook carrots according to package directions. Drain.

2. Stir in honey to coat carrots. Stir in mint. Serve.

Nutrient Analysis per Serving

48 calories
19 grams carbohydrate
1 gram protein
0 grams fat
3 grams fibre

Key Nutrients

167% vitamin A

Diabetic Exchanges

1 vegetable
¼ starch

Ratatouille

My husband introduced me to this wonderful and versatile dish. You can serve it over rice with cheese as a main dish, as a side dish, or as a topping on your pizza or potato. In Europe, ratatouille is often served topped with a fried egg.

Makes: 8 servings

1 aubergine, peeled and cut into 25-mm (1-in) cubes

1 teaspoon olive oil

4 garlic cloves, crushed

8 tomatoes, cut into quarters

3 courgettes, sliced

75 g (3 oz) mushrooms, sliced

1 teaspoon oregano

1 teaspoon basil

1 teaspoon salt

¼ teaspoon pepper

1. Brown aubergine in oil in non-stick pan. Add garlic and cook until tender.

2. Add remaining ingredients. Cook over medium heat until vegetables are tender, stirring frequently.

3. Reduce heat, cover, and simmer 10 to 15 minutes.

4. Remove cover and continue cooking until most of liquid has evaporated.

Variations

Add chopped red and green peppers and sliced black olives.

Quick Method: Use 450-g (16-oz) tin of tomatoes and 4 tbsp tomato paste instead of fresh tomatoes.

Nutrient Analysis per Serving

58 calories
12 grams carbohydrate
2 grams protein
1 gram fat
4 grams fibre

Key Nutrients

40% vitamin C
29% potassium
6% folic acid

Diabetic Exchanges

2 vegetables

Roasted New Potatoes/Home Fries

Do you like fried foods, but not the fat in them? Try these crispy roasted potatoes. Their secret is a high oven temperature.

Makes: 4 servings

450 g (1 lb) new potatoes or baking potatoes, well scrubbed

1 tablespoon olive oil

1 to 2 cloves garlic, crushed

½ teaspoon salt

Rosemary, 1 teaspoon dried or 2 teaspoons fresh, chopped

1. Preheat oven to 230°C/450°F/Gas mark 8.

2. Cut potatoes into 25-mm (1-in) pieces. Toss in bowl with oil, garlic, salt, and rosemary.

3. Spread potatoes on baking sheet. Roast about 30 minutes until potatoes are tender and brown, turning once halfway through cooking.

Variations

All should cook in about 20 minutes.

Oven Home Fries: Slice white potatoes, sweet potatoes, or yams into 6-mm (¼-in) slices to make home fries, or slice thinner for homemade potato crisps.

Sweet Crisps: Thinly sliced sweet potatoes dusted with cinnamon or pumpkin spice makes a sweet snack crisp.

French Fries: Cut into thin, long strips for French fries.

Nutrient Analysis per Serving

144 calories
26 grams carbohydrate
2 grams protein
4 grams fat
3 grams fibre

Key Nutrients

24% vitamin C
19% vitamin B_6
11% riboflavin

Diabetic Exchanges

2 starches
1 fat

Vegetables in Vinaigrette

A starting course of raw vegetables in vinaigrette dressing is a French tradition.

Makes: 4 servings

Use one or more of the following vegetables:

7 carrots, finely grated

½ celery root, finely grated (also called celeriac)

2 cucumbers, thinly sliced

⅓ head red cabbage, finely grated

Add

125 ml (4 fl oz) fat-free or low-fat vinaigrette dressing (Strong-flavoured is best.)

4 tbsp parsley, finely chopped

Salt and pepper to taste

1. Combine all ingredients. Marinate at least 30 minutes.

Variation

Add 1 to 2 tablespoons fat-free or light soured cream to vinaigrette dressing.

Nutrient Analysis per Serving

30 calories
7 grams carbohydrate
1 gram protein
0 grams fat

Key Nutrients
(for carrots)

194% vitamin A
Small amounts of other nutrients

Diabetic Exchanges

1 vegetable

Apricot-Glazed Chicken

You can cook this chicken in a flash and serve it to family or friends.

Makes: 4 servings

*4 chicken breast halves,
    skinned and boned*

2 teaspoons margarine

Salt and pepper to taste

*6 tbsp apricot or peach all-fruit
    spread*

*1½ tbsp tarragon wine vinegar or
    other flavoured vinegar*

2 teaspoons ginger

4 tbsp cashews, chopped

1. Rinse chicken and pat dry with kitchen paper towels.

2. Melt margarine in non-stick pan.

3. Sauté chicken over medium heat for 8 to 10 minutes. Remove chicken and keep warm. Sprinkle with salt and pepper. Set aside pan juices.

4. Stir preserves, vinegar, and ginger into pan juices. Cook over medium heat until hot.

5. Spoon glaze over chicken breasts. Sprinkle with cashews.

**Nutrient Analysis
per Serving**

240 calories

11 grams carbohydrate

28 grams protein

9 grams fat

Key Nutrients

66% niacin

28% vitamin B₆

13% magnesium

Diabetic Exchanges

4 lean meats

1 fruit

Bean and Corn Bread Bake

This one-dish meal is easy to make, and it's high in fibre, too!

Makes: 6 servings

Beans

**1 450-g (16-oz) tin pinto beans,
drained**

**1 450-g (16-oz) tin kidney
beans, black beans, or
black-eyed beans, drained
(Any combination will work!)**

**4 tbsp each chopped green
pepper, onion, and celery**

2 tbsp ketchup

1 225-g (8-oz) tin tomato sauce

1 teaspoon dry mustard

Oil or cooking spray

Corn Bread Topping

**200 to 230 g (7 to 8½ oz) corn
bread mix**

**4 tbsp reduced-fat or fat-free
Cheddar cheese, grated**

4 tbsp green chillies (optional)

1. Preheat oven to 190°C/375°F/Gas mark 5.

2. Mix together beans and vegetables. Pour into baking
dish that has been lightly oiled or sprayed with
cooking spray.

3. Prepare corn bread according to package directions,
adding cheese and chillies if desired. Pour over beans.

4. Bake for 30 to 35 minutes or until corn bread is
golden brown.

5. Serve with spinach salad and fresh fruit.

Nutrient Analysis
per Serving

360 calories
53 grams carbohydrate
16 grams protein
10 grams fat
7 grams fibre

Key Nutrients

29% potassium
25% folic acid
21% magnesium
11% iron

Diabetic Exchanges

3½ starches
1½ fats
1 lean meat

Black Bean Enchilada Casserole

This quick and easy casserole was modified from Janet Boyd's recipe.

Makes: 4 servings

1 425-g (15-oz) tin spicy black beans, undrained

1 425-g (15-oz) tin tomatoes with chillies

4 tbsp picante sauce

Cooking spray

3 corn tortillas

100 to 175 g (4 to 6 oz) fat-free or low-fat cheese, grated

1. Preheat oven to 180°C/350°F/Gas mark 4.

2. In bowl, mix beans, tomatoes, and sauce. Spray 2-l (3½ pt) round casserole dish with cooking spray.

3. Place 1 corn tortilla in bottom of dish. Add ⅓ of bean mixture, ⅓ of cheese, another tortilla, ⅓ of bean mixture, another tortilla, and rest of bean mixture.

4. Bake 20 minutes. Sprinkle remaining 2 tablespoons cheese on top during last 5 minutes of cooking.

Low-Sodium Variation

Cook 1 sliced onion, 1 teaspoon chopped garlic, and 1 sliced pepper until tender. Add 425-g (15-oz) tin stewed tomatoes and 200 ml (6.5 fl oz) picante sauce. Use plain black beans with 1½ teaspoons cumin and 1 teaspoon chilli powder.

Nutritional Analysis per Serving

269 calories
35 grams carbohydrate
20 grams protein
8 grams fat
10 grams fibre

Key Nutrients

28% folic acid
28% magnesium
26% vitamin C
18% copper

Diabetic Exchanges

2 starches
1½ lean meats
1 vegetable
½ fat

Broccoli Quiche

This recipe, from the book *Quick and Healthy Volume II* by Brenda Ponichtera, is great for a luncheon or brunch. Serve with a fruit cup or orange wedges.

Makes: 6 servings

Cooking spray

3 flour tortillas (200-mm [7½-in] diameter)

450 g (1 lb) broccoli, cooked, drained, and chopped into bite-size pieces

8 tbsp spring onion, sliced

100–125 g (4 oz) reduced-fat Cheddar cheese, grated

8 eggs

4 tbsp skimmed milk

¼ teaspoon paprika

Salt and pepper (optional)

6 tomato slices

1. Preheat oven to 180°C/350°F/Gas mark 4.

2. Spray 225-mm (9-in) pie pan with cooking spray.

3. Cut 2 tortillas in half and place each half in pan so that rounded edge is 6 mm (¼ in) above rim. Place remaining tortilla in centre of pan. Add broccoli, onion, and cheese.

4. In separate bowl, mix eggs with milk and add salt and pepper (if desired). Pour into pan; sprinkle with paprika.

5. Bake 45 minutes or until knife inserted in centre comes out clean. Let sit 10 minutes before cutting into 6 wedges.

6. Top each piece with tomato slice.

Source: Adapted with permission from *Quick and Healthy Volume II* by Brenda Ponichtera, R.D. (ScaleDown Publishing, Inc.).

Nutrient Analysis per Serving

213 calories

14 grams carbohydrate

16 grams protein

11 grams fat

Key Nutrients

33% vitamin A

31% riboflavin

28% vitamin C

20% calcium

Diabetic Exchanges

2 medium-fat meats

½ starch

½ vegetable

Cheese-Topped Fish

This recipe is from *Simply Colorado,* a cookbook by the Colorado Dietetic Association. Using this recipe, you can serve dinner in 15 to 20 minutes!

Makes: 6 servings

900 g (2 lb) orange sole, cod, or red snapper

Cooking spray

Topping

6 tbsp light mayonnaise

6 tbsp Parmesan cheese, grated

4 tbsp spring onion, sliced

½ teaspoon lemon juice

¼ to ½ teaspoon garlic powder

Hot sauce to taste (optional)

1. Preheat oven to 180°C/350°F/Gas mark 4.

2. Place fish in shallow metal pan coated with cooking spray; bake 8 minutes or until fish flakes easily when tested with fork.

3. Meanwhile, mix topping ingredients. Spread topping evenly over cooked fish fillets. Grill 150 mm (6 in) from heat for 5 minutes or until topping is lightly browned.

Source: Reprinted with permission from Simply Colorado, Inc.

Nutrient Analysis per Serving

164 calories

2 grams carbohydrate

27 grams protein

5 grams fat

Key Nutrients

102% vitamin B_{12}

18% potassium

17% magnesium

12% niacin

Diabetic Exchanges

3 very lean meats

½ fat

Chicken and Prawns with Fruit Salsa

My friend Debbie Russell is a wizard in the kitchen. She has won several regional and national cooking contests in America, and this recipe is one of her winners.

Makes: 6 servings

450 g (1 lb) large prawns, shelled and deveined

450 g (1 lb) boneless, skinless chicken breasts, cut into pieces

Marinade

4 tbsp mild picante sauce

1 tbsp lime or lemon juice

1 tbsp soy sauce

½ teaspoon coriander, ground

½ teaspoon fresh ginger root, grated

1 clove garlic, crushed

Fruit Salsa

8 tbsp peaches, diced

8 tbsp pineapple, diced

8 tbsp green apple, diced

8 tbsp red bell pepper, diced

2 tbsp green onion, chopped

1 teaspoon lime or lemon juice

1 teaspoon sugar

Garnish

12 thin slices pineapple or peaches

Coriander or parsley sprigs

1. In dish or plastic bag, combine marinade ingredients.

2. Add prawns and chicken, turning to coat pieces well. Cover dish or close bag and marinate at least 30 minutes in refrigerator.

3. In small bowl, combine salsa ingredients. Cover and set aside.

4. Drain prawns and chicken, reserving marinade for basting. Thread prawns and chicken alternately on skewers.

5. Grill chicken and prawns over medium-hot coals or grill at 200°C/400°F/Gas mark 6 until prawns turn pink and chicken is well cooked (7 to 10 minutes), basting often with marinade.

6. Serve with fruit salsa on the side. Garnish with pineapple or peach slices and coriander or parsley.

(continued on next page)

Chicken and Prawns with Fruit Salsa
(continued)

Variations

• Stir-fry the chicken and prawns instead of grilling.

• Serve with Peanut-Butter Sauce instead of Fruit Salsa:

8 tbsp natural non-fat yogurt

2 teaspoons peanut butter

½ teaspoon Dijon mustard

⅛ teaspoon Worcestershire sauce

Nutrient Analysis per Serving
(with Fruit Salsa)

256 calories

18 grams carbohydrate

37 grams protein

4 grams fat

1 gram fibre

Key Nutrients

90% selenium

64% niacin

30% vitamin C

30% vitamin B_6

Diabetic Exchanges

5 very lean meats

1 fruit

½ vegetable

Nutrient Analysis per Serving
(with Peanut-Butter Sauce)

223 calories

4 grams carbohydrate

38 grams protein

5 grams fat

Key Nutrients

92% selenium

64% niacin

28% vitamin B_6

15% magnesium

Diabetic Exchanges

5 very lean meats

Colorado Stuffed Peppers

Makes: 4 servings

3 small tomatoes or 2 medium tomatoes, chopped coarsely

2 spring onions, chopped

¼ medium red onion, finely chopped

1 clove garlic, crushed

½ sweet red pepper, chopped

2 teaspoons olive oil

250 ml (8 fl oz) cooked brown rice or bulgur

375 ml (12 fl oz) cooked black beans

8 tbsp plus 2 teaspoons reduced-fat Cheddar cheese, grated

4 peppers, cored and seeded

1. Sauté tomatoes, both onions, garlic, and red pepper in oil until cooked to desired tenderness. (The less the tomato and pepper are cooked, the more vitamin C they retain.)

2. Add brown rice, black beans, and 8 tbsp cheese to pan and gently stir until warm and cheese is melted.

3. Meanwhile, steam whole peppers in microwave until tender-crisp; then fill with bean mixture.

4. Sprinkle remaining 2 teaspoons of cheese on top before serving. (To increase protein content, add some lean meat, chicken, tofu, or more cheese to the filling.)

Nutrient Analysis per Serving

237 calories
37 grams carbohydrate
12 grams protein
6 grams fat
5 grams fibre

Key Nutrients

106% vitamin C
32% selenium
25% magnesium
20% folic acid

Diabetic Exchanges

2 starches
1½ vegetables
1 lean meat
½ fat

Country Brunch Casserole

This recipe is from *Simply Colorado,* a cookbook by the Colorado Dietetic Association. It's perfect to serve to house guests; just prepare the dish the night before, and enjoy a leisurely brunch.

Makes: 8 servings

8 tbsp onion, chopped

2 tbsp water

3 cups bread cubes

Cooking spray

150 g (⅓ lb) bacon, thinly sliced and cut into bite-size pieces (you can also use very lean ham)

100–125 g (4 oz) reduced-fat Cheddar cheese, grated

3 eggs

2 egg whites

500 ml (17 fl oz) skimmed milk

½ teaspoon dry mustard

½ teaspoon onion salt

1. Microwave onion and water on high for 2 minutes, stirring occasionally.

2. Place bread cubes in bottom of 300-by-200-by-50-mm (12-by-8-by-2-in) baking dish that has been coated with cooking spray.

3. Sprinkle pan with microwaved onion, sliced ham, and grated cheese.

4. In separate bowl, mix eggs, egg whites, milk, and seasonings; pour over stuffing mixture. Cover and refrigerate overnight.

5. Bake uncovered at 160°C/325°F/Gas mark 3 for 1 hour. Let stand 10 minutes before serving.

Source: Reprinted with permission from Simply Colorado, Inc.

Nutrient Analysis per Serving

202 calories

13 grams carbohydrate

18 grams protein

9 grams fat

Key Nutrients

19% vitamin B$_{12}$

19% calcium

17% riboflavin

12% vitamin A

Diabetic Exchanges

1½ medium-fat meats

1 starch

Crab Marinara

This is a quick, delicious meal. If tomato sauce gives you heartburn, you may be able to tolerate this dish because the soured cream reduces the acidity of the sauce. You can keep the sauce on hand in the freezer for those times when you have no time to cook. Freeze leftovers for lunch.

Makes: 6 servings

350 g (12 oz) spaghetti, uncooked

1 200-g (7-oz) or 400-g (14-oz) tin artichoke hearts (depending on how well you like artichokes)

1 l (1¾ pt) prepared marinara sauce

200 ml (6.5 fl oz) fat-free soured cream

¼ cup olives, sliced

½ teaspoon tarragon

¼ teaspoon dill

350 g (12 oz) imitation crab or other shellfish, cooked

1. Cook spaghetti according to package directions.

2. Meanwhile, drain artichokes and chop into 12-mm (½-in) pieces.

3. In saucepan, combine marinara sauce with soured cream, olives, artichokes, and herbs.

4. Break crab into bite-size pieces, add to sauce, and stir until thoroughly combined. Heat over medium heat until warm.

5. Serve sauce over pasta with salad and wholemeal garlic bread.

Nutrient Analysis per Serving

351 calories
64 grams carbohydrate
17 grams protein
3 grams fat

Key Nutrients

50% thiamin
30% vitamin C
23% magnesium

Diabetic Exchanges

3½ starches
1½ vegetables
1 very lean meat
½ fat

Hoppin' John

This southern American classic dish can be prepared in a flash with tinned beans and quick-cooking brown rice or bulgur.

Makes: 4 servings

2 450-g (16-oz) tins red kidney beans or black-eyed beans, undrained

500 ml (17 fl oz) cooked brown rice or bulgur

175 g (6 oz) lean ham, chopped

¼ teaspoon onion powder

Pepper and salt to taste

Garnish

Fresh parsley and red onion, chopped (optional)

1. Combine undrained beans with rice, ham and spices. Cook over medium heat, stirring frequently.

2. Serve topped with parsley and chopped onion, if desired. If you can't tolerate raw onion, cook onion with beans.

Nutrient Analysis per Serving

262 calories
39 grams carbohydrate
17 grams protein
4 grams fat
2 grams fibre

Key Nutrients

89% selenium
19% vitamin B$_6$
17% zinc

Diabetic Exchanges

2½ starches
1½ lean meats

Mock Egg Foo Yung

This recipe provides a good way to incorporate soya into your diet.

Makes: 4 servings

450 g (16 oz) firm, low-fat tofu

2 eggs, beaten

4 spring onions, finely chopped

50 g (2 oz) mung bean sprouts,
   cut into 25-mm (1-in) pieces

1 garlic clove, crushed,
   or ¼ teaspoon garlic powder

1 tbsp soy sauce

1 teaspoon salt

2 tbsp old-fashioned oatmeal

1 carrot, finely grated

½ teaspoon sesame oil

1. Stir all ingredients together until well blended.

2. Form into 75-mm (3-in) patties and cook in small amount of oil until lightly browned.

Nutrient Analysis per Serving

119 calories

7 grams carbohydrate

13 grams protein

5 grams fat

4 grams fibre

Key Nutrients

73% vitamin A

42% iron

35% magnesium

25% calcium

Diabetic Exchanges

2 lean meats

1 vegetable

Oat-Nut Burgers

This recipe is modified from a recipe in *Meatless Meals for Working People*. When my picky friends ate these, they wanted seconds! If you have hamburger lovers at your house, you can put just about any type of burgers between the buns, and they'll be happy.

Makes: 3 to 4 servings

50 g (2 oz) rolled oats

175 g (6 oz) cashews (or other nuts), chopped

1 onion, chopped

3 stalks celery, chopped

2 carrots, grated (or use 1 carrot and ½ small courgette, grated)

4 tbsp wholemeal flour

4 tbsp water

1 teaspoon soy sauce (optional)

Salt and pepper to taste

Oil or cooking spray

1. Mix all ingredients. Season to taste with salt, pepper, or soya sauce.

2. Shape into 6 burgers.

3. Cook in lightly oiled pan (or pan sprayed with cooking spray) until brown on both sides; or grill burgers in oven.

4. Serve on toasted buns with lettuce, tomato, and so on. Oven-fried potatoes (page 329) go well with these burgers.

Nutrient Analysis per Serving

189 calories
25 grams carbohydrate
7 grams protein
8 grams fat
4 grams fibre

Key Nutrients

49% vitamin A
23% magnesium
11% zinc

Diabetic Exchanges

1½ fats
1½ starches
1 vegetable

Quick Grilled Fish

I never enjoyed thick cuts of fish until I started marinating them. Marinating adds flavour and keeps fish moist. We enjoy fish cooked this way at least twice a month!

450 g (1 lb) halibut, salmon, or other fish steaks

8 tbsp vinaigrette or fat-free Italian dressing (Experiment with different dressings.)

1. Pour fish and dressing into Ziploc bag. Marinate in refrigerator at least 1 hour; the longer the better.

2. Grill approximately 10 minutes per 25 mm (inch) of thickness at thickest part; or grill at 230°C/450°F/Gas mark 8 for same amount of time. Fish is cooked when opaque and flakes easily with fork.

Nutrient Analysis per Serving
(4 ounces)

158 calories
less than 1 gram carbohydrate
23 grams protein
6 grams fat

Key Nutrients

81% selenium
47% vitamin B_{12}
27% magnesium

Diabetic Exchanges

3 lean meats

Sesame Beef

This recipe was modified from a recipe in the 1991 US National Beef Cookoff.

Makes: 6 servings

900 g (2 lb) boneless top sirloin

Marinade

**4 tbsp rice wine or white wine
 vinegar**

4 tbsp soy sauce

2 tbsp dark sesame oil

1 tbsp granulated sugar

1 teaspoon fresh ginger, minced

1 teaspoon baking soda

2 teaspoons cornflour

Sauce

250 ml (8 fl oz) beef stock

2 tbsp cornflour

8 tbsp light brown sugar, packed

4 tbsp hoisin sauce

1½ tbsp sesame seeds

1 tbsp teriyaki sauce

½ tbsp molasses

1 clove garlic, minced

1 tbsp dark sesame oil

Garnish

**1 large head cos lettuce,
 shredded**

Sesame seeds

**Crushed red-pepper pods
 or hot chilli paste (optional)**

1. Slice beef into 25-mm (1-in) strips; remove all fat.

2. Mix together marinade ingredients. Toss with beef and store in plastic bag, turning occasionally. Marinate in refrigerator at least 30 minutes, preferably overnight.

3. Drain marinade. Cook beef quickly in non-stick pan, adding small amount of oil if needed. Keep warm.

4. Mix 2 tablespoons stock with cornflour; set aside. Mix remaining stock with next 5 sauce ingredients.

5. Add garlic and ½ teaspoon oil to same pan in which you cooked beef. Sauté 1 minute.

6. Add sauce mixture; bring to the boil. Add stock-cornflour mixture. Cook over medium heat until thickened, stirring occasionally.

7. Arrange lettuce on platter. Top with meat and drizzle with sauce or serve sauce on side. Sprinkle with sesame seeds and optional crushed red pepper.

Diabetic Variation

Follow directions for sauce, omitting brown sugar and molasses.

Diabetic Exchanges

6 lean meats
1 vegetable

Nutrient Analysis per Serving

451 calories
30 grams carbohydrate
42 grams protein
17 grams fat

Key Nutrients

65% zinc
36% vitamin B$_6$
22% iron
11% folic acid

Nutrient Analysis (meat and lettuce)

357 calories
6 grams carbohydrate
42 grams protein
17 grams fat

Spinach-Stuffed Shells

I recently discovered large pasta shells. Shells can be the busy cook's elegant meal! They freeze well, so try doubling the recipe and freezing half.

Makes: 4 servings

1 275-g (10-oz) package frozen spinach, cooked or thawed and well drained

250 ml (8 fl oz) low-fat or fat-free cottage cheese

6 tbsp Parmesan cheese, preferably freshly grated

8 tbsp mozzarella cheese, grated

¼ teaspoon garlic powder or to taste

225 g (½ lb) large pasta shells, cooked until still slightly firm (al dente) and drained

600 ml (20 fl oz) prepared low-fat marinara sauce

Garnish

Mozzarella and Parmesan cheese, grated

1. Preheat oven to 180°C/350°F/Gas mark 4.

2. Mix all ingredients except shells until well blended.

3. Stuff shells with spinach mixture. Cover with marinara sauce. Bake 30 minutes.

4. Sprinkle with a bit of extra cheese just before serving.

Variation

Double the amounts of pasta and spinach. Drain 450 g (1 lb) of firm tofu and squeeze out excess water. In food processor, blend tofu, 2 cloves fresh garlic, and a bunch of fresh basil leaves until smooth. Add cottage cheese and blend until smooth. Remove from processor and stir in spinach. Stuff and cook shells as directed above.

Nutrient Analysis per Serving

388 calories
58 grams carbohydrate
25 grams protein
7 grams fat

Key Nutrients

78% vitamin A
54% calcium
42% vitamin C
34% folic acid

Diabetic Exchanges

3 starches
2 lean meats
2 vegetables

Tofu Loaf

This recipe is from Norma Robinson. The pecans give it an interesting texture and flavour.

Makes: 8 servings

450 g (16 oz) low-fat tofu, firm

4 tbsp pecans, chopped

125 ml (4 fl oz) tinned tomatoes, chopped

2 egg whites

4 tbsp skimmed milk

75 g (3 oz) dry seasoned bread crumbs or old-fashioned oatmeal

½ teaspoon salt

½ teaspoon each onion and garlic powder

1 teaspoon thyme, cumin, oregano, or Italian seasoning

Optional seasonings: finely chopped parsley, spring onion, or celery

Cooking spray

1. Preheat oven to 180°C/350°F/Gas mark 4.

2. Squeeze out excess liquid from tofu and crumble. With spoon, mix with rest of ingredients until well blended.

3. Pour into loaf pan that has been sprayed with cooking spray. Bake 50 to 60 minutes.

4. Serve like meat loaf with ketchup, salsa, or pasta sauce, or on a bun like a burger. Leftovers are great as sandwiches.

Nutrient Analysis per Serving

86 calories
5 grams carbohydrate
8 grams protein
4 grams fat

Key Nutrients

26% iron
20% magnesium
14% calcium

Diabetic Exchanges

1 lean meat
1 vegetable
1 fat

Veal Piccata with Roasted Red Pepper Sauce

The sauce makes this dish tasty and colourful.

Makes: 4 servings

450 g (16 oz) veal loin

3 tbsp lemon juice

½ to 1 clove garlic, crushed

Sauce

*½ spring onion, chopped
(If you can't tolerate onions,
just use green tops.)*

*1 110 g (4 oz) roasted
red peppers*

*2 tbsp white wine vinegar
(can be flavoured)*

*6 tbsp parsley (or 2 fresh
spinach or lettuce leaves)*

*6 tbsp non-fat yogurt or
reduced-fat soured cream*

Dash cayenne pepper (optional)

1. Marinate veal in lemon juice and garlic in refrigerator for at least 1 hour.

2. Cook over medium-high heat or grill to desired doneness.

3. Purée all sauce ingredients except yogurt in food processor or blender. Place in microwave-safe dish and heat on medium-high 2 minutes.

4. Fold in yogurt or soured cream. Return to microwave for 30 seconds on high. Stir and serve over meat. (The sauce can be made ahead of time and refrigerated.)

Variation

Turkey tenderloin or chicken breast can also be used.

Nutrient Analysis per Serving

301 calories
5 grams carbohydrate
39 grams protein
12 grams fat

Key Nutrients

44% vitamin C
32% zinc
22% vitamin B$_6$

Diabetic Exchanges

5½ lean meats
1 vegetable

Vegetable-and-Tofu Stir-Fry

You won't even miss the meat!

Makes: 4 servings

2 tbsp vinegar

½ teaspoon sesame oil

2 tbsp hoisin sauce

4 tbsp light soy sauce

4 tbsp water

450 g (1 lb) low-fat, firm tofu, cubed

2 tbsp chicken stock

1 to 2 teaspoons ginger

2 cloves garlic, crushed

3 spring onions, chopped

450 g (16 oz) mixed vegetables (carrots, peppers, bean sprouts, cabbage, broccoli, snow peas) or frozen vegetable mixture

1. Mix together vinegar, sesame oil, hoisin sauce, soy sauce, and water. Add tofu and marinate 10 to 20 minutes.

2. Heat chicken stock in non-stick pan. Add ginger, garlic, and spring onions. Sauté 2 minutes.

3. Add vegetables (except broccoli) and stir-fry until tender-crisp. Add more chicken stock or water to pan if necessary.

4. Add tofu and cook, turning until brown on all sides. Remove from pan and set aside.

5. Add broccoli to pan along with remaining marinade and stir-fry until broccoli is tender-crisp.

6. Add tofu and continue cooking until warm.

Serving Suggestion

This dish is great served over brown rice, bulgur, or noodles.

Nutrient Analysis per Serving

117 calories

11 grams carbohydrate

15 grams protein

3 grams fat

3 grams fibre

Key Nutrients

133% vitamin C

29% vitamin A

19% potassium

Diabetic Exchanges

2 very lean meats

2 vegetables

Vegetarian Breakfast Tacos

Linda Hood developed this recipe, which won first place for entrées in a local American recipe contest. The term *Mexican food* often brings to mind high fat content, but this recipe is low in fat and full of flavour. It is not spicy, and you may make it even milder by reducing garlic and onion and using mild salsa (or chopped tomatoes with lemon juice and onion powder). You can also use parsley instead of coriander.

2 teaspoons olive oil

1 small clove garlic

8 tbsp onion, chopped

8 tbsp green pepper, chopped

1 medium potato, chopped

1 small courgette, chopped

*1 egg, plus 2 egg whites
(or 3 whole eggs)*

1 medium tomato, chopped

*1 tbsp coriander or parsley,
chopped*

Salt and pepper to taste

*4 wholemeal flour
or corn tortillas*

250 ml (8 fl oz) Mexican salsa

*100–125 g (4 oz) part-skimmed
mozzarella cheese, grated*

Makes: 4 servings

1. In oil, sauté garlic, onion, and green pepper.

2. Add potato and courgette. Stir until tender.

3. Push veggies aside and scramble eggs in middle of pan; gradually stir in vegetables.

4. Add tomato and heat thoroughly.

5. Season with coriander, salt and pepper.

6. Steam tortillas on top of mixture in covered pan. Fill tortillas with vegetable-egg mixture. Fold over.

7. Spoon salsa over folded tortilla and sprinkle cheese on top.

**Nutrient Analysis
per Serving**

255 calories

27 grams carbohydrate

16 grams protein

10 grams fat

3 grams fibre

Key Nutrients

51% vitamin C

20% calcium

14% vitamin B$_{12}$

**Diabetic
Exchanges**

1½ lean meats

1½ starches

1 fat

1 vegetable

Favourite Snack Cake

This is one of my son's favourite snacks. Unfortunately, it's also our dog's favourite – the first time I made this cake, he climbed on the counter and finished it off!

Makes: 12 servings

175 g (6 oz) wholemeal flour

75 g (3 oz) rolled oats

4 tbsp cornflour

1 teaspoon baking soda

1 teaspoon each ground ginger and cinnamon

½ teaspoon ground cloves

½ teaspoon salt

1 large egg

2 tbsp corn/vegetable oil

125 ml (4 fl oz) blackstrap molasses

450 ml (¾ cup) applesauce (see page 264)

Margarine and flour (for greasing)

1. Preheat oven to 160°C/325°F/Gas mark 3.

2. Mix together all dry ingredients and spices.

3. In separate bowl, combine egg, oil, molasses, and applesauce.

4. Gradually add egg mixture to dry ingredients.

5. Pour batter into greased and floured 225-by-225-mm (9-by-9-in) pan. (In a pinch you can also use a 225-mm/9-in pie plate.)

6. Bake 45 minutes, or until knife inserted in middle comes out clean. Let cool on wire rack.

Nutrient Analysis per Serving

129 calories

25 grams carbohydrate

2 grams protein

3 grams fat

2 grams fibre

Key Nutrients

23% potassium

10% calcium

9% iron

Diabetic Exchanges

1½ starches

½ fat

Fruit Crisp

This recipe from the US National Heart, Lung, and Blood Institute is full of fibre and vitamins. Try the summer and winter variations, or come up with your own.

Makes: 6 servings

Winter Variation

Filling

8 tbsp sugar

3 tbsp all-purpose flour

1 teaspoon lemon peel, grated

¼ teaspoon lemon juice

750 g (1¼ lb) apples, unpeeled, sliced

100–125 g (4 oz) fresh cranberries or 65 g (2½ oz) raisins

Topping

50 g (2 oz) rolled oats

6 tbsp brown sugar, packed

4 tbsp wholemeal flour

2 teaspoons ground cinnamon

1 tbsp soft margarine, melted

1. To prepare filling, in medium bowl, combine sugar, flour, and lemon peel; mix well. Add lemon juice, apples, and cranberries and stir to mix.

2. To prepare topping, in small bowl, combine oats, brown sugar, flour, and cinnamon. Add melted margarine and stir to mix.

3. Pour apple mixture into baking pan and sprinkle oat mixture on top.

4. Bake in 190°C/375°F/Gas mark 5 oven for approximately 40 to 50 minutes. Serve warm or at room temperature. It's delicious with low-fat yogurt!

Summer Variation

Instead of apples and cranberries, substitute fresh or unsweetened frozen (thawed) peaches and fresh or frozen (unthawed) blueberries. If frozen, thaw peaches completely (do not drain). Do not thaw blueberries before mixing or they will be crushed.

Note: This dish contains a significant amount of carbohydrate, and women with diabetes should eat it only in very small amounts.

Nutrient Analysis per Serving
(winter variation)

283 calories
62 grams carbohydrate
4 grams protein
4 grams fat
5 grams fibre

Key Nutrients

13% magnesium
10% vitamin C
8% chromium

Nutrient Analysis per Serving
(summer variation)

309 calories
68 grams carbohydrate
5 grams protein
4 grams fat
7 grams fibre

Key Nutrients

37% manganese
24% vitamin C
21% potassium
11% vitamin A

Diabetic Exchanges

Winter	*2 fruits*
	2 starches
Summer	*2½ fruits*
	2 starches

Fruit Pizza for a Crowd

This recipe is adapted from the book *Quick and Healthy Recipes and Ideas* by Brenda Ponichtera. The secret to this impressive dessert is to arrange the fruit in attractive patterns – try combinations of strawberries, raspberries, blueberries, and kiwi fruit. You can also add light whipped topping. (See notation below for using different-size pans.) This dessert is considered a 'somewhat healthy' splurge, so go easy on portion sizes!

Makes: 18 servings

Cooking spray

1 package 600 g (20 oz) Cookie Dough

1 large packet (150 g/5 oz) vanilla instant pudding

750 ml (1¼ pt) skimmed milk

175 g (6 oz) fat-free cream cheese, room temperature

1.3 kg (3 lb) strawberries (or other fresh fruit), washed and hulled

Source: Reprinted with permission from *Quick and Healthy Recipes and Ideas* by Brenda J. Ponichtera, R.D. (ScaleDown Publishing, Inc.).

1. Preheat oven to 180°C/350°F/Gas mark 4.

2. Spray pizza pan with cooking spray.

3. Slice cookie dough into 6-mm (¼-in) slices.

4. Arrange slices on pizza pan so that they are 12 to 25 mm (½ to 1 in) apart. Bake 18 to 20 minutes or until golden and set. Cool.

5. In small mixing bowl, combine pudding mix and milk. Beat on low to mix. Add cream cheese and beat until smooth and thickened.

6. Pour over cooled cookie crust. Arrange fruit on top.

Note: This amount will also make four 200-mm (8-in) pizzas or one 275-by-350-mm (11-by-14-in) and one 200-mm (8-in) pizza. 200-mm (8-in) cake tins work fine.

Diabetic Variation

Use sugar-free pudding instead of regular pudding. This diabetic variation still contains significant amounts of sugar. Women with diabetes should either skip this recipe or eat only in limited amounts.

Nutrient Analysis per Serving

191 calories
31 grams carbohydrate
5 grams fat
4 grams protein

Key Nutrients

27% vitamin C
Small amounts of many other nutrients

Nutrient Analysis per Serving
(Diabetic Variation)

167 calories
25 grams carbohydrate
5 grams fat
4 grams protein

Diabetic Exchanges

1½ starches
1 fat
½ very lean meat

Sunshine Sorbet

The beauty of this dessert is that it's made entirely of fruit, with no added sugar or thickener!

Makes: 5 servings

1 600-g (20-oz) tin crushed pineapple, in its own juice

1 ripe banana, sliced

3 nectarines, peeled and sliced, or 225 g (8 oz) tinned peaches, in their own juice

350 g (12 oz) strawberries, fresh or frozen, unsweetened

2 teaspoons orange or lemon rind, freshly grated

Garnish

Fresh mint

1. Freeze fruit before preparing. Thaw pineapple enough to slice into chunks.

2. Place all fruit in food processor, and process until smooth. Scrape down sides occasionally.

3. Serve immediately; garnish with mint sprigs or place in 200-by-200-mm (8-by-8-in) pan and freeze.

4. To serve after freezing: Thaw enough to break into chunks. Process again in food processor and store in airtight freezer container.

Nutrient Analysis per Serving

112 calories
1 gram protein
less than 1 gram fat
2 grams fibre

Key Nutrients

36% vitamin C
19% potassium
12% vitamin B_6

Diabetic Exchanges

2 fruits

References

Chapter 1

1. "Knowledge and Use of Folic Acid by Women of Childbearing Age–United States, 1995 and 1998." *Morbidity and Mortality Weekly Report,* 1999 Apr. 30; 48(16): 325–7.

2. Willett, W. C. "Folic Acid and Neural Tube Defects: Can't We Come to Closure." *American Journal of Public Health,* 82, 5, May 1992: 666.

3. Fall, C., et al. "Fetal and Infant Growth and Cardiovascular Risk Factors in Women." *British Medical Journal,* 310, 1995: 428–432.

4. Godfrey, K. M., et al. "Maternal Nutritional Status in Pregnancy and Blood Pressure in Childhood." *British Journal of Obstetrics and Gynæcology,* 101, 5, May 1994: 398.

5. Kitzmiller, J., et al. "Pre-Conception Care of Diabetes. Glycemic Control Prevents Congenital Anomalies." *Journal of the American Medical Association,* 265, 6, 1991: 731.

6. Achadi, E. L., et al. "Women's Nutritional Status, Iron Consumption and Weight Gain during Pregnancy in Relation to Neonatal Weight and Length in West Java, Indonesia." *International Journal of Gynæcology and Obstetrics,* 48, suppl., June 1995: S103.

7. Crawford, M. "The Role of Essential Fatty Acids in Neural Development: Implications for Perinatal Nutrition." *American Journal of Clinical Nutrition,* 57, suppl., 1993: S703.

8. Buchanan, T. A., and S. L. Kjos. "Gestational Diabetes: Risk or Myth." *Journal of Clinical Endocrinology and Metabolism,* 1999 Jun; 84(6): 1854–7.

9. Olds, D. "Intellectual Impairment in Children of Women Who Smoke Cigarettes during Pregnancy." *Pediatrics,* 93, 2, 1994: 221.

10. Sasco, A. J., and H. Vainio. "From in Utero and Childhood Exposure to Parental Smoking to Childhood Cancer: A Possible Link and the Need for Action." *Human Experimental Toxicology,* 1999 Apr.; 18(4): 192–201.

11. Wilkinson, C. E., et al. "Trends in Food and Nutrient Intakes by Adults: NFCS 1977-78, CSFI 1989-1991, and CSFII 1994-95." *Family Economics and Nutrition Review,* 1997 10(4).

12. Haines, P. S., et al. "Trends in Breakfast Consumption of U.S. Adults between 1965 and 1991." American Dietetic Association. 1996 May; 96(5): 464–70.

13. Cnattingius, S., et al. "Pre-pregnancy Weight and the Risk of Adverse Pregnancy Outcomes." *New England Journal of Medicine,* January 15, 1998, 338(3): 147–153.

14. Werler, M., et al. "Prepregnant Weight in Relation to Risk of Neural Tube Defects." *Journal of the American Medical Association,* 275, 14, April 10, 1996: 1089.

Shaw, G. "Risk of Neural Tube Defect Affected Pregnancies among Obese Women." Journal of the American Medical Association, 275, 14, April 10, 1996: 1093.

15. Clark, A. M., et al. "Weight Loss Results in Significant Improvement in Pregnancy and Ovulation Rates in Anovulatory Obese Women." *Human Reproduction,* 1995 Oct. 10(10): 2705–12.

16. Worthington-Roberts, Bonnie, and Sue Williams. *Nutrition in Pregnancy and Lactation,* 6th edition, Brown and Benchmark Publishers, 1997, p. 32.

17. Shen, H. M., et al. "Evaluation of Oxidative DNA Damage in Human Sperm and Its Association with Male Infertility." *Journal of Andrology,* 1999 Nov.–Dec.; 20(6): 718–23.

18. Fraga, C. G., et al. *Mutation Research,* 1996 Apr. 13; 351(2): 199–203.

19. Augood. C. "Smoking and Female Infertility: A Systematic Review and Meta-Analysis." *Human Reproduction,* 1998 Jun.; 13(6): 1532–9.

20. Bolumar, F., et al. "Caffeine Intake and Delayed Conception: A European Multicenter Study on Infertility and Subfecundity." European Study Group on Infertility and Subfecundity. *American Journal of Epidemiology,* 1997 Feb. 15; 145(4): 324–34.

21. Pirke, K., et al. "Dieting Influences the Menstrual Cycle: Vegetarian versus Nonvegetarian Diet." *Fertility and Sterility,* 46, 6, 1986: 1083.

22. Stewart, D. "Reproductive Functions in Eating Disorders." *Annals of Medicine,* 24, 1992: 287.

23. Ibid.

24. Rushton, D. "Ferritin and Fertility." Letter. *The Lancet,* 337, 1991: 1554.

25. Jensen, T. K., et al. "Does Moderate Alcohol Consumption Affect Fertility? Follow Up Study among Couples Planning First Pregnancy." *British Medical Journal,* 1998 Aug. 22; 317(7157): 505–10.

26. Cicero, T. J., et al. "Acute Alcohol Exposure Markedly Influences Male Fertility and Fetal Outcome in the Male Rat." *Life Science* 1994; 55(12): 901–10.

27. Dawson, E., et al. "Effect of Vitamin C Supplementation on Sperm Quality of Heavy Smokers." *Federation of the American Societies for Experimental Biology Journal,* 5, 4, 1991: A915.
   Dawson, E. "Effect of Ascorbic Acid on Male Fertility." Annals of the New York Academy of Science, 498, 1987: 312.

28. Werbach, M. *Nutritional Influences on Illness.* 2nd edition. Tarzana, Calif.: Third Line Press, 1993: 376–381.

29. Kemmann, E., et al. "Amenorrhea Associated with Carotenemia." *Journal of the American Medical Association,* 249, 7, 1983: 926.

30. Shortbridge, L. "Advances in the Assessment of the Effect of Environmental and Occupational Toxins on Reproduction." *Journal of Perinatal and Neonatal Nursing,* 3, 4, 1990: 1.

31. Fraga, C. "Ascorbic Acid Protects against Endogenous Oxidative DNA Damage in Human Sperm." Proceedings of the National Academy of Sciences, 88, December 1991: 11003.

32. U.S. Environmental Protection Agency, Office of Water. *Lead in Your Drinking Water,* June 1993, pub # EPA/810-F93-001.

33. Wilson, J. *The Pre-Pregnancy Planner.* Garden City, N.Y.: Doubleday & Co. Inc., 1986: 70.

34. Lindbohm, M. L., et al. "Effects of Paternal Occupational Exposure on Spontaneous Abortions." *American Journal of Public Health,* 81, 1991: 1029.

35. Shortbridge, L. "Advances in the Assessment of the Effect of Environmental and Occupational Toxins on Reproduction." *Journal of Perinatal and Neonatal Nursing,* 3, 4, 1990: 1.

36. *Food-Borne Risks in Pregnancy,* March of Dimes Birth Defects Foundation, 1998, Pub # 09-1305-99 8/99.

37. Center for Disease Control. "Recommendations for the Use of Folic Acid to Reduce the Number of Cases of Spina Bifida and Other Neural Tube Defects." *Morbidity and Mortality Weekly,* 11, 41 (RR-14), September 1992: 1, 3.

38. Ries, C., et al. "Impact of Commercial Eating on Nutrient Adequacy." *Journal of the American Dietetic Association,* 87, 1987: 463.

39. American College of Obstetricians and Gynecologists. *Planning for Pregnancy, Birth, and Beyond.* Washington, D.C.: ACOG, 1990: 10.

Chapter 2

1. International Food Information Council and the American Dietetic Association. "How Are Kids Making Food Choices?" July 1991.

2. Cong, K., et al. "Calcium Supplementation during Pregnancy for Reducing Pregnancy-Induced Hypertension." *Chinese Medical Journal,* 108, 1, January 1995: 57.

3. Committee on Diet and Health, National Research Council. *Diet and Health: Implications for Reducing Chronic Disease Risk.* Washington, D.C.: National Academy Press, 1989: 514–515.

4. Scholl, T.O. "Anemia vs. Iron Deficiency: Increased Risk of Preterm Delivery in a Prospective Study." *American Journal of Clinical Nutrition,* 1992 May; 55 (5): 985–8.

5. Duyff, R. L. *The American Dietetic Association's Complete Food and Nutrition Guide.* Wylie, N.Y.: 1998, page 106.

6. Committee on Diet and Health, National Research Council. *Diet and Health: Implications for Reducing Chronic Disease Risk.* Washington, D.C.: National Academy Press, 1989: 678.

7. Carmichael, S. L., and B. A. Abrams. "Critical Review of the Relationship between Gestational Weight Gain and Preterm Delivery." *Obstetrics and Gynecology,* 1997 May; 89 (5 pt. 2): 865–73.

8. Office of Public Information, University of California-Berkeley. News Release. May 1992.

9. Committee to Study the Prevention of Low Birth Weight, Division of Disease Prevention and Health Promotion, Institute of Medicine. *Preventing Low Birth Weight.* Washington, D.C.: National Academy Press, 1985: 1.

10. Hickey, C., et al. "Relationship of Psychosocial Status to Low Prenatal Weight Gain among Nonobese Black and White Women Delivering at Term." *Obstetrics and Gynecology,* 86, 2, August 1995: 177.

11. Tuthill, D. P., et al. "Maternal Cigarette Smoking and Pregnancy Outcome." *Pædiatric Perinatology and Epidemiology,* 1999 July; 13 (3): 245–53.

12. Lichtenstein, A. H., et al. "Dietary Fat Consumption and Health." *Nutrition Reviews.* 1998 May; 56 (5 pt. 2): S3–19; discussion S19–28.

13. Stender, S., et al. "The Influence of Trans-Fatty Acids on Health: A Report from the Danish Nutrition Council." *Clinical Science* (Colch) 88, 4, April 1995: 375.

14. American Heart Association. *The American Heart Association Diet–An Eating Plan for Healthy Americans.* 1998.

15. NIH Consensus Conference. "NIH Consensus-Development Panel on Optimal Calcium Intake." *Journal of the American Medical Association,* 272, 24, December 28, 1994: 1942.

16. Committee on Diet and Health, National Research Council. *Diet and Health: Implications for Reducing Chronic Disease Risk.* Washington, D.C.: National Academy Press, 1989: 515.

17. Rothman, K. "Teratogenicity of High Vitamin A Intake." *New England Journal of Medicine,* 333, 21, November 1995: 1369.

18. Specker, B. "Do North American Women Need Supplemental Vitamin D during Pregnancy?" *American Journal of Clinical Nutrition,* 59, 2, suppl., February 1994: 484S.

19. Studzinski, G., and D. Moore. "Sunlight–Can It Prevent as well as Cause Cancer?" *Cancer Research,* 55, 18, September 1995: 4014.

20. Bailey, L. "The Role of Folate in Human Nutrition." *Nutrition Today,* September/October 1990: 12.

21. "Knowledge and Use of Folic Acid by Women of Childbearing Age–United States, 1995 and 1998." *Morbidity and Mortality Weekly Report,* 1999 April 30; 48(16): 325–7.

22. Committee on Diet and Health, National Research Council. *Diet and Health: Implications for Reducing Chronic Disease Risk.* Washington, D.C.: National Academy Press, 1989: 71.

23. Jameson, S. "Zinc Status in Pregnancy: The Effect of Zinc Therapy on Perinatal Mortality, Prematurity, and Placental Ablation." *Annals of the New York Academy of Science,* 15, 678, March 1993: 178.

24. Committee on Diet and Halth, National Research Council. *Diet and Health: Implications for Reducing Chronic Disease Risk.* Washington, D.C.: National Academy Press, 1989: 422.

25. Ibid: 73.

26. National Academy of Sciences Report: *Nutrition during Pregnancy:* 15.

27. Ibid: 16, 254.

28. Rothman, K. "Teratogenicity of High Vitamin A Intake." *New England Journal of Medicine,* 333, 21, November 1995: 1369.

29. Belizan, J., et al. "Calcium Supplementation to Prevent Hypertensive Disorders of Pregnancy." *New England Journal of Medicine,* 325, November 14, 1991: 1399.
   Yabes-Almirante, C. "Calcium Supplementation in Pregnancy to Prevent Pregnancy-Induced Hypertension (PIH)." *Journal of Perinatal Medicine,* 1998; 26(5): 347–53.
   Crowther, C. A., et al. "Calcium Supplementation in Nulliparous Women for the Prevention of Pregnancy-Induced Hypertension, Preeclampsia and Preterm Birth: An Australian Randomized Trial." FRACOG and the ACT Study Group. *Australia-New Zealand Journal of Obstetrics and Gynæcology,* 1999 Feb.; 39(1): 12–8.

30. Gulson, B. L. "Mobilization of Lead from the Skeleton during the Postnatal Period is Larger than during Pregnancy." *Journal of Laboratory and Clinical Medicine,* 1998 Apr.; 131(4): 324–9.
   McGowan, J. A. "Bone: Target and Source of Environmental Pollutant Exposure." *Otolaryngology Head and Neck Surgery,* 1996 Feb.; 114(2): 220–3.

31. Hallberg, L., et al. "Calcium Effect of Different Amounts on Nonheme and Heme Iron Absorption in Humans." *American Journal of Clinical Nutrition,* 53, 1991: 112.

32. Kahn, A. "Prenatal Exposure to Cigarettes in Infants with Obstructive Sleep Apnea." *Pediatrics,* 93, 5, May 1994: 778.

33. Olds, D. "Intellectual Impairment in Children of Women Who Smoke Cigarettes during Pregnancy." *Pediatrics,* 93, 2, February 1994: 221.

34. Kandel, D. B., and J. R. Udry. "Prenatal Effects of Maternal Smoking on Daughters' Smoking: Nicotine or Testosterone Exposure?" *American Journal of Public Health,* 1999 Sep.; 89(9): 1377–83.

Weissman, M. M., et al. "Maternal Smoking during Pregnancy and Psychopathology in Offspring Followed to Adulthood. *Journal of the American Academy of Child and Adolescent Psychiatry,* 1999 Jul.; 38(7): 892–9.

Brennan, P. A., et al. "Maternal Smoking during Pregnancy and Adult Male Criminal Outcomes." *Archives of General Psychiatry,* 1999 Mar.; 56(3): 215–9.

35. Wahlgren, D. R. "Involuntary Smoking and Asthma." *Current Opinions in Pulmonary Medicine,* 2000 Jan.; 6(1): 31–6.

36. Subcommittee on Nutritional Status and Weight Gain during Pregnancy. *Nutrition during Pregnancy.* Washington, D.C.: National Academy Press, 1990: 394.

37. Farley, D. "Dangers of Lead Still Linger." *FDA Consumer,* Jan.–Feb. 1998. 32(1).

38. *Consumer Reports Magazine.* "Lead in Water, Pipe Nightmares." *Consumer Reports Magazine,* July 1995: 463.

39. Farley, D. "Dangers of Lead Still Linger." *FDA Consumer,* Jan.–Feb. 1998. 32(1).

40. West, J. R. "Fetal Alcohol Syndrome: A Review for Texas Physicians." *Texas Medicine,* 1998 Jul.; 94(7): 61–7.

41. *Diet and Health:* 450.

42. "Update: Trends in Fetal Alcohol Syndrome: United States, 1979-1993." *Morbidity and Mortality Weekly Report,* 1995 Apr. 7; 44(13): 249–51.

43. Ibid.

44. Hinds, T. S., et al. "The Effect of Caffeine on Pregnancy Outcome Variables." *Nutrition Reviews,* 1996 July; 54 (7): 203–7.

45. Jacobson, M., et al. *Safe Food: Eating Wisely in a Risky World.* Los Angeles, Calif.: Living Planet Press, 1991: 45.

46. *The Boston Globe.* December 13, 1989: 1.

47. Sullivan, K. "Maternal Implications of Cocaine Use during Pregnancy." *The Journal of Perinatal and Neonatal Nursing,* 3, 4, 1990: 12.

48. Ibid.

49. Haines, P., et al. "Eating Patterns and Energy and Nutrient Intakes of U.S. Women." *Journal of the American Dietetic Association,* 92, 6, June 1992: 698.

50. Ibid.

Chapter 3

1. Subcommittee on Nutritional Status and Weight Gain during Pregnancy. *Nutrition during Pregnancy.* Washington, D.C.: National Academy Press, 1990: 430.

2. Food and Nutrition Board. *Recommended Dietary Allowances.* Revised 1989. Washington, D.C.: National Academy Press, 1998.

3. National Academy of Sciences. *Nutrition during Pregnancy.* Washington, D.C.: National Academy Press, 1990: 386.

4. Scholl, T. "Low Zinc Intake during Pregnancy: Its Association with Preterm and Very Preterm Delivery." *American Journal of Epidemiology,* 137, 10, May 15, 1993: 1115.

5. Slavin, J. L., et al. "Plausible Mechanisms for the Protectiveness of Whole Grains." *American Journal of Clinical Nutrition,* 1999 Sep.; 70(3 suppl.): 459S–463S.

6. Anderson, J. W., et al. "Effects of Psyllium on Glucose and Serum Lipid Responses in Men with Type II Diabetes and Hypercholesterolemia." *American Journal of Clinical Nutrition,* 1999 Oct.; 70(4): 466–73.

Cohen, L. A. "Dietary Fiber and Breast Cancer." *Anticancer Research,* 1999 Sep.–Oct.; 19(5A): 3685–8.

7. National Center for Nutrition and Dietetics, The American Dietetic Association. "Whole Grain Goodness–Three Are Key." Nutrition Fact Sheet.

8. Committee on Diet and Halth, National Research Council. *Diet and Health: Implications for Reducing Chronic Disease Risk.* Washington, D.C.: National Academy Press, 1989: 678.

9. Aikins, Murphy P. "Alternative Therapies for Nausea and Vomiting of Pregnancy." *Obstetrics and Gynecology,* 1998 Jan. 91(1): 149–55.

Chapter 4

1. Subcommittee on Nutritional Status and Weight Gain during Pregnancy. *Nutrition during Pregnancy.* Washington, D.C.: National Academy Press, 1990: 12.

2. American Dietetic Association. "Position of the American Dietetic Association: Vegetarian Diets." *Journal of the American Dietetic Association,* 93, 11, November 1993: 1317.

3. Anderson, J., et al. "Meta-Analysis of the Effects of Soy Protein Intake on Serum Cholesterol." *New England Journal of Medicine,* 333, 5, August 3, 1995: 276.

4. Widhalm, K. "Effect of Soy Protein Diet versus Standard Low-Fat, Low-Cholesterol Diet on Lipid and Lipoprotein Levels in Children with Familial or Polygenic Hypercholesteroloemia." *Journal of Pediatrics,* 123, 1, July 1993: 30.

5. Scheiber, M. D., and R. W. Rebar. "Isoflavones and Postmenopausal Bone Health: A Viable Alternative to Estrogen Therapy?" *Menopause,* 1999 Fall; 6(3): 233–41.

6. Food and Nutrition Board. *Recommended Dietary Allowances.* 10th edition. Washington, D.C.: National Academy Press, 1989.

7. Szilagyi, A., et al. "Lactose Handling by Women with Lactose Malabsorption Is Improved during Pregnancy." *Clinical and Investigative Medicine,* 1996 Dec; 19(6): 416–26.

8. Solomons, N., et al. "Dietary Manipulation of Postprandial Colonic Lactose Fermentation: Effect of Solid Foods in a Meal." *American Journal of Clinical Nutrition,* 41, 1985: 199.

9. Lee, C., and C. Hardy. "Cocoa Feeding and Human Lactose Intolerance." *American Journal of Clinical Nutrition,* 49, 5, 1989: 840.

10. Recker, R., et al. "Calcium Absorbability from Milk Products, an Imitation Milk-and-

Calcium Carbonate." *American Journal of Clinical Nutrition,* 47, 1988: 93.

11. Whitney, E., and F. Sizer. *Nutrition: Concepts and Controversies.* Saint Paul, Minn.: West Publishing Company, 1988: 248.

12. CSPI Staff. *Nutrition Action Healthletter,* May 1992: 11.

Chapter 5

1. Food and Nutrition Board, Institute of Medicine. *Dietary Reference Intakes: Recommended Intakes for Individuals,* Washington, D.C.: National Academy of Sciences, 1999.

2. Subcommittee on Nutritional Status and Weight Gain during Pregnancy. *Nutrition during Pregnancy.* Washington, D.C.: National Academy Press, 1990: 265.

3. Wolraich, M. L., et al. "The Effect of Sugar on Behavior or Cognition in Children: A Meta-Analysis." *Journal of the American Medical Association,* 1995 Nov. 22–29; 274(20): 1617–21.
     Overgaard, C., and A. Knudsen. "Pain-Relieving Effect of Sucrose in Newborns during Heel Prick." *Biology of the Neonate,* 1999 May; 75(5): 279–84.

4. U.S. Department of Agriculture. *Report of the Dietary Guidelines Committee on the Dietary Guidelines for Americans 2000,* March 2000.
     American Dietetic Association. "Position of the American Dietetic Association: Use of Nutritive and Non-Nutritive Sweeteners." *Journal of the American Dietetic Association,* 98, 1998, 580–587.

Chapter 6

1. Key T. J., et al. "Health Benefits of a Vegetarian Diet." *Proceedings of the Nutrition Society,* 1999 May; 58(2): 271–5.

2. Sacks, F. M., et al. "A Dietary Approach to Prevent Hypertension: A Review of the Dietary Approaches to Stop Hypertension (DASH) Study." *Clinics in Cardiology,* 1999 Jul.; 22(7 suppl.): III6–10.)
     "Position of the American Dietetic Association: Vegetarian Diets." *Journal of the American Dietetic Association,* 1997; 97: 1317.

3. Ornish, D. "Intensive Lifestyle Changes for Reversal of Coronary Heart Disease." *Journal of the American Medical Association,* 1998 Dec. 16; 280(23): 2001–7.

4. "Position of the American Dietetic Association: Vegetarian Diets." *Journal of the American Dietetic Association,* 1997; 97: 1317.

5. Janelle, K., and S. Barr. "Nutrient Intakes and Eating Behavior Scores of Vegetarian and Nonvegetarian Women." *Journal of the American Dietetic Association,* 95, 2, February 1995: 180.

6. Craig, W. J. "Iron status of Vegetarians." *American Journal of Clinical Nutrition,* 1994 May; 59(5 suppl.): 1233S–1237S.
     Food and Nutrition Board. *Recommended Dietary Allowances,* Revised 1989. Washington, D.C.: National Academy Press, 1998.

7. "Position of the American Dietetic Association: Vegetarian Diets." *Journal of the American Dietetic Association,* 1997; 97: 1317.

8. Messina, Mark and Virginia. *The Dietitian's Guide to Vegetarian Diets.* Gaithersburg, Md.: Aspen Publishers, 1996. 110–112.

9. "Position of the American Dietetic Association: Vegetarian Diets." *Journal of the American Dietetic Association,* 1997; 97: 1317.

10. Glerup, H., et al. "Commonly Recommended Daily Intake of Vitamin D Is Not Sufficient if Sunlight Exposure Is Limited." *Journal of Internal Medicine,* 2000 Feb.; 247(2): 260–8.

11. Freeland-Graves, J., et al. "Zinc Status of Vegetarians." *Journal of the American Dietetic Association,* 80, 12, December 1980: 655.

12. Messina, Mark and Virginia. *The Dietitian's Guide to Vegetarian Diets.* Gaithersburg, Md.: Aspen Publishers, 1996. 28.

13. "Position of the American Dietetic Association: Vegetarian Diets." *Journal of the American Dietetic Association,* 1997; 97: 1317.

Chapter 7

1. Rosenn, B., et al. "Glycemic Thresholds for Spontaneous Abortion and Congenital Malformations in Insulin-Dependent Diabetes Mellitus." *Obstetrics and Gynecology,* 84, 4 October 1994: 515–20.

2. American Diabetes Association. Clinical Practice Recommendations. *Diabetes Care,* 23, (Suppl. 1), January 2000.

3. American Diabetes Association. *Diabetes and Pregnancy: What to Expect.* American Diabetes Association, 1989: 15.

4. Remsberg, K. E., et al. "Diabetes in Pregnancy and Cesarean Delivery." *Diabetes Care,* 22, 9, September 1999: 1561–7.
　　Berkowitz, G. S., et al. "Risk Factors for Preterm Birth Subtypes." *Epidemiology,* 9, 3 May 1998: 279–85.
　　American Diabetes Association. "Proceedings of the Fourth Annual Workshop Conference on Gestational Diabetes." *Diabetes Care,* 21 (Suppl. 2), August 1998.
　　Sibai, B. M., et al. "Risks of Pre-eclampsia and Adverse Neonatal Outcomes among Women with Pregestational Diabetes Mellitus." *American Journal of Obstetrics and Gynecology,* 182, 2, February 2000: 364–9.

5. American College of Obstetricians and Gynecologists. *Planning for Pregnancy, Birth, and Beyond.* Washington, D.C.: ACOG, 1990: 133.

6. American Diabetes Association. "Proceedings of the Fourth Annual Workshop Conference on Gestational Diabetes." *Diabetes Care,* 21 (Suppl. 2), August 1998.

7. American Diabetes Association. "Position Statement of the American Diabetes Association on Preconception Care of Women with Diabetes." American Diabetes Clinical Practice Recommendations. *Diabetes Care,* 21 (Suppl. 1), 1998.

8. California Department of Health Services. California Diabetes and Pregnancy Program: Sweet Success Guidelines for Care, 1999.

9. Krall, L., and R. S. Beaser. *Joslin Diabetes Manual.* 12th edition. Philadelphia, Pa.: Lea and Febiger, 1989: 236.

10. Ruggiero, L., et al. "Impact of Social Support and Stress on Compliance in Women with Gestational Diabetes Mellitus." *Diabetes Care,* 13, 1990: 441.

11. American Diabetes Association. "Why Worry About Gestational Diabetes?" in Diabetes Info [on-line publication]. Alexandria, Va.: 1999 [cited 31 March 2000 from www.diabetes.org].

12. Finney, L. S., and J. M. Gonzalez-Campoy. "Dietary Chromium and Diabetes: Is There a Relationship?" *Clinical Diabetes,* 15, 1 January/February 1997.

13. Ibid: 16.

14. Ibid: 14–15.

15. Langer, O., et al. "Intensified versus Conventional Management of Gestational Diabetes." *American Journal of Obstetrics and Gynecology,* 170, 4, April 1994: 1036.

16. American Diabetes Association. "Proceedings of the Fourth Annual Workshop Conference on Gestational Diabetes." *Diabetes Care,* 21 (Suppl. 2), August 1998.

17. King, H. "Epidemiology of Glucose Intolerance and Gestational Diabetes in Women of Childbearing Age." Proceedings of the Fourth Annual Workshop Conference on Gestational Diabetes. *Diabetes Care,* 21 (Suppl 2), August 1998.

18. American Diabetes Association. "Clinical Practice Recommendations 1998." *Diabetes Care,* 21 (Suppl. 1), 1998.

19. American Diabetes Association. *Gestational Diabetes and Pregnancy: What to Expect.* Alexandria, Va.: American Diabetes Association Inc., 1989: 13.

20. *Sweet Success Diabetes and Pregnancy Program Guidelines for Care.* Sacramento, Calif.: State of California Department of Health Services, Maternal and Child Health, 1992.

21. Spears, B. Telephone interview. April 1992.

22. Jovanovic-Peterson, L., and C. Peterson. "Is Exercise Safe or Useful for Gestational Diabetic Women?" *Diabetes,* 40, Suppl. 2: 179.

23. Jovanovic-Peterson, L. *Managing Your Gestational Diabetes.* Minneapolis, Minn.: Chronimed Publishing Inc., 1994: 55–56.

24. Powers, M. "Guidelines for Making Food Adjustments for Exercise for People," "Nutrition Guide for Professionals," and "Diabetic Education and Meal Planning." American Dietetic Association and American Diabetes Association, 1988, 41.

25. American Dietetic Association. "Position of The American Dietetic Association: Use of Nutritive and Nonnutritive Sweeteners." *Journal of the American Dietetic Association,* 98, 1998: 580–587.

26. Ibid.

27. Ibid.

28. *Chemical Cuisine: CSPI's Guide to Food Additives.* Center for Science in the Public Interest, 2000.
    California Diabetes and Pregnancy Program Sweet Success Guidelines for Care. California Department of Health Services, 1999.

29. *Chemical Cuisine: CSPI's Guide to Food Additives.* Center for Science in the Public Interest, 2000.

30. Huggins, C. E. "Natural Sweetener Not Yet Ready for FDA Approval." In Reuters Health Information [online publication]. New York: 27 March 2000 [cited 3 April 2000 from www.reutershealth.com].

31. DiGiacomo, J. E., and W. W. Hay, Jr. "Fetal Glucose Metabolism and Oxygen Consumption during Sustained Hypoglycemia." *Metabolism,* 39, 2, February 1990: 193.

32. Stenninger, E., et al. "Long-Term Neurological Dysfunction and Neonatal Hypoglycemia after Diabetic Pregnancy." *Archives of Diseases in Children: Fetal and Neonatal Edition,* 1998 Nov; 79(3): F174–9.

33. American Diabetes Association. "Clinical Practice Recommendations: Position Statement on Gestational Diabetes Mellitus." *Diabetes Care,* Volume 21, Supplement 1. 1998.

34. U.S. Department of Health and Human Services. *Working Group Report on High Blood Pressure in Pregnancy, High Blood Pressure Education Program.* Washington, D.C.: NIH Publication 91-3029, 1991.

35. Ibid: 6.
    Eskenazl, B., et al. "A Multivariate Analysis of Risk Factors for Preeclampsia." *Journal of the American Medical Association,* 266, 2, July 10, 1991: 237.

36. Villar, J., and J. Repke. "Calcium Supplementation May Reduce Preterm Delivery in High Risk Populations." *American Journal of Obstetrics and Gynecology,* 1124, 1990: 103.

Cong, K., et al. "Calcium Supplementation during Pregnancy for Reducing Pregnancy-Induced Hypertension." *Chinese Medical Journal,* 108, 1, January 1995: 57.

37. Marcoux, S., et al. "Job Strain and Pregnancy-Induced Hypertension." *Epidemiology,* 1999 Jul.; 10(4): 376–82.

38. U.S. Department of Health and Human Services. *Working Group Report on High Blood Pressure in Pregnancy.* Washington, D.C.: NIH Publication: 14.

39. Ibid: 2–3.

40. Ibid: 29.

41. Ibid: 6.

42. National Vital Statistics Report, Births: Final Data for 1997. 47,18, April 1999.
    Brown, J. "Nutrition and Multifetal Pregnancy." *Journal of the American Dietetic Association,* 100, 3, March 2000.

43. National Vital Statistics Report, Births: Final Data for 1997. 47,18, April 1999.

44. Brown, J. "Nutrition and Multifetal Pregnancy." *Journal of the American Dietetic Association,* 100, 3, March 2000.

45. Subcommittee on Nutritional Status and Weight Gain during Pregnancy. *Nutrition during Pregnancy.* Washington, D.C.: National Academy Press, 1990: 12.

46. Pederson, A. L. "Weight Gain Patterns during Twin Gestation." *Jounal of the American Dietetic Association,* 89, 5, May 1989: 642.

47. Luke, B., et al. "The Importance of Early Weight Gain in the Intrauterine Growth and Birth Weight of Twins." *American Journal of Obstetrics and Gynecology,* 1998 Nov.; 179(5): 1155–61.

48. Lantz, M. E., et al. "Maternal Weight Gain Patterns and Birth Weight Outcome in Twin Gestation." *Obstetrics and Gynecology,* 1996 Apr.; 87(4): 551–6.

49. Smith, L. G. Jr. "Calcium Homeostasis in Pregnant Women Receiving Long-Term Magnesium Sulfate Therapy for Preterm Labor." *American Journal of Obstetrics and Gynecology,* 1992 Jul.; 167(1): 45–51.

50. Levav, A. L., et al. "Long-Term Magnesium Sulfate Tocolysis and Maternal Osteoporosis in a Triplet Pregnancy: A Case Report." *American Journal of Perinatology,* 1998 Jan.; 15(1): 43–6.

51. Okah, F. A. "Bone Turnover and Mineral Metabolism in the Last Trimester of Pregnancy: Effect of Multiple Gestation." *Obstetrics and Gynecology,* 1996 Aug.; 88(2): 168–73.

52. Foreman-van Drongelen, M. M., et al. "Essential Fatty Acid Status Measured in Umbilical Vessel Walls of Infants Born after a Multiple Pregnancy." *Early Human Development,* 1996 Nov. 21; 46(3): 205–15.

Zeijdner, E. E., et al. "Essential Fatty Acid Status in Plasma Phospholipids of Mother and Neonate after Multiple Pregnancy." *Prostaglandins Leukotrienes and Essential Fatty Acids,* 1997 May; 56(5): 395–401.

53. Ollis, T. E., et al. "Australian Food Sources and Intakes of Omega-6 and Omega-3 Polyunsaturated Fatty Acids." *Annals of Nutrition and Metabolism,* 1999 Nov.; 43(6): 346–355.

54. Luke, B., et al. "Improving Outcomes in Twin Pregnancies: Obstetric, Neonatal and Healthcare Cost Implications." *American Journal of Obstetrics and Gynecology,* in press.

55. Dubois, S., et al. "Twin Pregnancy: The Impact of the Higgins Nutrition Intervention Program on Maternal and Neonatal Outcomes." *American Journal of Clinical Nutrition,* 53, 1991: 1397.

56. Cambell, D., et al. "Maternal Nutrition in Twin Pregnancy." *Acta Genetica Gemellologica,* 32, 1982: 221.

57. Cnattingius, S., et al. "Delayed Childbearing and Risk of Adverse Perinatal Outcome: A Population-Based Study." *Journal of the American Medical Association,* 1992 Aug. 19; 268(7): 886–90.

58. Cnattingius, S., et al. "Do Delayed Childbearers Face Increased Risks of Adverse Pregnancy Outcomes after the First Birth?" *Obstetrics and Gynecology,* 1993 Apr.; 81(4): 512–6.

59. Van Katwijk, C., and L. L. Peeters. "Clinical Aspects of Pregnancy after the Age of 35 Years: A Review of the Literature." *Human Reproductive Update,* 1998 Mar.-Apr.; 4(2): 185–94.

60. Cnattingius, S., et al. "Obstacles to Reducing Cesarean Rates in a Low-Cesarean Setting: The Effect of Maternal Age, Height, and Weight." *Obstetrics and Gynecology,* 1998 Oct.; 92(4 Pt. 1): 501–6.

61. Gilbert, W. M., et al. "Childbearing beyond Age 40: Pregnancy Outcome in 24,032 Cases." *Obstetrics and Gynecology,* 1999 Jan.; 93(1): 9–14.

62. Worthington-Roberts, S., and S. R. Williams. *Nutrition in Pregnancy and Lactation,* 6th edition. Dubuque, Iowa: Times Mirror Higher Education Group, Inc., 1997. 33–34.

63. Prysak, M., et al. "Pregnancy Outcome in Nulliparous Women 35 Years and Older." *Obstetrics and Gynecology,* 1995 Jan.; 85(1): 65–70.

64. National Vital Statistics Report. Births: Final Data for 1997. Volume 47, Number 18, April 1999.

65. Scholl, T., et al. "Maternal Growth during Pregnancy and the Competition for Nutrients." *American Journal of Clinical Nutrition,* 60, August 1994: 183.

66. Hediger, M. L., et al. "Implications of the Camden Study of Adolescent Pregnancy: Interactions among Maternal Growth, Nutritional Status, and Body Composition." *Annals of the New York Academy of Science,* 1997 May 28; 817: 281–91.

67. Munoz, K. A., et al. "Food Intakes of U.S. Children and Adolescents Compared with Recommendations." *Pediatrics,* 1997 Sep.; 100 (3 Pt. 1): 323–9.

68. Krebs-Smith, S. M., et al. "Fruit and Vegetable Intakes of Children and Adolescents in the United States." *Archives of Pediatric and Adolescent Medicine,* 1996 Jan.; 150(1): 81–6.

69. Guthrie, J. F., and J. F. Morton. "Food Sources of Added Sweeteners in the Diets of Americans." *Journal of the American Dietetic Association,* January 2000, 100(1): 43–51, quiz 49–50.

70. "Guidelines for School Health Programs to Promote Lifelong Healthy Eating." *Morbidity and Mortality Weekly Report,* June 14, 1996. Volume 45, Number RR-9.

71. American Academy of Pediatrics Committee on Adolescence. "Adolescent Pregnancy: Current Trends and Issues 1998." *Pediatrics,* Volume 103(2) February 1999. 516–520.

72. Casanueva, E., et al. "Weight Gain during Pregnancy in Adolescents: Evaluation of a Non-Nutritional Intervention." *Reviews of Investigative Clinics,* 1994 Mar.–Apr.; 46(2): 157–61.

73. Ibid.

74. Desjardins, E., and D. Hardwick. "How Many Visits by Health Professionals Are Needed to Make a Difference in Low Birth Weight? A Dose-Response Study of the Toronto Healthiest Babies Possible Program." *Canadian Journal of Public Health,* 1999 July–August; 90(4): 224–8.

75. Lenders, C. M., et al. "Effect of High Sugar Intake by Low-Income Pregnant Adolescents on Infant Birth Weight." *Journal of Adolescent Health,* 1994 Nov.; 15(7): 596–602.

76. Subcommittee on Nutritional Status and Weight Gain during Pregnancy. *Nutrition during Pregnancy.* Washington, D.C.: National Academy Press, 1990: 10.

77. Hediger, M., et al. "Patterns of Weight Gain in Adolescent Pregnancy: Effects on Birth Weight and Preterm Delivery." *Obstetrics and Gynecology,* 74, 1, July 1989: 6.

78. Rees, J. M., et al. "Weight Gain in Adolescents during Pregnancy: Rate Related to Birth-Weight Outcome." *American Journal of Clinical Nutrition,* 1992 Nov.; 56(5): 868–73.

79. Scholl, T. O., et. al. "Low Zinc Intake during Pregnancy: Its Association with Preterm and Very Preterm Delivery." *American Journal of Epidemiology,* 1993 May 15; 137(10): 1115–24.

80. Goldenberg, R. L. "The Effect of Zinc Supplementation on Pregnancy Outcome." *Journal of the American Medical Association,* 1995 Aug. 9; 274(6): 463–8.

81. Worthington-Roberts, B. S., and S. R. Williams. *Nutrition in Pregnancy and Lactation,* 6th edition. Dubuque, Iowa: Times Mirror Higher Education Group, Inc., 1997.

Chapter 8

1. Lanting, C., et al. "Neurological Differences between Nine-Year-Old Children Fed Breast Milk or Formula Milk as Babies." *The Lancet,* 344, 1994: 1319.

Cunnane, S. C., et al. "Breast-Fed Infants Achieve a Higher Rate of Brain and Whole Body Docosahexaenoate Accumulation than Formula-Fed Infants Not Consuming Dietary Docosahexaenoate." *Lipids,* 35, 1, January 2000: 105–11.

2. Gordon, A. E., et al. "The Protective Effect of Breast Feeding in Relation to Sudden Infant Death Syndrome (SIDS): III. Detection of IgA Antibodies in Human Milk That Bind to Bacterial Toxins Implicated in SIDS." *FEMS Immunology and Medical Microbiology,* 1999, Aug. 1; 25(1-2): 175–82.

3. American Academy of Pediatrics, Work Group on Breastfeeding. Policy Statement: "Breastfeeding and the Use of Human Milk." *Pediatrics,* 100, 6, December 1997: 1035–1039.

4. Potischman, N., and R. Troisi. "In-Utero and Early Life Exposures in Relation to Risk of Breast Cancer." *Cancer Causes Control,* 1999, Dec.; 10(6): 561–73.

Newcomb, P. A., et al. "Lactation in Relation to Postmenopausal Breast Cancer." *American Journal of Epidemiology,* 1999 Jul., 15; 150(2): 174–82.

Labbok, M. H. "Health Sequelae of Breastfeeding for the Mother." *Clinics in Perinatology,* 262, 2, viii–ix June 1999; 491–503.

5. American Academy of Pediatrics, Work Group on Breastfeeding. Policy Statement: "Breastfeeding and the Use of Human Milk." *Pediatrics,* 100, 6, December 1997: 1035–1039.

Labbok, M. H. "Health Sequelae of Breastfeeding for the Mother." *Clinics in Perinatology,* 26, 2, viii–ix , June 1999; 491–503.

6. U.S. Department of Health and Human Services. *Healthy People 2000 Progress Review: Maternal and Infant Health.* May 5, 1999.

7. Crase, B. Personal communication. May 1996, 1992.

8. Ibid.

9. Ibid.

10. Krebs, N., M.D. Presentation; Colorado Dietetic Association Annual Meeting. May 14, 1992.

11. Nafziger, S., M.D. Reprinted with permission of author from *Community Network Newsletter,* 1st quarter, 1992; Pueblo, Colo.

12. Modified from the Colorado Breast-Feeding Task Force.

13. Schanler, R. J. "Pediatricians' Practices and Attitudes Regarding Breastfeeding Promotion." *Pediatrics,* Volume 103, Number 3, March 1999, e35.

14. Colorado Breast-Feeding Task Force.

15. Krebs, N. Personal communication. June 1992.

16. Modified from the Colorado Breast-Feeding Task Force.

17. Subcommittee on Nutritional Status during Lactation, et al. *Nutrition during Lactation.* Washington, D.C.: National Academy Press, 1990: 74.

18. Dewey, K. G. "Energy and Protein Requirements during Lactation." *Annual Review of Nutrition,* 17, 1997: 19–36.

19. Strode, M. A., et al. "Effects of Short-Term Caloric Restriction on Lactational Performance in Well-Nourished Women." *Acta Pædiatrica Scandinavica,* 75, 1986: 222.

Butte, N., et al. "Effect of Maternal Diet and Body Composition on Lactational Performance." *American Journal of Clinical Nutrition,* 39, February 1984: 296.

20. Food and Nutrition Board. *Recommended Dietary Allowances.* 10th edition. Washington, D.C.: National Academy Press, 1989.

21. Subcommittee on Nutritional Status during Lactation, et al. *Nutrition during Lactation.* Washington, D.C.: National Academy Press, 1990: 219.

22. Gulson, B. L., et al. "Impact of Diet on Lead in Blood and Urine in Female Adults and Relevance to Mobilization of Lead from Bone Stores." *Environmental Health Perspectives,* 107, 4, April 1999: 257–63.
Gulson, B. L., et al. "Relationships of Lead in Breast Milk to Lead in Blood, Urine, and Diet of the Infant and Mother." *Environmental Health Perspectives,* 106, 10, October 1998: 667–74.

23. Food and Nutrition Board. "Dietary Reference Intakes: Recommended Intakes for Individuals." Washington, D.C.: National Academy Press, 1999.

24. Sanders, T. A. "Essential Fatty Acid Requirements in Pregnancy, Lactation, and Infancy." *American Journal of Clinical Nutrition,* 70, 3 Suppl, September, 1999: 55s-59s.

25. Marcus, P. M., et al. "Adolescent Reproductive Events and Subsequent Breast Cancer." *American Journal of Public Health,* 89, 8, August 1999: 1244–7.

26. Schanler, R. J., and S. A. Atkinson. "Effects of Nutrients in Human Milk on the Recipient Premature Infant." *Journal of Mammary Gland Biology and Neoplasia,* 1999 Jul.; 4(3): 297–307.

27. Hattevig, G., et al. "Effects of Maternal Dietary Avoidance during Lactation on Allergy in Children at 10 Years of Age." *Acta Pædiatrica,* 1999 Jan.; 88(1): 7–12.

28. Chandra, R. K., et al. "Five-Year Follow-Up of High-Risk Infants with Family History of Allergy Who Were Exclusively Breast-Fed or Fed Partial Whey Hydrolysate, Soy, and Conventional Cow's Milk Formulas." *Journal of Pediatric Gastroenterology Nutrition,* 24, 4, April 1997: 380–8.

29. Subcommittee on Nutritional Status during Lactation, et al. *Nutrition during Lactation.* Washington, D.C.: National Academy Press, 1990: 168.

30. Ibid: 14.

31. Schanler, R. J., and S. A. Atkinson. "Effects of Nutrients in Human Milk on the Recipient Premature Infant." *Journal of Mammary Gland Biology and Neoplasia,* 1999 Jul.; 4(3): 297–307.

32. Lucas, A., et al. "Breast Milk and Subsequent Intelligence Quotient." *The Lancet,* 339, 1992: 261.

33. Little, R., et al. "Maternal Alcohol Use during Breastfeeding and Infant Mental and Motor Development at One Year." *New England Journal of Medicine,* 321, 7, August 1989: 425.

34. Mennella, J. "The Transfer of Alcohol to Human Milk." *New England Journal of Medicine,* 325, 14, October 1991: 981.

35. Mennella, J. A., and C. J. Gerrish. "Effects of Exposure to Alcohol in Mother's Milk on Infant Sleep." *Pediatrics,* 101, 5, E2, May 1998.

36. Subcommittee on Nutritional Status during Lactation, et al. *Nutrition during Lactation.* Washington, D.C.: National Academy Press, 1990: 177.

37. Von Kries, et al. "Breastfeeding and Obesity; A Cross-Sectional Study." *British Medical Journal,* 319, 7203, July 1999: 147–150.

38. McCrory, M. A., et al. "Randomized Trial of the Short-Term Effects of Dieting Compared with Dieting plus Aerobic Exercise on Lactation Performance." *American Journal of Clinical Nutrition,* 69, 5, May 1999: 959–67.
Lovelady, C. A. "The Effect of Weight Loss in Overweight Lactating Women on the Growth of Their Infants." *New England Journal of Medicine,* 342, 2000: 449-53.

39. Merchant, K., et al. "Maternal and Fetal Responses to the Stresses of Lactation Concurrent with Pregnancy and Short Recuperative Intervals." *American Journal of Clinical Nutrition,* 52, 1990: 280.

40. Melton, L. J., III, et al. "Influence of Breastfeeding and Other Reproductive Factors on Bone Mass Later in Life." *Osteoporosis International,* 3, 2, March 1993: 76–83.
Lopez, J. M., et al. "Bone Turnover and Density in Healthy Women During Breastfeeding and After Weaning." *Osteoporosis International,* 6, 2, 1996: 153–154.

41. Villalpando, S., and M. del Prado. "Interrelation Among Dietary Energy and Fat Intakes, Maternal Body Fatness and Milk Total Lipid in Humans." *Journal of Mammary Gland Biology and Neoplasia,* 4, 3, July 1999: 285–295.

Piccianoo, M. F., et al. "Human Milk: Nutritional Aspects of a Dynamic Food." *Biology of the Neonate,* 74, 2, 1998: 84–93.

Innis, S. M., and D. J. King. "Trans Fatty Acids in Human Milk Are Inversely Associated with Concentration of Essential c0s-n-6 and n-3 Fatty Acids in Plasma Lipids of Breastfed Infants." *American Journal of Clinical Nutrition,* 70, 3, September 1999: 383–390.

Hayat, L., et al. "Fatty Acid Composition of Human Milk in Kuwait Mothers."

42. Worthington-Roberts, B., and S. R. Williams. *Nutrition in Pregnancy and Lactation,* 6th edition. Dubuque, Iowa: Brown and Benchmark Publishers, 1997.

43. Patandin, S. "Effects of Environmental Exposure to Polychlorinated Biphenyls and Dioxins on Cognitive Abilities in Dutch Children at 42 Months of Age." *Journal of Pediatrics,* 134, 1, January 1999: 33–41.

44. Crase, B. Personal communication. May 1992.

45. Rogan, W. J., et al. "Pollutants in Breast Milk." *Archives in Pediatric and Adolescent Medicine,* 150, 9, September 1996: 981–90.

46. La Leche League International Staff. *The Womanly Art of Breastfeeding.* 4th revised edition. Franklin Park, Ill.: La Leche League International, 1987: 348.

47. Nafziger, S., M.D. Personal communication. June 1992.

48. Dewey, K. G., et al. "A Randomized Study of the Effects of Aerobic Exercise by Lactating Women on Breast-Milk Volume and Composition." *New England Journal of Medicine,* 330, 7, February 1994: 449–53.

49. Food and Nutrition Board. *Dietary Reference Intakes: Recommended Intakes for Individuals.* National Academy Press, 1999.

50. Potischman, N., and R. Troisi. "In-Utero and Early Life Exposures in Relation to Risk of Breast Cancer." *Cancer Causes Control,* 1999, Dec.; 10(6): 561–73.

Newcomb, P. A., et al. "Lactation in Relation to Postmenopausal Breast Cancer." *American Journal of Epidemiology,* 1999 Jul., 15; 150(2): 174–82.

Labbok, M. H. "Health Sequelae of Breastfeeding for the Mother." *Clinics in Perinatology,* 262, 2, viii–ix June 1999; 491–503.

51. Freudenheim, J., et al. "Exposure to Breast Milk in Infancy and the Risk of Breast Cancer." *Epidemiology,* 5, 1994: 324.

52. Committee on Nutrition. "Iron-Fortified Infant Formulas." *Pediatrics,* 84, 6, December 1989: 114.

53. American Academy of Pediatrics. "Infant Feeding Practices and Their Possible Relationship to the Etiology of Diabetes Mellitus." *Pediatrics,* 94, 5, November 1994: 752.

54. Shannon, M., and J. Graef. "Hazards of Lead in Infant Formula." Letter. *New England Journal of Medicine,* 326, 2, January 9, 1992: 137.

Chapter 9

1. Gerlin, A. "Workplace Nursing Becoming a Benefit." *The Wall Street Journal,* December 29, 1994.

2. Brownell, K. D. "The Central Role of Lifestyle Change in Long-Term Weight Management." *Clinical Cornerstone,* 2, 3, 1999: 43–51.

3. Wing, R. R., and R. W. Jeffery. "Benefits of Recruiting Participants with Friends and Increasing Social Support for Weight Loss and Maintenance." *Consulting Clinical Psychology,* 67, 1, February 1999, 132–8.

4. Williams, G. C., et al. "Motivational Predictors of Weight Loss and Weight-loss Maintenance." *Journal of Personal Social Psychology,* 70, 1, January 1996: 115–26.

5. Brownell, K. D. "The Central Role of Lifestyle Change in Long-Term Weight Management." *Clinical Cornerstone,* 2, 3, 1999: 43–51.

6. International Food and Information Council. *Food Insight: Current Topics in Food Safety and Nutrition,* March/April 1992.

7. Greene, G., et al. "Postpartum Weight Change: How Much of the Weight Gained in Pregnancy Will Be Lost after Delivery?" *Obstetrics and Gynecology,* 71, 5, May 1988: 701.

8. Fuentes-Afflick, E., and N. A. Hessol. "Interpregnancy Interval and the Risk of Premature Infants." *Obstetrics and Gynecology,* 95, 3, March 2000: 383–90.

Chapter 10

1. American College of Obstetricians and Gynecologists. *Planning for Pregnancy, Birth, and Beyond.* Washington, D.C.: ACOG, 1990: 77, 82.

2. Jovanovic-Peterson, L., and C. Peterson. "Is Exercise Safe or Useful for Gestational Diabetic Women?" *Diabetes,* 40, suppl. 2, December 1991: 179.

3. American College of Obstetricians and Gynecologists. *Exercise during Pregnancy and the Postnatal Period.* ACOG Home Exercise Programs. Washington, D.C.: ©1985. Reprinted with permission.

4. Ibid.

5. Grediagin, A., et al. "Exercise Treatment Does Not Effect Body Composition Change in Untrained Moderately Overfat Women." *Journal of the American Dietetic Association,* 95, 6, June 1995: 661.

6. American College of Obstetricians and Gynecologists. *ACOG Guide to Planning for Pregnancy, Birth, and Beyond.* Washington, D.C.: ACOG ©1990. Reprinted with permission.

Chapter 11

1. The Food and Drug Administration. "The New Food Label." *FDA Backgrounder,* April 1994.

2. Ibid.

3. *Consumer Reports on Health,* March 1992: 18.

4. Whitmire, D. Telephone interview. June 1992.

5. Food Marketing Institute. *Food Safety and the Microwave: A Consumer Guide to Food Quality and Safe Handling.*

6. Sharara, F. I., et al. "Environmental Toxicants and Female Reproduction." *Fertility and Sterility,* 70(4) Oct. 1998: 613–22.

7. Groth, Edward III, and Mark Silbergeld. *Report to the FDA with Results of Recent Tests Conducted by Consumers Union.* June 1998.

8. Groth, Edward III, Project Director. *Do You Know What You're Eating? An Analysis of U.S. Government Data on Pesticide Residues in Foods,* Consumers Union, February 1999.

9. U.S. Department of Agriculture, Agriculture Marketing Service. *National Organic Program Proposed Rule,* December 1997.

10. Jacobson, M., et al. *Safe Food: Eating Wisely in a Risky World.* Los Angeles, Calif.: Living Planet Press, 1991: 72.

11. Reprinted from *Safe Food,* © 1991, available for $9.95 at CSPI, 1875 Connecticut Ave. NW #300, Washington, DC 20009.

12. Dairy Industry Coalition. "Facts about BST and Milk Safety."

13. Daughaday, W. H., and D. M. Barbano. "Bovine Somatotropin Supplementation of Dairy Cows: Is the Milk Safe?" *Journal of the American Medical Association,* 264, 8, 1990: 1003.

14. Kendall, P. Telephone interview. June 1992.

15. National Pork Producers Council. *Today's Pork in Foodservice,* 1988: 6.

16. Wilson, L. "Producing Leaner Beef More Efficiently." Presentation at Pennsylvania State University, 1989.

17. Texas A & M University. *Growth Promoting Hormones: A Scientific Review,* January 1989.

18. EPA Fact Sheet. *Polychlorinated Dibenzo-p-dioxins and Related Compounds Update: Impact on Fish Advisories,* September 1999.
   EPA Fact Sheet. *PCB Update: Impact on Fish Advisories,* September 1999.

19. EPA Fact Sheet. *Mercury Update: Impact on Fish Advisories,* September 1999.

20. Connor, W. E. "Impact of Omega 3 Fatty Acids in Health and Disease." *American Journal of Clinical Nutrition,* 71, (1 Suppl.): 171s–175s.
   Carlson, S. E. "Long-Chain Polyunsaturated Fatty Acids and Development of Human Infants." *Acta Pædiatrica,* 88, 430: 72–77.

21. National Fisheries Institute. *Omega 3 Content of Fish and Shellfish.*

22. Ollis, T. E., et al. "Australian Food Sources and Intakes of Omega-6 and Omega-3 Polyunsaturated Fatty Acids." *Annals of Nutrition and Metabolism,* 1999 Nov.; 43(6): 346–355.

23. Makrides, M., and R. A. Gibson. "Long-Chain Polyunsaturated Fatty Acid Requirements During Pregnancy and Lactation." *American Journal of Clinical Nutrition,* 71, (1 Suppl.): 1308s–311s.

24. Vanderbeek, C. Telephone interview. May 1996.

25. *Consumer Reports Magazine,* 57, 2, February 1992: 106.
   Harsila, J. Telephone interview. May 1992.
   Jacobson, M., et al. *Safe Food: Eating Wisely in a Risky World.* Los Angeles, Calif.: Living Planet Press, 1991: 13.

26. U.S. Department of Agriculture, Food Safety and Inspection Service. *Focus on Beef: From Farm to Table,* revised May 1998.
   U. S. Department of Agriculture and Food Safety and Inspection Service. *Minimum Internal Temperatures: Use a Meat Thermometer,* June 1997.

Chapter 15

1. American Dry Bean Board. *Good Health Is Habit-Forming: Commit to the Bean Routine.*

Recommended Resources

As you may know, there are many, many good books about health and nutrition. I had a hard time picking only a few.

Pre-pregnancy Planning

Lauersen, Niels H., M.D., and Colette Bouchez. *Getting Pregnant: What Couples Need to Know Right Now*. Fireside.

Sussman, John R., M.D., and B. Blake Levitt. *Before You Conceive: The Complete Prepregnancy Guide*. Bantam.

Tannenhaus, Norra. *Pre-Conceptions: What You Can Do Before Pregnancy to Help You Have a Healthy Baby*. Contemporary Books.

Pregnancy

Bard, Maureen. *Getting Organized for Your New Baby*. Meadowbrook.

Brott, Armin A., and Jennifer Ash. *The Expectant Father: Facts, Tips, and Advice for Dads-to-Be*. Abbeville Press.

Curtis, Glade B., M.D. *Your Pregnancy Week by Week* and *Your Pregnancy After 30*. Fisher Books.

Erick, Miriam. *No More Morning Sickness: A Survival Guide for Pregnant Women*. Plume. *Take Two Crackers and Call Me in the Morning: A Real-Life Guide to Surviving Morning Sickness*. Grinnen-Barrett.

Graham, Janis. *Your Pregnancy Companion*. Pocket Books.

Hotchner, Tracy. *Pregnancy Pure and Simple*. Avon Books.

Nilsson, Lennart. *A Child Is Born*. Dell.

Noble, Elizabeth. *Essential Exercises for the Childbearing Year*. New Life Images.

Sears, William, M.D., and Martha Sears. *The Birth Book*. Little, Brown.

Shapiro, Howard, M.D. *The Pregnancy Book for Today's Woman*. HarperCollins.

Simkin, Penny, Janet Whalley, and Ann Keppler. *Pregnancy, Childbirth, and the Newborn*. Meadowbrook.

Spencer, Paula, et al. Parenting *Guide to Pregnancy and Childbirth*. Ballantine Books.

Stone, Joanne, M.D., Keith Eddleman, M.D., and Mary Murray. *Pregnancy for Dummies*. IDG Books.

Stoppard, Miriam, M.D. *New Pregnancy and Birth Book*. Ballantine Books.

Baby Names

Lansky, Bruce. *The Very Best Baby Name Book*. Meadowbrook.

High-Risk Pregnancy/Birth

Rich, Laurie. *When Pregnancy Isn't Perfect*. Larata Press.

Diabetes and Gestational Diabetes

American Diabetes Association. *Diabetes: What to Expect* and *Gestational Diabetes: What to Expect*. The American Diabetes Association.

Cryer, Philip. *American Diabetes Association Complete Guide to Diabetes: The Ultimate Home Diabetes Reference*. Bantam Books.

Franz, Marion. *Exchanges for All Occasions*. International Diabetes Center.

Hayes, Marcia, Jane Stephenson, and Jackie Boucher. *No Fuss Diabetes Recipes for 1 or 2*. Chronimed Publishing.

Hess, Mary Abbott. *The Art of Cooking for the Diabetic*. Signet.

Jovanovic-Peterson, Lois, M.D., with Morton Stone. *Managing Your Gestational Diabetes: A Guide for You and Your Baby's Good Health*. Chronimed Publishing.

Marks, Betty. *The Microwave Diabetes Cookbook*. Surrey Books.

Palumbo, P.J., M.D., and Joyce Daly Margie. *The All-In-One Diabetic Cookbook*. New American Library.

Polin, Bonnie Sanders, and Frances Towner Giedt. *The Joslin Diabetes Gourmet Cookbook*. Bantam Books.

Multiple Births

Agnew, Connie, et al. *Twins! Expert Advice from Two Practicing Physicians on Pregnancy, Birth, and the First Year of Life with Twins*. HarperCollins.

Baglivi Tinglof, Christina. *Double Duty: The Parents' Guide to Raising Twins, from Pregnancy through the School Years*. Contemporary Books.

Luke, Barbara and Tamara Eberlein. *When You're Expecting Twins, Triplets or Quads: The Complete Resource*. HarperCollins.

Noble, Elizabeth. *Having Twins: A Parent's Guide to Pregnancy, Birth, and Early Childhood*. Houghton Mifflin.

Rothbart, Betty. *Multiple Blessings: From Pregnancy through Childhood, a Guide for Parents of Twins, Triplets, or More.* Hearst Books.

Prematurity
Tracy, Amy and Dianne Maroney. *Your Premature Baby and Child: Helpful Answers and Advice for Parents.* Berkley Publishing Group.

Teen Pregnancy
Arthur, Shirley. *Surviving Teen Pregnancy: Your Choices, Dreams, and Decisions.* Morning Glory Press.

Hammerslough, Jane. *Everything You Need to Know about Teen Motherhood.* Rosen Publishing Group.

Lindsay, Jeanne Warren. *School-Age Parents: The Challenge of Three Generation Living,* and *Teens Parenting: Your Pregnancy and Newborn Journey,* and *Your Baby's First Year.* Morning Glory Press.

Infertility
Aronson, Diane and Resolve (organization). *Resolving Infertility: Understanding the Options and Choosing Solutions When You Want to Have a Baby.* HarperCollins.

Levitt, B. Blake. *50 Essential Things to Do When the Doctor Says It's Infertility.* Plume.

Miller, Manya Deleon, and Ronald Clisham. *The Complete Fertility Organizer: A Guidebook and Record-Keeper for Women.* John Wiley and Sons.

Raab, Diana. *Getting Pregnant and Staying Pregnant: Overcoming Infertility and Managing Your High-Risk Pregnancy.* Hunter House.

Rosenberg, Helane S., and Yakov M. Epstein. *Getting Pregnant When You Thought You Couldn't.* Warner Books.

Rosenthal, M. Sara. *The Fertility Sourcebook: Everything You Need to Know.* Lowell House.

Stone, Frances and Philip. *Pennies from Heaven: 101 Meditations for Couples Trying to Get Pregnant.* Penguin.

Weschler, Toni. *Taking Charge of Your Fertility.* Harper Perennial.

Breastfeeding
Behan, Eileen. *Eat Well, Lose Weight While Breastfeeding.* Villard Books.

Gotsch, Gwen and Judy Torgus. *The Womanly Art of Breastfeeding.* Plume.

Gotsch, Gwen. *Breast Feeding Your Premature Baby.* La Leche League International.

Gromada, Karen Kerkhoff. *Mothering Multiples: Breastfeeding and Caring for Twins or More.* La Leche League International.

Huggins, Kathleen. *The Nursing Mother's Companion.* 4th Edition. Harvard Common Press.

Moran, Elaine. *Bon Appetit, Baby! The Breastfeeding Kit.* Treasure Chest Books.

Pryor, Gale. *Nursing Mother, Working Mother: The Essential Guide for Breastfeeding and Staying Close to Your Baby After You Return to Work.* Harvard Common Press.

Sears, William. *The Breastfeeding Book.* Little, Brown.

Parenthood
Black Fatherhood: The Guide to Male Parenting. Impact! Publications.

Brazelton, T. Berry, M.D. *Touchpoints: Your Child's Emotional and Behavioral Development.* Perseus Press.

Cline, Foster W., and Jim Fay. *Parenting with Love and Logic: Teaching Children Responsibility.* Navpress.

Crary, Elizabeth. *Without Spanking or Spoiling: A Practical Approach to Toddler and Preschool Guidance.* Parenting Press.

Einzig, Mitchell J., M.D., ed. *Baby and Child Emergency First Aid Handbook.* Meadowbrook.

Eisenberg, Arlene, et al. *What to Expect the First Year.* Workman Publishing.

Hart, Terril H., M.D., ed. *The Parent's Guide to Baby and Child Medical Care.* Meadowbrook.

Hunter, Brenda. *Home by Choice.* Multnomah Books.

Huntley, Becky. *The Sleep Book for Tired Parents.* Parenting Press.

Johnson, Spencer, M.D. *The One Minute Mother.* William Morrow.

Kelly, Paula, M.D., ed. *First-Year Baby Care.* Meadowbrook.

Lague, Louise. *The Working Mom's Book of Hints, Tips, and Everyday Wisdom.* Petersons Guides.

Lansky, Vicki. *Getting Your Child to Sleep...and Back to Sleep: Tips for Parents of Infants, Toddlers, and Preschoolers.* Book Peddlers. *Practical Parenting Tips.* Meadowbrook.

Saavedra, Beth Wilson. *Meditations for New Mothers.* Workman Publishing.

Any books by parenting experts Penelope Leach, T. Berry Brazelton, or William Sears.

Baby Products

Fields, Denise and Alan. *Baby Bargains*. Windsor Peak Press.

Jones, Sandy, and the editors of Consumer Reports. *Guide to Baby Products, 6th Edition*. Consumer Reports Books.

Pregnancy and Parenting Books with a Touch of Humor

Atalla, Bill. *Thirteen Months of Pregnancy: A Guide for the Pregnant Father*. Oddly Enough.

Bernard, Susan. *The Mommy Guide: Real-Life Advice and Tips from Over 250 Moms and Other Experts*. NTC Publishing.

Glick, Eunice. *Expect the Unexpected When You're Expecting!* HarperTrade.

Gookin, Sandra Hardin and Dan, eds. *Parenting for Dummies*. IDG Books.

Hill, Thomas. *What to Expect When Your Wife Is Expanding*. Andrews McMeel Publishing.

Justice, Jeff. *The Pregnant Husband's Handbook*. Strawberry Patch.

Justice, Jeff, and Diane Pfeifer. *You Know You're a New Parent When...*. Strawberry Patch.

Lovine, Vicki. *The Girlfriends' Guide to Pregnancy: Or Everything Your Doctor Won't Tell You*. Pocket Books.

Feeding Your Infant and Child

Lansky, Vicki. *Feed Me! I'm Yours*. Meadowbrook.

Nissenberg, Sandra, et al. *How Should I Feed My Child? From Pregnancy to Preschool*. John Wiley and Sons.

Satter, Ellyn. *Child of Mine: Feeding with Love and Good Sense* and *How to Get Your Kid to Eat...But Not Too Much*. Bull Publishing.

Swinney, Bridget. *Healthy Food for Healthy Kids*. Meadowbrook.

General Nutrition

Donkersloot, Mary. *The Fast-Food Diet: Quick and Healthy Eating at Home and on the Go*. Fireside.

Duyff, Roberta Larson. *The American Dietetic Association's Complete Food and Nutrition Guide*. John Wiley and Sons.

Evers, Connie L. *How to Teach Nutrition to Kids*. 24 Carrot Press.

Finn, Susan, and Linda Stern Kass. *The Real Life Nutrition Book: Making the Right Choices Without Changing Your Life-Style*. Penguin Books.

Lambert-Lagacé, Louise. *The Nutrition Challenge for Women*. Bell Publishing.

Tribole, Evelyn. *Eating on the Run*. Human Kinetics Publishing. *Stealth Health: How to Sneak Nutrition Painlessly into Your Diet*. Penguin.

Warshaw, Hope. *The Restaurant Companion: A Guide to Healthier Eating Out*. Surrey Books.

Cookbooks

General-Healthy

The American Diabetes Association and the American Dietetic Association Family Cookbook. Simon & Schuster.

Colorado Dietetic Assocation staff. *Simply Colorado: Nutritious Recipes for Busy People*. Colorado Dietetic Association.

Cull, Julie Metcalf. *The Quality Time Family Cookbook*. Chronimed Publishing.

Fletcher, Anne. *Eating Thin for Life: Food Secrets and Recipes from People Who Have Lost Weight and Kept It Off*. Houghton Mifflin.

Gadia, Madhu. *Lite and Luscious Cuisine of India*. Piquant Publishing.

Mycoskie, Pam. *Butter Busters: The Cookbook*. Warner Books.

Oxmoor House. *Cooking Light Cookbook Series*. Oxmoor House.

Ponichtera, Brenda. *Quick & Healthy Recipes and Ideas*. ScaleDown Publishing.

Smith, M.J. *366 Low-Fat Brand-Name Recipes in Minutes!* John Wiley and Sons.

Tribole, Evelyn. *Healthy Homestyle Cooking*. Rodale Press. *Healthy Homestyle Desserts*. Viking.

Seafood

Hansen, Evie and Cindy Snyder. *Seafood Twice a Week*. National Seafood Educators.

Harsila, Janis, and Evie Hansen. *Light-Hearted Seafood: Tasty, Quick, Healthy*. National Seafood Educators.

Ver Ploeg, Marcie, et al. *Seafood Cooking for Dummies*. IDG Books.

Vegetarian

Callan, Ginny. *Beyond the Moon Cookbook*. Harper Perennial.

Crocker, Betty. *Betty Crocker's Vegetarian Cooking.* Simon and Schuster.

Elliot, Rose. *The Vegetarian Mother and Baby Book.* Pantheon Books.

Havala, Suzanne. *Simple, Lowfat and Vegetarian.* Vegetarian Resource Group. *Being Vegetarian.* John Wiley and Sons.

Hinman, Bobbie, and Millie Snyder. *Lean and Luscious and Meatless.* Prima Communications.

Katzen, Mollie. *Moosewood Cookbook,* and *The Enchanted Broccoli Forest,* and *Still Life with Menu Cookbook.* Ten Speed Press.

Kirchner, Bharti. *Vegetarian Burgers.* HarperCollins.

Lakhani, Mrs. *Indian Recipes for a Healthy Heart.* Fahil Publishers.

Mangum, Karen. *Life's Simple Pleasures.* Harvest Press. *Vegetarian Pleasure Revised.* Millenium Group.

Robertson, Laurel, et al. *The New Laurel's Kitchen.* Ten Speed Press.

Wasserman, Debra. *Meatless Meals for Working People* and *Simply Vegan.* Vegetarian Resource Group.

Weight Control/Weight Maintenance/ Low-Fat Eating

Bailey, Covert. *The Ultimate Fit or Fat* and *Smart Exercise.* Houghton Mifflin.

Berry, Frank, and Bridget Swinney. *Make the Change for a Healthy Heart.* Fall River Press.

Connor, Sonja, and William Connor, M.D. *The New American Diet.* Fireside.

Ferguson, Cassandra and James, M.D. *Habits Not Diets.* Bell Publishing.

Fletcher, Anne. *Thin For Life.* Houghton Mifflin.

Goor, Ron and Nancy. *Choose to Lose.* Houghton Mifflin.

Katahn, Martin and Jamie Pope. *The T-Factor 2000 Fat Gram Counter.* R.S. Means.

Lund, JoAnna. *Healthy Exchanges Cookbook.* Putnam.

McDougall, Mary and John, M.D. *The McDougall Program for Maximum Weight Loss.* Plume.

Moquette-Magee, Elaine. *Fight Fat and Win!* Chronimed Publishing.

Nash, Joyce. *Maximize Your Body Potential.* Bull Publishing.

Pope, Jamie. *The Last Five Pounds.* Pocket Books.

Stevens, Tree. *Living and Loving Low Fat.* Northwest.

Tribole, Evelyn, and Elyse Resch. *Intuitive Eating.* St. Martin's Press.

Ulene, Art. *Lose Weight with Dr. Art Ulene.* Ulysses Press.

Waterhouse, Debra. *Outsmarting the Female Fat Cell.* Warner Books.

Other Resources

American Dietetic Association Consumer Nutrition Hotline, 800-366-1655, www.eatright.org.

Confinement Line: a support network for women on bed rest, 703-941-7183.

Consumer Product Safety Commission, 800-638-2772.

National Organization of Mothers of Twins Clubs, 877-540-2200.

Sidelines: support for those experiencing a high-risk pregnancy, www.sidelines.org.

Triplet Connection, 209-474-0885.

Twin Services (counseling and referrals), 510-524-0863.

Vegetarian Resource Group, 410-366-8343, www.vrg.org.

Newsletters and Magazines

American Health Magazine.

Cooking Light Magazine.

Diet and Nutrition Letter, Tufts University.

Environmental Nutrition, The Professional Newsletter of Diet, Nutrition, and Health.

Health Magazine.

Nutrition Action Health Letter, Center for Science in the Public Interest, Washington, D.C.

Vegetarian Journal, Vegetarian Resource Group.

Wellness Letter, University of California, Berkeley.

Index

abdomen, after the birth 173
acesulfame K 119, 120
additives, food 197-9
air travel 44-5
alcohol 11
  and birth defects 5, 42
  and breastfeeding
    162-3
  and fertility 10
  and unknown pregnancy
    5, 15
alitame 121
allergies, food 161
amenorrhoea 10
Ames, Bruce 11
anaemia 33 *see also* iron
  and low birth weight
    baby 19
  preventing 69-71
ankle swelling 85
anorexia nervosa 10
antimicrobials 198
antioxidants 198
artificial flavourings 198
artificial sweeteners 119-21,
    197, 198
ascorbic acid *see* vitamin C
aspartame 119, 120
aspirin 11, 43, 159
aversions 57-8

baby's development
  first trimester 47-8
  second trimester 61-2
  third trimester 79-80
baby, the first weeks with
    169-80

backache 85
  and the pelvic tilt 189
bacteria
  in fish 217
  in food 218
  in poultry 213, 215
beans *see also* Beans *in*
    Recipe Index
  beating bean bloat 316
  nutritional value 316
bed rest
  eating while on 136-7
  entertainment during 137-8
  exercise and 138
  and fitness 188
  for high blood pressure
    126-7
  setting up the room 135-6
  survivial tips 138-9
Before-Baby Eating Plan 8,
    11
Best-for-Baby Breastfeeding
    Eating Plan 154-8
beta-carotene 31
beverages 241
  caffeine content 43
  calcium content 67, 68
  high-energy drink 84
  milk 69
biotin 29
birth control pill 14-15
birth defects 4-5
  and alcohol 5, 42
  and diabetes 5, 108
  and diet 11
  and drugs 43-4
  and eating disorders 10

and folic acid 33
and high blood sugar 104
birth, the first weeks after
    169-80
birth weight 17-18 *see also*
    low birth weight
blood glucose *see* blood
    sugar
blood pressure, high
    see high blood pressure
blood sugar 104, 106-7
    see also diabetes
body changes, after the birth
    172-80
bonding 167-8
bottlefeeding (formula milk)
    167
bovine somatotropin (BST)
    210
breakfast, importance of
    178-9 *see also* menus
breast cancer risk, and
    breastfeeding 166
breast changes 58
breastfeeding 145-68
  and alcohol use 162-3
  benefits of 147-8
  and bonding 167-8
  and breast cancer risk 166
  and caffeine 162
  decision about 146
  and drugs 159
  during next pregnancy
    163-4
  Eating Plan 154-8
  effects of diet on milk 161,
    162-3, 164

environmental pollutants in milk 164-5

and exercise 166

father's support 151-2

and food poisoning 166

going back to work 171-2

help with 149, 150-1, 154, 161

multiple babies 159

nutrition during 154-8

and osteoporosis risk 164

possible obstacles 148-52

premature babies 160-1, 162

preparing for 152-4

smoking and 163

teens 160

vegetarians 159-60, 166

weight-loss during 163

bulimia 10

caffeine 12, 13, 42-3

and breastfeeding 162

content of beverages and foods 43

and fertility 9

calcium 19, 30

content of animal-based foods and beverages 67

content of vegetarian foods and beverages 68

importance of 66-9

and lactose intolerance 69

requirement during breastfeeding 157, 158

supplements 37, 38-9

third trimester 81

in vegetarian diet 91, 92-3

calories

adding to diet

amount needed for breastfeeding 156

amount needed for pregnancy 48, 62, 80-1

Campylobacter bacteria in poultry 213, 215

car, travel by 45

carrots, effects on fertility 10

cats, and toxoplasmosis 218

chemicals *see* environmental contaminants

chickenpox (varicella) 11, 41

choline 30

chromium 35, 64

chronic hypertension 124

cobalamin 30

cocaine 44

colouring agents 198

Connor, Sonja 27

constipation 75

convenience food *see also* fast food

cost of 201

fifty quick-and-easy meals or snacks 234, 236-7

for the whole family 230

healthy menus 230-3

last-minute meals from the cupboard 233, 235

meals for one 228-30

tips for choosing 227-8

vegetarian 100

cooking *see* food preparation; food safety; kitchen; menus

copper 34-5

counselling, pre-pregnancy 3-4, 17

Crase, Betty 165

cravings 57-8

Crawford, Michael 5, 7

Crohn's disease 147

curing agents 198

cytomegalovirus (CMV) 41

dairy products 50, 66-7, 69

dehydration 107-8

deep-freeze 199

diabetes 15

and birth defect risk 5

exercise and 118-19

gestational 7, 110-13, 114-23

labour and delivery 110

possible effects on baby 108,

pre-existing 104-10, 114-23

questions about 121-3

risk factors 112

using sweeteners 119-21

testing for 112-13

type II 112

Diabetic Eating and Exercise Plan 114-23

diabetic food exchanges 102, 116, 242

diabetic snacks 117-18

diet *see also* Eating Plans; menus; nutrition; weight-loss

checking against Eating Plan 62-4

healthy 18-20

check, third trimester 81-2

diet foods 121

drugs 11, 43-4

and breastfeeding 159

residues in meat 212

eating, after the birth 100-1, 101-2, 169-70

eating disorders
  and fertility 10
  and low weight gain 25

Eating Expectantly Eating Plan 53-4

Eating Expectantly for Teens Plan 142-4

Eating Expectantly Vegetarian Eating Plan 94-102

eating out 237-40
  choosing wisely 237-40
  food safety 205
  vegetarian-style 98-100

Eating Plans,
  Before-Baby 8, 11
  Best-for Baby Breastfeeding 154-8
  comparing your diet with 62-4
  Diabetic Eating and Exercise Plan 114-23
  Eating Expectantly 53-4
  Lose That Baby Fat 178
  Teens 142-4
  Thrive on Five 71-3
  Vegetarian 94-102

eclampsia 124

eggs 28
  food safety for 211-12
  protein from 50
  storage 212, 214

emotions, dealing with 103-4

emulsifiers 198

endocrine disruptors, in food 207

energy levels
  how to help 84-5

energy needs
  first trimester 48
  second trimester 62
  third trimester 80-1

environmental contaminants 11-12
  in fish/seafood 217-19
  pesticides 206-8
  in the workplace 12-13

Erick, Miriam 54-6

Escherichia coli (E. coli) bacteria 208-9

estrogen levels in food 213

exercise 19, 85
  back strengthening 189
  during bed rest 188
  benefits of 181-2
  and breastfeeding 166
  consulting your doctor first 184-5
  and diabetes 109, 118-19
  to help fatigue 57
  effects on fertility 10
  fitting it in 185-6
  guidelines for pregnant women 182-5
  on-line resources 188
  post partum 182, 186-8
  videos 188
  weight loss and 186-7

fast food 13-14, 59 see also convenience food
  eating in 227-37
  eating out 237-40
  making healthy choices 239-40

fat (dietary) 25-8
  omega-3 oils 25-6, 81, 94, 219

omega-6 oils 26
  substitutes and replacers 198
  in vegetarian diet 94, 101
  and weight gain 21

fathers
  pre-pregnancy diet 11
  support from 151-2

fatigue 57, 84-5

feeding, infants 168

fertility, factors affecting 8-11

fibre 20, 51-3
  content of foods 52
  and diabetes 109
  in diet during breastfeeding 157

figs 53

first trimester 48-60
  fibre intake 51-3
  foetal growth 47-8
  menus 241, 243-7
  morning sickness 54-6
  nutrient needs 50
  protein needs 48-50
  recipes 249-73
  snack ideas 246
  weight gain 48

fish and seafood
  bacteria 217, 218
  buying 219-20
  cooking 221-2
  fish oils 25, 26
  omega-3 fats 219
  pollutants 217-18
  storage and handling 216, 220-1

fitness 181-9 see also exercise

flavour enhancers 198

flavouring agents 198
fluids
  and breastfeeding 150
  and diabetes 107-8
  drinking enough 20
  after labour 170
  and morning sickness 55-6
fluoride 35
Foetal Alcohol Effect (FAE)
  42
Foetal Alcohol Syndrome
  (FAS) 42
foetal growth
  first trimester 47-8
  second trimester 61-2
folacin see folic acid (folacin)
folic acid (folacin) 4-5, 13,
  14, 32-3
  and birth defects 33
  supplements 12, 37
  first trimester 50
  sources of 158
food
  eating on a budget
    199-201
  organic 208
  smart shopping 200
  stocking the kitchen 193-
    226
food additives 197-9
food allergies, and
  breastfeeding 161
food cravings and aversions
  57-8
food exchanges, diabetic
  102, 116, 242
Food Guide Pyramid 18-19
  and vegetarian eating
    89-90
food labels 195-99

food planning see also menus
  first trimester 59-60
  second trimester 77
  third trimester 87
food poisoning 166
food preparation, hygiene
  204-5
food safety 13
  beef and pork 212-13
  cooking times 206
  daily products 210-11
  essential guide 204-26
  eating away from home
    205
  eggs 211-12
  fish and seafood 216-22
  fruits 208-10
  grains and nuts 208-10
  poultry 213-15
  storage guides 205, 211,
    214-15, 216
  summary 223-6
  vegetables 208-10
food safety reports 222-3
formula milk feeding 167
fruit
  adding to meals 72-3
  benefits of 71-2
  food safety and 208-10
  in snacks 73, 74

gas-causing foods 161
genetic counselling 4
German measles (rubella)
  11, 41
gestational diabetes mellitus
  (GDM) 7, 64, 110-13,
  114-23
  and vegetarian diet 101,
    102

gestational hypertension
  see pregnancy-induced
  hypertension
glucose see blood sugar
grains 8, 14, 19, 51, 52
growth hormones in meat
  212-13

haemorrhoids 75-6
health care team 104-5
health claims for foods
  196-7
healthy snacks 73-4
heartburn 86
hepatitis B
herbal teas 43
Higgins Nutrition
  Intervention Programme
  133
high blood pressure 23,
  123-8
high blood sugar 104, 107
  see also diabetes
high-risk pregnancies
  103-44
  dealing with emotions
    about 103-4
  gestational diabetes
    mellitus (GDM) 110-13,
    114-23
  high blood pressure 123-8
  multiple births 128-35
  older mothers 139-40
  pre-existing diabetes
    104-110, 114-23
  sick day rules 107-8
  teen pregnancy 140-4
high temperatures, and
  fertility 12
holidays 44-6

hospital
  breastfeeding in 152, 153-4
  food for vegetarians 100,
    101-2
human immunodeficiency
  virus (HIV) 41
human parvovirus B19 41
hyperglycaemia (high blood
  sugar) 104, 107
hypertension *see* high blood
  pressure
hypoglycaemia (low blood
  sugar) 106-7

illness, during pregnancy
  41, 107-8
immunization 11, 41
infant feeding 168
infertility 8-11
ingredients list, on food
  labels 197-8
inherited disorders 4
insomnia 86
insulin resistance 106
  see also diabetes
internet resources
  see websites
iodine 35
iron 19, 69-71
  preventing anaemia 33
  content of animal-based
    foods 70
  and infertility 10
  and multiple births 131
  in the second trimester 64
  supplements 38-9
  teen pregnancy and 144
  content of vegetarian foods
    71
  in vegetarian diet 91, 92

junk food 13-14
Johnston, Richard B. 42

ketoacidosis 106
kitchen
  example lists of foods
    stocked 194-5
  stocking 193-226
  tools 201-3
Krebs, Nancy 153

labour and delivery
  eating after 100 1, 101-2,
    169-70
  for diabetic women 110
lacto-ovo vegetarian diet 91
lactose intolerance 69
laxatives 75-6
lead exposure 40-1
Listeria monocytogenes bacteria
  in food 13, 218
Listeriosis 218
lochia 172-3
Lose That Baby Fat Eating
  Plan 178
low birth weight 5, 7
  anaemia and 19
  caffeine and 42
  multiple births and 129-30
  poor nutrition and 17-18
  teen pregnancy and 141
low blood sugar
  (hypoglycaemia) 106-7
low-fat food substitutions
  177
Luke, Barbara 130

macrosomia 111
magnesium 30-1
  sources of 158

male fertility
  and alcohol 10
  and high temperatures 12
  and selenium 10
  and vitamin C 10
  and zinc 10
manganese 35
  first trimester 50
mannitol 119
meals, skipping 59
meat
  food safety and 212-13
  nutrient content 36
medications 43
menu planning 210
menus *see also* convenience
    foods; fast foods
  about 241
  first trimester 241, 243-7
  second trimester 275-8
  third trimester 307-16
  A Month of Breakfast Ideas
    275-6
  Best Bite Snacks 311
  Blender Breakfasts (or
    Snacks to Go) 245
  Company's Coming! 277-8
  Don't Feel Like Cooking
    243-4
  Don't Feel Like Cooking or
    Eating 244
  Don't Feel Like Eating 243
  Feel Full Meals 310-11
  Feel Great 245
  Feel Like Staying in Bed
    but Can't 244-5
  High Energy Snack Ideas
    247
  for a Hungry Appetite
    276-7

I Could Cook All Day 277
Meals in Minutes 309-10
Snack Ideas 245-7
Using Leftovers with Flair
  307-9
Vegetarian on a Budget
  311-16
mercury 217
microwave cooking, safety
  206
milk, lactose intolerance 69
minerals 28
  first trimester needs 50
  second trimester needs 64,
   66-71
  third trimester needs 81-3
  chromium 35, 64
  copper 34-5
  fluoride 35
  iodine 35
  magnesium 30-1, 158
  manganese 35, 50
  molybdenum 35
  phosphorus 30, 121
  potassium 30, 64
  selenium 10, 35
  sodium 34, 126, 228
see also calcium; folic acid;
   iron; zinc
molybdenum 35
monosodium glutamate
  (MSG) 198
morning sickness 50, 54-6,
  59
  survival tips 55-6
multiple births, 128-35
  birth weights 129-30
  breastfeeding 159
  Higgins Programme 133
  nutrient requirements 131-2

resources for parents 134-5
statistics 128-9
weight gain and 130-4

Nafziger, Steven 151
nausea 50
neural tube defects 4-5, 12,
  37
niacin 29
nutrient content of protein
  foods 36
nutrients 198
  for building 30-3
  for energy release 29
  support 34
  trace elements 34
nutrition
  and fertility 9-10
  importance of 4-5
  poor 5, 7, 8
  ten steps to a healthy diet
   18-20

oedema (swelling) 85
older mothers 15, 139-40
oligomenorrhoea 10
omega-3 oils (fats) 25-6, 81
  sources of 219
  in vegetarian diet 94
omega-6 oils (fats) 26
organic food 208
osteoporosis risk, and
  breastfeeding 164
overweight
  and fertility 9
  risks associated with 8

pantothenic acid 29
PCBs, in breast milk 164-5
pelvic tilt exercise 189

perineum, after the birth
  173
pesticides, in food 206-8
  see also environmental
   contaminants
phosphorus 30, 121
pizza 234
polyols (sugar alcohols) 119
pork, food safety 212-13
postpartum
  body changes 172-3
  eating during 170
  going back to work 171-2
  preparing for next
   pregnancy 180
  weight loss 173-80
  what to expect 169-70
potassium 34, 64
poultry, food safety 213-15
pre-eclampsia 23, 124
  signs of 127-8
pre-existing diabetes see
  diabetes
pregnancy
  changing your mindset 28
  counselling before 3-4, 17
  older women 15
  planning 3-8, 11-15
  positive aspects 46
  preparing for the next one
   180
  and vegetarian diet 90-102
pregnancy-induced
  hypertension (PIH) 123-8
premature babies see also
  low birth weight
  breastfeeding 160-1, 162
pre-pregnancy counselling
  3-4, 17
pre-pregnancy planning 3-8

preservatives 198
protein
  first trimester needs 48-50
  second trimester needs 64
  third trimester needs 81,
    82
  complete and incompelete
    64
  content of foods 49, 65
  during breastfeeding 156
  in vegetarian diet 94, 96
  quality of 49
pyridoxine 32

quiz
  how's your diet? 62-4, 81-2
  pre-pregnancy 6-7
  weight gain 23

radiation, in the
    environment 12
recipes
  diabetic exchanges 242
  first trimester 249-73
  nutrient analysis 242
  second trimester 279-306
  third trimester 317-54
Recommended Daily
  Allowance (RDA) 29
rest, during pregnancy 125,
    127
restaurants see also eating out
  choosing wisely 237-9
Retin-A 31
riboflavin 29
rubella (German measles)
    11, 41

saccharin 120
salad bars 238, 239

salads, main dishes 237
Salmonella bacteria in poultry
    213, 215
sandwiches 236
sauna 12
seafood see fish and seafood
second trimester
  calcium 66-9
  constipation 75
  how's your diet? 62-4
  energy needs 62
  foetal growth 61-2
  food planning 77
  haemorrhoids 75-6
  iron 69-71
  menus 275-8
  nutrient needs 64-71
  protein needs 64, 65
  recipes 279-306
  snacks 73-4, 246-7
  soya 66
  stress 76
  'Thrive on Five' 71-3
  vaginal discharge 75
  weight gain 62
selenium 35
  and fertility 10
shopping see food
sick day rules 107-8
sleepless nights 86
smoking 12
  and breastfeeding 163
  effects on the baby 39
  and infertility 9
  and low weight gain 25
  during pregnancy 7
snacks
  to help energy levels 84-5
  healthy options 73-4
  ideas for 245-7

most nutritious 311
  to help weight gain 25
sodium 34, 126, 228
soft drinks 7
sorbitol 119
soya protein, benefits of 66
Spears, Bev 115
spina bifida 4-5, 12, 37
stabilizers 198
stevia 121
storing food see food safety,
    storage guides
stress
  coping with 76
  and fertility 12
sucralose 120-1
sucrose 119
sudden infant death
    syndroms (SIDS) 147
sugar, facts about 83-4
sugar alcohols 119
surgery, eating after 100-1
sweeteners 119-21, 197, 198
swelling 85

teas, herbal 43
teen pregnancy 140-4
  breastfeeding 160
  eating plan 142-3
  getting support 141
  nutrient needs 141, 142-3,
    144
  weight gain during 143-4
teeth and gum changes 58-9
ten steps to a healthy diet
    18-20
textured vegetable protein
    (TVP) 66
thiamin 29
third trimester 79-87

backache 85
energy needs 80-1, 84-5
exercise 85
food planning 87
growth of baby 79-80
heartburn 86
menus 307-16
nutrient needs 81-3
oedema (swelling) 85
recipes 317-54
sleepless nights 86
snack ideas 246-7
sugar 83-4
Thrive on Five 71-3
vitamin B6 82
weight gain 80-1
zinc 81, 82-3
tocopherol 34
tofu 66
toxaemia 124
Toxoplasma gondii in food 218
toxoplasmosis 13, 41, 218
trans fatty acids (trans fat) 26
travelling during pregnancy 44-6
trichinosis 212
triplets *see* multiple births
twins *see* multiple births
Tyler, Varro 43
type II diabetes 112
   see also diabetes

underweight 10
  and fertility 9
urinary tract infection 111
urination, frequent 56-7
uterus, changes after birth 172

vagina, after the birth 173
vaginal discharge 75
vegan diet 90-1
vegetables
  adding to meals 72-3
  benefits of 71-2
  food safety 208-10
  heathiest cooking methods 203-4
  in snacks 73, 74
  storage and preparation 203
vegetarian diet 89
  and breastfeeding 159-60, 166
  and fertility 9
  and good health 90
  getting enough protein 49
  types of 90-1
  to help weight loss 177-8
Vegetarian Eating Plan 94-102
videos, exercise 188
vitamin A 31
  first trimester 50
vitamin B1 29
vitamin B2 29
vitamin B3 29
vitamin B6 32, 81, 82
  and protein intake 93
  sources 82, 158
vitamin B12 30
  fortified cereal 92
  in vegetarian diet 91, 92
vitamin C 33
  and male fertility 10
  in the second trimester 64
  supplements 37
vitamin D 31-2
  and multiple births 132

  in vegetarian diet 91, 93
vitamin E 34
vitamin K 31
vitamins 28-34 *see also* names of individual vitamins
  first trimester needs 50
  second trimester needs 64, 70
  third trimester needs 81-2
  supplements 12, 36-9
  vegetarian diet and

water 50
  lead in 40-1
websites
  breastfeeding 161
  diabetes 104
  fitness 188
  food additives 199
  food safety 218, 226
  food-borne illnesses 218, 226
  infant feeding 168
  multiple births 104
  pregnancy 76
  sweeteners 119
  vegetarian resources 100
weight
  and fertility 9
  guidelines for adults 21
weight gain
  excessive 23-4
  first trimester 48
  and health of baby 21
  and multiple births 130-4
  not enough 24-5
  during pregnancy 20-5
  second trimester 62
  third trimester 80-1

weight loss
  and breastfeeding 163
  diets 8
  and exercise 186-7
  plans, evaluating 175-6
  post partum 173-80
  tips for success 175
  and vegetarian eating 177-8
  what to expect 179-80

whole grains 8, 14, 19, 51, 52
Wilson, Lowel L. 212-13
work
  breastfeeding and 171-2
  environmental contaminants at 12-13
  going back to 171-2

zinc 33, 34
  and fertility 10
  first trimester 50
  food sources 83
  importance of 81, 82-3
  sources of 158
  teen pregnancy 144
  third trimester 81, 82-3
  in vegetarian diet 91, 93

Recipe Index

Beans

Aspen Black Bean Soup 321
Basic Black Beans 287
Bean and Corn Bread Bake 332
Beans 101 288
Black Bean and Corn Salad 254
Black Bean Enchilada Casserole 333
Bridget's Garden Salad 255
Colorado Stuffed Peppers 338
Hoppin' John 341
Lentil Soup 322
Minute Minestrone 284
Vegetarian Chilli 324

Beef

Sesame Beef 345
Spanish Steak Roll with Sautéed Vegetables 299
Stuffed Aubergine Creole 300

Beverages

High Energy Drink 84

Breads and Muffins

Apple-Date Bran Muffins 262
Bean and Corn Bread Bake 332
French French Toast 280
Greek Island Pitta Pockets with Cucumber Yogurt Sauce 296
Pumpkin Muffins 262
Strawberry Bread 264
Thrive-on-Five Bread 265

Cakes and Pies

see Sweets

Cheese

Boursin Cheese Spread 318
Caramel Dip 319
Cheese-Topped Fish 335
Country Brunch Casserole 339
Creamy Pesto Pasta 293
Delightful Spinach 250
Rocky Mountain Quesadillas 261
Salmon Pâté 251
Spinach-Stuffed Shells 346

Chicken

Apricot-Glazed Chicken 331
Chicken and Prawns with Fruit Salsa 336-7
Chicken-and-Spinach Salad 256
Chicken Roll-ups 291

Creole

Stuffed Aubergine Creole 300

Desserts

see Sweets

Dips and Spreads

Basic Black Beans 287
Boursin Cheese Spread 318
Caramel Dip 319
Delightful Spinach 250
Salmon Pâté 251

Eggs

Broccoli Quiche 334
French French Toast 280
Mock Egg Foo Young 342

Fish and Seafood

Cheese-Topped Fish 335
Chicken and Prawns with Fruit Salsa 336-7
Crab Marinara 340
Quick Grilled Fish 344
Salmon en Papillote 298
Salmon Pâté 251
Stuffed Aubergine Creole 300

Fondue

Company Fondue 292

Fruits

Apple Pie à la Mode Shake 266
Apple-Date Bran Muffins 262
Banana-Orange Flip 267
Berry Mousse Parfait 303
Chicken-and-Spinach Salad 256
Favourite Snack Cake 351
Fruit Crisp 352
Fruit Pizza for a Crowd 353
Pancakes with Raspberry Sauce 281

Peach Pops 268

Piña Colada Frappé 270

Quick and Easy Blueberry
  Cobbler 306

Raspberry Surprise Shake
  271

Salsa 336

Strawberry Bread 264

Sunshine Sorbet 354

Tangy Salad 286

Tropical Pudding 272

Very Berry Shake 273

Grains

Bulgur-and-Veggie Mix 325

Colorado Suffed Peppers
  338

Hoppin' John 341

Mushroom-and-Barley Soup
  285

Oat-Nut Burgers 343

see also Breads and Muffins

Lamb

Leg of Lamb 297

Mexican Dishes

Black Bean Enchilada
  Casserole 333

Mexican Kale-and-Pork
  Soup 323

Rocky Mountain Quesadillas
  261

Vegetarian Breakfast Tacos
  350

Muffins

see Breads and Muffins

Nuts

Oat-Nut Burgers 343

Pancakes

Crepe Dinner 294-5

Pancakes with Raspberry
  Sauce 281

Quick and Healthier
  Pancakes 282

Pasta

Crab Marinara 340

Creamy Pesto Pasta 293

Pasta with Quick Alfredo
  Sauce 260

Spinach-Stuffed Shells
  346

Peanut Butter

Peanut-Butter-Chocolate-
  Shake 269

Pork

Basic Black Beans 287

Country Brunch Casserole
  339

Greek Island Pitta Pockets
  with Cucumber Yogurt
  Sauce 296

Hoppin' John 341

Mexican Kale-and-Pork
  Soup 323

Poultry

Apricot-Glazed Chicken
  331

Chicken and Prawns with
  Fruit Salsa 336-7

Chicken Roll-Ups 291

Chicken-and-Spinach Salad
  256

Turkey Pot Pie 301

Turkey with Hoisin Sauce
  302

Salads

Asian Salad 253

Black Bean and Corn Salad
  254

Bridget's Garden Salad 255

Chicken-and-Spinach Salad
  256

Tangy Salad 286

Salsa

Fruit Salsa 336

Sauces

Company Fondue 292

Cream Sauce 259

Creamy Pesto Pasta 293

Cucumber Yogurt Sauce
  296

Dijon Sauce 320

Hoisin Sauce 302

Pasta with Quick Alfredo
  Sauce 260

Raspberry Sauce 281

Roasted Red Pepper Sauce
  348

Sesame Beef Sauce 345

Shakes

Apple Pie à la Mode Shake
  266

Banana-Orange Flip 267

Peanut-Butter-Chocolate
  Shake 269

Piña Colada Frappé 270
Raspberry Surprise Shake
 271
Very Berry Shake 273

Snacks
Baked Tortilla Chips 251
Berry Mousse Parfait 303
Carrots Antibes 257
Favourite Snack Cake 351
Rocky Mountain Quesadillas
 261

Soups
Aspen Black Bean Soup 321
Basic Black Beans 287
Creamy Asparagus Soup
 252
Leek and Potato Soup 283
Lentil Soup 322
Mexican Kale-and-Pork
 Soup 323
Minute Minestrone 284
Mushroom-and-Barley Soup
 285

Sweets
Apple Pie à la Mode Shake
 266
Banana-Orange Flip 267
Berry Mousse Parfait 303
Favourite Snack Cake 351
Fruit Crisp 352
Fruit Pizza for a Crowd 353
Mocha Java Cake 304
Peach Pops 268
Peanut-Butter-Chocolate
 Shake 269

Piña Colada Frappé 270
Pumpkin Roll 305
Quick and Easy Blueberry
 Cobbler 306
Raspberry Surprise Shake
 271
Sunshine Sorbet 354
Tropical Pudding 272
Very Berry Shake 273

Tofu
Mock Egg Foo Young 342
Spinach-Stuffed Shells
 346
Stuffed Aubergine Creole
 300
Tofu Loaf 347
Vegetable-and-Tofu Stir-Fry
 349

Turkey
Turkey Pot Pie 301
Turkey with Hoisin Sauce
 302

Veal
Veal Piccata with Roasted
 Red Pepper Sauce 348

Vegetable Side Dishes
Basic Black Beans 287
Beans 101 288
Bulgur-and-Veggie Mix 325
Carrots Antibes 257
Delightful Spinach 250
Easy Microwave Potatoes
 326
Kids' Carrots 327

Oven-Fried Courgette Sticks
 258
Potatoes Marie Louise 289
Ratatouille 328
Roasted New
 Potatoes/Home Fries 329
Spring Vegetables in Cream
 Sauce 259
Thanksgiving Sweet Potatoes
 290
Vegetables in Vinaigrette
 330

Vegetarian Dishes
Black Bean Enchilada
 Casserole 333
Bean and Corn Bread Bake
 332
Broccoli Quiche 334
Colorado Stuffed Peppers
 338
Creamy Pesto Pasta 293
Crepe Dinner 294-5
Minute Minestrone 284
Mock Egg Foo Young 342
Oat-Nut Burgers 343
Pasta with Quick Alfredo
 Sauce 260
Ratatouille 328
Spinach-Stuffed Shells 346
Tofu Loaf 347
Vegetable-and-Tofu Stir-Fry
 349
Vegetarian Breakfast Tacos
 350
Vegetarian Chilli 324